Botanical Medicine

A European Professional Perspective

Dan Kenner, L.Ac. and Yves Requena, M.D.

Paradigm Publications   Brookline, Massachusetts

1996

Botanical Medicine

A European Professional Perspective

Dan Kenner and Yves Requena
Copyright © 1996 Paradigm Publications

Library of Congress Cataloging-in-Publication Data:

Kenner, Dan, 1950-
    Botanical medicine : a European professional perspective / Dan
Kenner, Yves Requena.
        p.   cm.
    Includes bibliographical references and index.
    ISBN 0-912111-48-8
    1. Herbs--Therapeutic use--Europe.   I. Requena, Yves.   II. Title.
RM666.H33K45 1996
615'.321'094--dc21   96-45883
                                        CIP

Library of Congress Catalog Card Number: 96-45883
International Standard Book Number (ISBN): 0-912111-48-8
Printed in the United States of America

Paradigm Publications
44 Linden Street
Brookline, Massachusetts 02146 USA.

TABLE OF CONTENTS

PREFACE

This book is designed to provide the herbal practitioner with information about botanical substances, how they are used in Western Europe today, and the necessary tools for developing clinical insights. By presenting the basics of three whole-system models – the neuroendocrine, the five phase and the diathetic – the practitioner can gain perspective from each system, even if choosing to use only one as a main paradigm. The five-phase model tends to be more physiological, or functional, in that the organs – liver, heart and so on, are not so much thought of as actual organs, but as sets of functions that are linked according to the classical Chinese medical paradigm. The neuroendocrine model is more anatomical, rooted in physiological systems which at the same time are discrete anatomical divisions of the body: the nervous system and endocrine glands. The diathetic model of Ménétrier is a classification of types based on research into the medical histories of a large population of patients, which are then grouped according to basic constitutional pathological tendencies or diatheses.

Our purpose is not to develop a single and unified universal paradigm combining Eastern and Western patterns of thought. Nor is it our purpose to establish firm, irrefutable classifications for plant substances to which future students of herbalism can adhere. Rather, it is to help practitioners in their quest to create their own internalized systems of understanding for developing the clinical skills that will ultimately allow judgments to be instinctive rather than intellectual.

It would be a satisfactory outcome of using this book if conventionally-trained practitioners were to feel at ease prescribing botanicals based on how plant substances influence the neuroendocrine system outlined herein. It would likewise be satisfactory if acupuncturists, or other practitioners familiar with East Asian schools of thought, could comfortably prescribe botanicals based on the five phase model we have described. However, studying both systems will optimally yield new levels of insight, and shorten the time necessary to gain familiarity with the plants, so that clinical usage can be undertaken more rapidly. In the final analysis, it is our conviction that what matters is clinical effectiveness, not theoretical rectitude.

The most successful use of this book would be as a template for developing a rapid, intuitive and sophisticated understanding of the plant substances as they are administered therapeutically, while developing an individual therapeutic system based on experience. Practitioners may develop their own system a little differently, while using it as a tool, not as a law.

Once the theory is familiar, it is important to translate it into experience. It is always a useful exercise to attempt to determine one's own type according to the sections on typologies, and experiment on oneself. For example, the person who is predominantly a Metal yin type should begin by trying Metal yin herbs. The sympathetic-dominant type of individual, when confronted with different herbs indicated for the same condition (for example, cough), should choose one having sympatholytic properties over one that may likewise be indicated for cough, but have the effect of further exciting the sympathetic nervous system function (which would be classified as "sympathomimetic").

In the section on plant substance profiles, one should study all indications as part of a physiological context, or "terrain." Keep in mind that a single plant does not yield to a simple classification any more than an individual does. Some plants are easily classified as a single phase classification, or for a single property by other classification methods. Many are complex, however, which can make a single classification appear arbitrary. The many uses of oil of thyme, for example, or eleutherococcus (Siberian ginseng) defy a single classification. Therefore classifying oil of thyme as predominately Metal yin, or eleutherococcus as Fire yin, is a result of the authors' bias regarding how the substance might be most profitably conceptualized from the viewpoint of the clinician.

The Symptom Listings in Part Three are neither a collection of prescriptions, nor recipes for disease conditions, nor a textbook of clinical medicine. We hope that the listings will stimulate the thought processes of the practitioner and be helpful in developing creative solutions to the ever-changing conditions of clinical practice, conditions that so often do not conform to even the most sophisticated theoretical prognostications. Therapeutic strategies are discussed in this section, along with general principles of phytotherapeutic practice. The appendices can be consulted for additional information which can be used in the context of the Symptom Listings, especially the section on the Oligoelements, or trace elements, which are often used in Western Europe as an adjunct to botanical substances.

INTRODUCTION

Phytotherapy is the use of plants and plant extracts for healing. The incorporation of phytotherapy into European medicine began with the physicians Henri Leclerc, the "father of phytotherapy," and Jean Valnet, who developed aromatherapy as a modality. Phytotherapy is the technical term used most often in Europe to distinguish it from herbalism, which is generally devoted to the folklore and mystical aspects of plant use. In the U.S., phytotherapy is becoming a word that refers exclusively to European botanical medicine. The distinction between phytotherapy and herbalism in Europe is an artificial one, but it does delineate the extent of formalism in the proper use of plant substances. This is especially true in the context of recommending herbal substances as a professional service based on a formal theoretical paradigm, which would be called phytotherapy. Herbalism, in contrast, would be considered the prescription of plant substances based strictly on oral tradition and folklore, particularly folklore in its more mystical aspects.

The use of plants for healing is as ancient and universal as medicine itself. Continuous traditions of phytotherapy methodologies exist throughout the third world, especially in the Orient, where numerous mineral and animal substances are also still in common use. Yet in the West, since the Middle Ages, the use of herbs for healing has gone through several cycles of ascendancy and decline.

The first decline of herbalism in the West was a result of the separation between herbalism and formalized theoretical professional medicine, which occurred as the use of mineral poisons including mercury and antimony increased. These substances were popularized to a large degree by the influence of Paracelsus. Before Paracelsus, the authority of Galen (AD 131-200) was undisputed. Galen, however, was always identified with botanical medicines. Even today, botanical medicines are sometimes referred to as Galenicals. Galen, an eminent surgeon and personal physician to Emperor Marcus Aurelius, created an elaborate system of medical practice based on the "humoral" model of Socrates. He wrote in rigorous detail of the properties not only of single herbs or simples, but also their interaction with different constitutional types. The four temperaments – sanguine, phlegmatic, melancholic and choleric – were based on the four fundamental "humors," or body fluids (blood, phlegm, "black bile" and bile). These temperaments constituted typologies with which herbs were considered to interact in diverse modes. He reasoned that the properties of herbs did not exist in isolation, abstracted from their field of activity. His classifications of the "simples" (single herbs) resembled the Chinese approach, delineating herbs as hot or cold, wet or dry, etc. This systematic approach likewise led to elaborate formulations with complex theoretical designs.

Paracelsus (Phillipus Aureolus Theophrastus Bombastus von Hohenheim 1493-1541), a Swiss physician and alchemist, a man of encyclopedic knowledge, idiosyncratic genius and forceful manner, was unpopular with the medical establishment of his day. A legendary practitioner with an expert knowledge of botanicals (he originally formulated laudanum), Paracelsus developed a system that adapted alchemy to the application of medicine. The use of Galenical herbal preparations began to decline as Paracelsus' influence strengthened.

Paracelsus' theories were supplanted numerous times by subsequent schools of thought. The use of mineral substances like mercury, lead, arsenic, and sulfur, which he introduced, lasted for three centuries. For most of the 19th century, the use of calomel, along with bloodletting, comprised nearly the full extent of "allopathic" medical practice, save for a handful of virulent mineral-based emetics and purges and, of course, tincture of opium, better known as laudanum, that brightest of stars in the 19th century galaxy of nostrums. Calomel, the toxic mercury salt that was the universal remedy for all afflictions from asthma to yellow fever, induced a severe fetid salivation and classic mercury poisoning symptoms. In the early 19th century, British physicians had suggested that repeated dosing of mercury could create a vulnerability and/or tendency toward contracting tuberculosis, but its use continued unrestrained for another century.

By the beginning of the twentieth century, herbalism was no longer in decline. Over a century of "heroic" medicine – blistering, bleeding, purging and vomiting – had disenchanted the public. For a time, they turned to the gentle ministrations of the eclectics: "root doctors," chiropractors and homeopaths.

With the ascension of Western biomedicine, however, the popularity of herbalism again declined, reaching a point where it was all but eradicated. The term "allopathy" fell into disuse for lack of recognition of the existence of any type of medical thought other than the conventional "scientific" model.

The system of Paracelsus, using toxic chemicals and heavy metals in accordance with alchemical theories, foreshadowed the trends of the later 20th century, in which challenging the human physiological systems with toxic chemicals played a central role in the theory and practice of medicine. Coal tar and petroleum derivatives had been used in medicine since the 1880's and the resulting focus on the chemistry of these compounds created a new frame of reference for medical therapeutics. An approach was generated with aspirations of altering the functioning of biological systems based on purely technical, and thus more detached, insights into the functioning of the organic microcosm.

This exploration of biological systems divided into ever smaller units, promising a "brave new world" of technology that could operate entirely at an invisible microscopic level. Symptoms and signs, which had been the fundamental diagnostic criteria for clinical practice from antiquity, were now considered to be the results of invisible warfare in the micro-world. The nature of this war could only be discerned by technicians with micro-scopes or by chemical laboratories performing assays of body fluids. Thus the authority of the clinical practitioner was usurped by the laboratory researcher. The observation of actual patients, hour by hour, day by day, by dedicated medical practitioners was trivialized as "anecdotal," and dispar-aged as lacking any scientific merit.

As we near the end of the twentieth century, more people are becoming aware of the limited resolving power of a solely analytical and "micro-scopic" viewpoint. Macroscopic observation, palpation, auscultation and interrogation to obtain a description of subjective symptoms, are once again gaining credibility with a public increasingly suspicious of a mechanistic approach to human problems. Although "science" as we know it must always be objective, particle physicists have discovered that even within their cold and inanimate field of observation, participation is a critical fac-tor. Increasingly, scientists who are concerned with research methodology are concluding that research results are not so much laws of Nature as they are the response of Nature to our methods of questioning, which are sub-ject to our own limitations and biases. It seems that in a quantum universe, objectivity is unattainable.

A fatal flaw of conventional medicine is the omission of the patient from the process. Patient participation cannot be supplanted by specimens of vital fluids, measurements or disembodied images in an attempt to pur-sue an illusory objectivity. In this "perspective universe," theories merely attempt to solve problems within certain parameters, rather than "uncover" the ultimate truths underlying pathological phenomena. The limitations of a singular attempt at pure objectivity have set the stage for the renewed interest in holistic medical models, in which the practitioner's skill in pat-tern recognition, observation and the ability to make meaningful correla-tions takes precedence over accumulating data for its own sake.

In traditional healing practices, the patients' subjective symptoms and the practitioners' direct observations together result in a diagnosis and ther-apeutic strategy. Today, many practitioners of East Asian and Ayurvedic medicine have developed palpation, pulse taking, tongue observation and the like to a high art. This refined level of personal development and acquired skill cannot be transformed into an objective science. It has always been taught through direct discipleship and not through reading. This is especially true of manual techniques and herbal prescription. In this book we will explore how different systems have been developed for solving problems in the context of direct observation of the patient as a unique entity, and how they use plant substances for therapy.

Herbal treatment is the ideal form of treatment for humankind. Plants act gently to stimulate and supplement the body's healing forces; they are the natural food for human beings. The great advantage of using herbs for medicine is that they are composed of the same stable chemical compo-nents as our daily food. In fact, "herbs" are a part of our diet that has been neglected in recent decades. It is difficult to say where and when this imag-inary line distinguishing foods from herbs was drawn, but the fact is that our bodies are well adapted for absorbing vitamins and minerals in this form. The omission of herbs from our daily diets is perhaps one reason for the popularity of vitamin and mineral supplements. The compatibility of plants with humans is illustrated by the fact that chlorophyll, the green essence of plants, and hemoglobin from our own red blood cells, have an almost identical molecular structure, magnesium being at the core of chlorophyll and iron at the heart of hemoglobin. The natural buffers, fibers, latexes, starches and other bulk materials in herbs help the body's ability to absorb nutrients and "biologically active" components.

Traditional treatment methods have almost universally included "hands-on" techniques like manipulation, massage, bleeding and of course herbal treatment. Even with herbal treatments, the "heroic" methods have had their role to play. In the East Asian medical tradition, purging, sweating and vomiting were prominent features of treating the first stage of illness in a robust individual. However, the experienced and intelligent healer, East or West, has had to develop a high level of skill and personal judgment that cannot be translated into an objective centralized medical theory or conveyed accurately in books or by quantitative methods.

The reader will note tables and comparisons throughout the book in which terms are interchanged or translated between the paradigms. This is intended to add perspective and to develop familiarity with more than one form of system modeling. One cannot expect to be able to "translate" one system completely. There are many similarities between systems, but it may not always be possible to find precise equivalents for concepts in the different systems, just as most languages have characteristic phrases that defy meaningful translation into other languages. The intent is to open new insights into constitutional types, pathological phenomena and plant substances and to stimulate the practitioner's curiosity and creative powers.

It is inherent in the use of whole-system models such as these that clinicians will, over time, develop their own observations and interpretations of theory. Ultimately, practitioners develop their own system, because the proper use of such systems is to provide access to all the unconsciously observed and stored data that accumulate through study, clinical experience and observation. The paradigms given here represent a starting point and, hopefully, the tools by which practitioners can begin to develop meaningful methodologies for their own use by integrating what is familiar, and also by critiquing our interpretations according to their own experience.

The message of this book is, in part, that the analytical approach to biological problems has inherent flaws that can be remedied by using a whole-system model. However, there is still useful information to be gained by understanding the types of constituents in plants. Although we must not depend entirely on this type of knowledge, much of the knowledge obtained through the analytical approach can still be more useful when placed in the context of a whole-system design. Here, we will examine the characteristics of some of the most important plant constituents. Later, we will examine the assumptions built into this approach by observing these characteristics in the whole-system context.

PART ONE
SYSTEMS OF PHYTOTHERAPY

PLANT SUBSTANCES IN A REDUCTIONIST PERSPECTIVE

For all the apparent intricacy of drugs designed by the methods of modern molecular biochemistry, the organized complexity of a single plant extract is of a much higher order. In addition to starches, fibers, latexes, vitamins and minerals, plants contain numerous other substances that have been isolated for medical uses. Alkaloids have such striking biological effects that pharmaceutical companies have long concentrated their plant investigations on them. A single plant can contain numerous alkaloids. The peyote cactus (*Lophophora williamsii*) contains seven psychoactive alkaloids in addition to mescaline. The (Eastern) Indian snakeroot (*Rauwolfia serpentina*) is an ancient Ayurvedic remedy for mental illness. Chemists at the CIBA Research Laboratories in Switzerland isolated reserpine in 1952, which was the first pharmaceutical tranquilizer. Also used as an antihypertensive drug, the value of reserpine inspired further research to seek other useful sedative agents. Over the following years thirty more alkaloids were extracted from *Rauwolfia serpentina*; yet these represent merely a fraction of its potentially extractable contents.

Glycosides include cardioglycosides such as digitalis, cyanhydric glycosides and thioglycosides. Saponins are substances that are soap-like, as their name implies, having emulsifying properties. Saponins produce foam in water and can act as a poison by destroying red blood cells. Navajo native Americans have traditionally used yucca leaves as soap and shampoo. Sapogenins, which can be isolated from saponins by removing the sugar part of molecule, are the starting materials for manufacturing sexual and cortical hormones. Ginseng is notably rich in saponins. Tannins coagulate albumins, heavy metals and alkaloids. Many plants are rich in aromatic substances such as phenylpropane, coumarins and naphthoquinones. Plants also contain essential oils, fatty oils, glucoquinines (vegetal insulins), vegetable mucilage, phytohormones, bitter principles, pigments, glucosides, amino acids, salts, vegetable sterols, resins, gum resins, oleoresins, balsams, waxes, starches, sugars and polyphenols such as flavones and flavonoids.

The reductionistic approach of attempting to understand a thing by breaking it into its components has resulted in a bias toward perceiving a plant in terms of its "active principle." Reconstructing this fragmented approach has promoted an atmosphere of ongoing "discovery." Science discovered, for example, that removing B vitamins from grains and refining them into white flour resulted in deficiency diseases such as beri beri and pellagra. Thus, it was discovered that these diseases could be cured by supplying these nutrients as medications. Wheat germ became a health food item, and subsequently, it was deemed necessary to put back the fiber to protect the bowel, eliminate fatty acids and allow the body to perform other functions. Wheat could be taken apart and sold to the consumer in pieces. The knowledgeable consumer could then reassemble it, at considerable additional cost.

Likewise in herbalism, each year there are new components "discovered" that have medical applications to help "combat" our seemingly increasing health problems. When cholesterol became a buzzword, herbs with cholesterol-lowering properties were "discovered." When immune deficiency became a popularized concept, the polysaccharides of reishi mushrooms and other adaptogenic herbs were similarly discovered. Bioflavonoids such as quercetin, catechin, rutin and other polyphenols are emerging favorites with strong antioxidant, anti-inflammatory and anticancer properties.

Plants are complex entities with properties that are not easily "reduced" to a list of components and their attributes. Understanding plant activity from a macroscopic point of view is essential. The complexity of the chemical structure of plants matches the complexity of our own biochemical environment. Despite the fact that reductionism is a flawed approach to understanding how whole systems operate, it can still be clinically useful. Because of the complex structures of plant substances, however, the current methods of pharmacology do not lend themselves to obtaining thorough analytical data about even a single herbal ingredient, much less the effects in combination. Thus, in the long run, chemical analysis is not usually decisive in making clinical choices about therapeutic plants.

EMPIRICAL CHARACTERISTICS OF PLANT COMPONENTS

ORGANIC ACIDS AND THEIR ESTERS

The simplest organic acid is formic acid, the substance that causes the sting in ant bites ("formic" comes from the Latin word for ant), and the sting in stinging nettles (*Urtica urens, Urtica dioica*). Formic acid and acetic acid (the acid in vinegar) are the first two acids of the series of monobasic acids called the "fatty acids." Another common monobasic or carboxylic acid is butyric acid, which gives the pungent odor to rancid butter. Oxalic acid is a poisonous substance found in spinach, nightshade vegetables, yellow dock and rhubarb. Citric acid is found in citrus fruits and promotes the flow of bile. Benzoic acid, found in balms such as Balsam of Peru, is the simplest aromatic acid and has antiseptic properties. Salicylic acid, a derivative of benzoic acid, is known for its pain relieving properties, acetylsalicylic acid being well-known as aspirin. Salicylic acid salts are found in plants including white willow, meadowsweet and viburnum (cramp bark).

Esters are the products of the combination of acids and alcohols or phenols. Many are fragrant. Amyl acetate has the odor of bananas, methyl butyrate the odor of pineapples and methyl salicylate, an ester of salicylic acid with methyl alcohol, is familiar as oil of wintergreen.

Unsaturated fatty acids are another important group of organic acids. Fats are esters of fatty acids. Several unsaturated fatty acids are known to be essential nutrients (essential fatty acids). Gamma-linolenic acid (GLA), found in abundance in the oils of black currant, borage and evening primrose, is an important anti-inflammatory agent useful in the treatment of rheumatoid arthritis, premenstrual syndrome and eczema. The most important and abundant fatty acids in human biochemistry are linoleic acid, linolenic acid and arachidonic acid. These three acids are common plant constituents.

PHENOLS AND POLYPHENOLS

The simplest phenol is phenol (hydroxybenzene or carbolic acid), which was the first surgical antiseptic used in modern medicine. Other phenols are eugenol (used as a dental analgesic and disinfectant), carvacrol and thymol, all potent antiseptics. They are found in essential oils of clove, cinnamon, thyme, oregano and savory. These "phenolic" oils are bactericidal, antifungal, immune-stimulating, invigorating and warming. Organic acids such as benzoic, cinnamic and salicylic can also be classified as phenols.

Other classes of phenols are xanthones, coumarins, naphthoquinones and bioflavonoids. Xanthone appears to inhibit thrombocyte aggregation and has antiallergic properties. Naphthoquinones include ubiquinone, also known as coenzyme Q, and vitamin K, the antihemorrhagic factor found in chloroplasts, the photosynthetic mechanism of plant cells.

Coumarins are vitamin K antagonists found in small amounts in many plants. Dicoumarol, a product of the fermentation of coumarin, is a powerful anticoagulant or "blood thinner."

Bioflavonoids are therapeutically the most important group of polyphenols. In 1936, Albert Szent-Gyorgyi discovered a complex of cofactors to vitamin C (ascorbic acid) which had properties capable of reducing capillary permeability. He called this complex citrin, and later vitamin P. The term "vitamin P" was replaced with "bioflavonoids" in 1950. There are twelve classes of bioflavonoids: flavans, flavones, flavanones, flavonols, flavanolols, isoflavones, leukoanthocyanins, chalcones, dihydrochalcones, aurones, anthocyanidins and catechins. They are often found as glycosides, e.g., rutin is the glycoside form of the flavonol quercitol. Several flavonoids, especially quercetin, luteolin, morin, fisetin and procyanidin, have been found to have antiviral activity *in vitro*.

Overall, bioflavonoids are potent antioxidants. Many have been found to be anticancer, antihepatotoxic, cardioprotective, anti-inflammatory, anti-infectious and immuno-stimulating. Some of the best known and therapeutically useful bioflavonoids found in numerous plants are quercetin, catechin, hesperidin, rutin, kaempferol, and silymarin (from milk thistle).

Tannins are a group of polyphenols that precipitate proteins. Therapeutically, they have an astringent quality and can be used to stop bleeding externally, and to dry mucus secretions in the treatment of digestive tract inflammations. In addition, they have healing properties for treating burns.

Anthraquinones are found in purgatives such as senna, rhubarb, cascara, sagrada, alder, buckthorn and aloes. Anthraquinones irritate the bowel wall and in some cases stimulate bile secretion.

GLYCOSIDES

Cardiac glycosides are found in a number of plants used for cardiac insufficiency, most notably digitalis, from the purple foxglove *(Digitalis purpurea)*. They are also found in black hellebore *(Helleborus niger)*, lily-of-the-valley *(Convallaria majalis)*, pheasant's eye *(Adonis vernalis)* and ouabain *(Strophanthus kombe)*. These types of plants are to be used with caution.

Cyanhydric glucosides have the characteristic odor of bitter almonds. The combination of these substances with water results in the formation of hydrocyanic acid. Hence, these can be extremely toxic substances, although varieties of almond and prune pits are used in Chinese medicine for the treatment of coughs, circulation problems and even tumors. Amygdalin, of which laetrile is one form, is a cyanogenic glycoside from the apricot pit. Other plants containing cyanogenic glycosides include red clover, hawthorn, both chamomiles *(Matricaria chamomilla* and *Anthemis nobilis)*, yarrow and black elder. Cyanhydric glycosides have sedative and antispasmodic properties, improve parasympathetic tonus and dissolve lipids.

Thioglycosides are found in mustards, horseradish, cabbage family plants (cruciferae include kale, broccoli, cauliflower, brussels sprouts and kohlrabi), turnips, parsnips, watercress and shepherd's purse. These sulphur-containing compounds inhibit thyroid function when taken internally. Externally, some of them can irritate the skin and mucous membranes.

SAPONINS

Saponins have a molecular structure similar to steroids. The importance of steroids to cell-wall integrity and as anti-inflammatory hormones is one explanation for the value of many of the plants that are rich in saponins. Plants rich in saponins generally have immune-boosting and anti-inflammatory properties. These include licorice, foenugreek, the Chinese herbs bupleurum, angelica sinensis, schizandra, black dates, polygala and akebia, horse chestnut, yarrow, maize, linden and different species of dioscorea. Ginsengs of the species panax, aralia and eleutherococcus are rich in triterpenoid saponins, which are thought to be responsible for some of their "adaptogenic" properties.

RESINS

Resins are semi-solid, amorphous substances that numerous plants exude when the plant is injured. In general, they are soluble in alcohol and ether. Three types of resins are oleoresins, gum resins and balsamic resins. Turpentine is an oleoresin; myrrh and frankincense are gum resins. Gum resins are soluble in alcohol and form emulsions with water. Balsam of Peru and benzoin are balsamic resins. Balsamic resins dissolve in alcohol but not in water. Resins are used as astringents and antiseptics, and seem to have immune-stimulating properties along with their antiseptic activity. They are traditionally used topically for wounds, both to seal and to disinfect.

GUMS

Gums dissolve in water, but form a thick, sticky liquid. They do not dissolve in alcohol (gum arabic, tragacanth).

ALKALOIDS

Alkaloids are clear, crystalline, bitter, nitrogen-containing substances that comprise various categories. There are quinolines such as quinine; iso-quinolines including morphine, codeine and papaverine, which come from the opium poppy *(Papavera somniferum)*, or berberine from barberry and goldenseal; indoles like ergotamine, ergometrine, ergonovine (from ergot, *Claviceps purpurea)* and some of the more commonly known such as mescaline (from peyote, *Lophophora williamsii)*, psilocin and psilocybin (from various psilocybe mushrooms); phenylalanines (colchicine from colchicum, capsaicine from capsicum); pyridine and piperidine (such as trigonelline from foenugreek and coniine from poison hemlock); tropanes such as scopolamine and atropine (from various nightshades); and steroids like aconitine (aconite) and veratrine (white hellebore).

The most common alkaloids are the methylxanthines, which are types of purine alkaloids. Caffeine is found in coffee, tea and guarana. Theo-bromine, theophylline and aminophylline are found in cocoa along with caffeine. These alkaloids have a characteristic bitter taste, and are fairly car-dioactive and sympathomimetic.

The recent controversy over the safety of the herbs comfrey and colts-foot (tussilago) is because of the presence of small amounts of the alkaloids pyrrolizidine and quinolizidine. The potential damage to the liver induced by these alkaloids, although found only in small amounts in these plants, was the reason they were recently banned by Canadian officials.

EMPIRICAL COMPONENTS OF ESSENTIAL OILS

TERPENES

Terpenes are found in all essential oils. They have strong penetrat-ing properties and a light aromatic fragrance. In one European study, the terpene d-limonene was administered orally to rats with tumors, and caused more than 80% of the tumors to regress. D-limonene is found in at least twenty common essential oils. Oil of lemon is 90% limonene. Other common terpenes include pinene, phellandrene, carene, cam-phene, dipentene, sabinene and cymene. Terpenes, also called monoter-penes, are composed of two isoprene units that are juxtaposed in chem-ical bonds.

THE ISOPRENE UNIT

Isoprene (C_5H_8) never occurs as a free molecule, but as the skeletal structure of all of the terpenoid compounds. Two isoprene units comprise a "monoterpene." Monoterpenes include ordinary terpenes, iridoids, which are bitter agents, and various other functional groups such as alco-hols and aldehydes.

Sesquiterpene hydrocarbons are made of three isoprene units. They are soothing and anti-inflammatory and are thought to speed wound healing. Sesquiterpene alcohols have liver-stimulating properties. Sesquiterpene lactones are anti-inflammatory and mucolytic for coughs, asthma and bronchitis.

Diterpenes are composed of four isoprene units. Resins, vitamin A and gibberellins (plant growth substances) are diterpenes. Triterpenes, composed of six isoprenes, are sterols, steroids and saponins. These include botanical saponins, cholesterol, ergosterol and squalene. Steroid hormones are closely related structures. Vitamin A is a tetraterpene (8 isoprenes). Further polymerization of isoprenes results in viscous substances such as gutta-percha (100 isoprenes) and India rubber (5000 isoprenes).

Monoterpenes have an immune-boosting and anti-inflammatory effect. Sesquiterpenes are antiallergic, antihistamine and calming.

FUNCTIONAL GROUPS

Alcohols – Monoterpene alcohols are anti-infectious and energizing, even for viral infections and viral fatigue. Sesquiterpene and diterpene alcohols have liver-stimulating and estrogen-like properties.

Aldehydes – Aldehydes have calming properties, and can dissolve mucus and even stones.

Esters – Esters are soothing and cooling, and have antispasmodic and often fungicidal properties.

Ethers – Ethers are soothing to the nervous system and to the digestive mucosa.

Ketones – Ketones dissolve mucus, prevent stone-formation and stimulate growth of epithelial tissue. They may cause irritation of the nerves or mucous membranes.

Phenols – Phenols are stimulating, warming, antiseptic, anti-infectious and detoxifying.

CHEMOTYPES

Some essential oils are known by their "chemotype," which is a variety rich in a certain component. An example of this is *Eucalyptus citriodora,* which contains citronellal. *Origanum vulgaris* is rich in thymol, but *Origanum compactum* (Moroccan oregano) is rich in carvacrol. Rosemary *(Rosmarinus officinalis)* has chemotypes rich in camphor, cineol or verbenone. Thyme, lavender, myrtle and numerous others have chemotypes that sometimes have significantly different properties. However, doctors practicing according to the terrain tend to place less emphasis on these distinctions. *Eucalyptus globulus,* for example, is often used without consideration of the other chemotypes. The reason for this is research that has demonstrated that essences can have identical effects regardless of the components (see "The Aromatogramme," in the therapeutic index).

GALENIC PREPARATIONS OF THERAPEUTIC PLANT SUBSTANCES

The global extract of a plant is the most common form of botanical medicine used clinically. Although many single herb products are said to be "standardized" to contain a consistent quantity of an "active principle," it can be argued that the healing qualities of a plant are most effective without any type of tampering. Certainly, essential oils are much more effective when they have not been falsified or fortified. Most essential oil producers in Europe try to use plants that have been wildcrafted or have been produced with non-chemical farming methods. Pharmaceutical grade products, used by health care practitioners, are tested by pharmacognosists who specialize in phytochemistry to assure a high grade of therapeutic extract or oil.

The various forms of plant substance in common use in phytotherapy for internal treatment are bulk herbs, tinctures, extracts, glycerin macerates, fresh plant suspensions, essential oils and plant bud extracts (gemmae).

BULK HERBS AND TEAS

Bulk herbs are usually crushed or cut and then dried, and prepared as infusions or decoctions. Infusions are prepared by "steeping" the herbs in boiled water for five to twelve minutes. An infusion is used for leaves and flowers, and is the preferred method of preparation when boiling the solution would result in the loss of useful aromatic substances from the plants. A decoction is prepared by boiling the herbs for several minutes, usually the roots, barks, stems, berries and sometimes the leaves. Prepared combinations of herbs in this form are available in natural food stores throughout Western Europe, but some pharmaceutical companies also supply them to practitioners for clinical use.

EXTRACTS

"Alcoholates" are obtained by maceration of the plant in alcohol and subsequent distillation of the macerate. When the dried plant is dissolved in alcohol, the result is a "tincture." Maceration of the fresh plant in alcohol obtains a "mother tincture." Buds, rootlets and young sprouting plants used for application in gemmotherapy are most often prepared in a glycerin macerate. Essential oils are extracted by means of steam distillation and separate precipitation of the water and the aromatic essences. Dry extracts are obtained by evaporation of the solvent, or "menstruum," usually water, alcohol or ether. Nebulizations are finely atomized dry extracts. Integrated fresh plant suspensions ("S.I.P.F." - *suspensions integrales des plantes frâiches*) are prepared from plants that are frozen at a carefully monitored rate, gradually at first and then more rapidly, to prevent destruction of enzymes and other plant components. After freezing, drying and cutting, the extracts are placed in gelatin capsules. Chromatography techniques show that the spectrum of the integral fresh plant suspension is almost identical to that of the unprocessed fresh plant.

Fluid extracts are obtained by evaporating a solution of plant material in water, alcohol or ether. The base plant materials are thoroughly extracted in two stages. The solutions derived from each stage are then blended in order to obtain a solution that is equivalent in strength to an equal amount of the original dried plant material. Thus one gram of the fluid extract is the equivalent of one gram of the dried raw plant material, whereas a tincture corresponds to one fifth of the weight of the plant material, and a mother tincture, made from the fresh plant, corresponds to one tenth of the weight of the dried plant. Therefore one gram of fluid extract equals five grams of tincture and ten grams of mother tincture of the extracted plant substance.

The relative advantages of each method of extraction depend on which methods are most appropriate for each plant. Some plants have different activities depending on whether the extract is a tincture, essential oil or glycerin macerate. Many plants are administered to greatest advantage by using them preferentially according to one method of extraction. For example, glycerin absorbs tannins very efficiently and prevents oxidation, thus preserving the freshness of buds which are growing and changing rapidly in the plant. Some plant components, such as saponins, dissolve more efficiently in alcohol than in water. Many aromatic substances ("camphors" like menthol and thymol) are soluble in alcohol but insoluble in water. Oleoresins also are soluble in alcohol but not in water. Using solvents prevents destruction by heat, and therefore oxidation of components that otherwise would be lost. The additional advantage of dry extracts, alcohol extracts and essential oils for the clinician is that they are highly concentrated; strong doses can thus be prescribed in an easily ingestible form.

FORMS OF APPLICATION

INTERNAL USAGE

Drops, pills, capsules and **syrups** for oral use can be stored and taken conveniently and in precise dosage. Teas and decoctions are taken in a less precise dosage, but are usually not as strong or as concentrated.

Suppositories are generally made with a base of a waxy or fatty material such as beeswax, paraffin or cocoa butter. Placement of the the plant substance in the rectum allows it to be absorbed directly into the bloodstream. The rectum is the preferred route for the treatment of pelvic congestion, including prostate, hemorrhoidal and gynecological complaints. Suppositories may be prescribed advantageously for infants, for patients who are unable to swallow or for patients whose digestive absorption is poor.

Enemas have the same advantages of suppositories but allow a larger dose of the plant extract. They are important for administrating essential oils in high doses to treat severe infections or even asthma attacks.

Ovules are prepared in the same fashion as vaginal suppositories to treat gynecological conditions including vaginitis and cervical dysplasia.

Douches are prepared by adding drops of extracts, especially essential oils, or decoctions in approximately a half pint or less of water, or sometimes a decoction of tea. The solution is introduced vaginally and retained from a few seconds up to ten minutes.

Inhalation therapy with diffusors or steam inhalers is used for the treatment of respiratory infections with essential oils.

EXTERNAL PREPARATIONS

A **cataplasm** is made from a fresh plant that is crushed, rolled and cut, then mixed with linseed, clay or flour. Sometimes clay is diluted with a little mineral water and an infusion or decoction of plants.

Oil extracts are made by crushing fresh or dried plants then infusing in a fatty oil such as olive oil. The fatty oil is used as both an extractant and a preservative. Olive oil, which is rich in chlorophyll, is extremely useful for this purpose.

Liniments are prepared in a base of oil or alcohol to use as a friction rub on an affected area.

Other forms of external application use different bases or excipients, including cerates (beeswax, carnuba wax), pommades, pastes, lotions and gels.

AROMATHERAPY

Aromatherapy is the use of aromatic plant essences, or aromatics, for healing. The prevailing notion of aromatherapy is as a treatment through the sense of smell. Therapy with fragrances is a branch of aromatherapy known as reflexotherapy, but the plant essences are actually administered in a variety of ways. These aromatics are used both externally and internally (including vaporizations and suppositories) for their healing benefits. Other terms for aromatics include essences, plant essences, vegetal essences, essential oils and volatile oils.

Essences were the backbone of ancient Egyptian medicine. A thirty-foot long papyrus written in 1552 B.C. classified seven hundred such substances. Biblical passages referenced heads anointed with oil. In ancient Egypt, mind-altering substances were rubbed into cranial sutures for ritual and ceremonial purposes.

Essential oils may also have rejuvenating properties, possibly because many of them supply hormone precursors that facilitate the body's manufacture of hormones. One oil, Canadian fleabane (*Coniza canadensis*), even contains small amounts of human growth hormone. According to Dr. Ivan Popov, former physician to King Peter II of Yugoslavia, and pioneer in the use of placenta and embryo extracts in cosmetics, "If anything is going to revolutionize the field of rejuvenation in the next few years, it's going to be aromatics (especially stimulating and tranquilizing aromatics). Alone, they have incredible properties. Used in conjunction with other treatments they often possess a powerful synergism, greatly accelerating and augmenting the regular beneficial effects."

When we think of oils, the highly viscous fatty oils (fixed oils, or non-volatile oils) like olive oil, corn oil and so on come to mind; but aromatic oils are very close to being gases, because plant essences are usually composed of a high proportion of hydrocarbon chains, called terpines. Unlike the shorter hydrocarbons which are gases, such as methane, ethane, propane and the like, essential oils are chains that are too long to remain in the gaseous state, and so they are liquid. As the hydrocarbon chains grow longer, they are in the form of resins, diterpenes like vitamin A, and gibberellins, which are types of plant hormones. Triterpenes include sterols (like cholesterol), steroids (anti-inflammatory hormones like cortisone) and saponins. India rubber is an example of a polyterpene.

Essential oils used internally are almost always those extracted by steam distillation. This extraction method uses finely chopped herbs placed in a container in which steam is produced, heating the herbs and extracting the aromatic portion. In turn, this is carried to condensation coils where the plant essence returns to the liquid state along with the water. Extraction may also be done chemically with solvents, where again the essences are separated out by distillation. Or a "hot" extraction method may be employed, using fatty oils, or fats that are heated along with the bulk herbs. The herbs are then strained out leaving the plant essences dissolved in the fat or oil.

The essences are highly concentrated. One hundred kilograms of thyme are required to make a single kilogram of oil of thyme. Two to three kilograms of hyssop are needed to make one hundred grams of essence. This is one reason why they can have such powerful physiological effects even at such low typical doses as nine to twelve drops a day, and sometimes much less.

GEMMOTHERAPY

Gemmotherapy is a branch of phytotherapy that uses the fresh buds and embryonic plant tissues: the channels of growth such as shoots, buds, sprouts, rootlets, stems and inner bark. These parts are rich in growth factors, vegetal hormones, auxins and gibberellins. The plant parts are crushed, then set in a five percent solution in a glycerin-alcohol mixture for about three weeks. The glycerine macerate is prepared homeopathically in a slight one decimal (1D) dilution to stabilize and activate the preparation. The five percent of vegetal material diluted to 1D contains about one-half gram of dried buds and vegetal material for each 100 grams of macerate. The resulting compound is used symptomatically or for drainage. Rather than a true therapeutic method, it is actually a method of medicine preparation.

Gemmotherapy is used as a complementary therapy to other forms of phytotherapy or methods of physical therapy. The glycerin macerate of a given plant has different properties from a mother tincture or essential oil of the same plant. Several macerates are exceptionally effective for allergic problems and for arthritis, rheumatism and their related pain.

OLIGOTHERAPY

Oligotherapy is not a type of phytotherapy, but has been adopted as a supplemental form of treatment by a majority of phytotherapy practitioners in France. The "oligoelements" are chemical elements electrolytically dispersed in distilled water and stabilized in glycerin at the proper concentration. In general, preparations of a single oligoelement or an oligoelement compound are prescribed for oral use, usually in combination with other types of therapy. The active levels of the trace elements are of the order of millionths of a gram.

The rationale of oligotherapy is the necessity of certain metallic ions to activate a number of enzymes. For example, alkaline phosphatase, an enzyme essential for bone formation, requires zinc ions to function. Zinc also plays a role in amino acid synthesis as a necessary cofactor for peptidase. Copper is part of superoxide dismutase that breaks down free radicals. Manganese is part of DNA polymerase, which is essential for DNA synthesis. The action of the trace elements is at the level of these and many other enzymes, which accelerate the biochemical reactions necessary for normal physiological function. Essentially, enzymes are regulators and catalysts that make most of the body's metabolic functions occur at a normal rate of speed and energy consumption. The action of many enzymes depends on their bond to metallic ions, and the metal-activated enzymes retain no catalytic power without this bond.

Oligotherapy addresses not only the quantitative deficiency of trace minerals, but their qualitative deficiency. By preparation of the minerals in a stable ionized form, the terrain is infused with metallic ions in the most assimilable form possible. The therapeutic result is to reactivate enzyme systems that can restore functions of metabolism and detoxification that may have been inert or latent for years. The fundamental purpose of the therapy is not to correct mineral deficiencies, because mineral deficiencies, according to oligotherapy proponents, are not so much a lack of mineral substance as a lack of activated metallic ions. These qualitative deficiencies can be rectified with very low doses of the elements.

FROM EMPIRICISM TO WHOLE-SYSTEM MODELS

THE DECLINE OF WESTERN HERBALISM

Throughout the 19th century in Europe or America, the skilled herbal practitioner could intelligently decide which herbs to use for a fever, based on whether it was worse at night or during the day, accompanied by sweating, constipation, dry cough, cough with clear or bloody sputum or any of a multitude of other signs. From generation to generation, rules of practice and the proper use of herbs were transmitted as an oral tradition through apprenticeship. Unfortunately, because the reductionist bias in Western cultures was so strong, concepts of differential diagnosis for herbal treatment were never formalized into a whole-system model. Much was lost as the population of herbalists dwindled and practitioners with a wealth of practical wisdom died out.

Notably, in the third world, living traditional whole-system models were not rejected with the introduction of the Western reductionist bias, and long traditions have survived somewhat more intact.

Western herbalism began its decline by its imitation of conventional medical thinking, using the logic of the "doctrine of specificity," in which a disease name is matched with a "remedy." The classical theories of herbal usage were taken out of their appropriate context and placed into an alien one of analytical, linear, reductionist thought. The proponents of herbalism silently accepted the conventional nosology – the method of disease classification – as being absolute and incontestable. Thus the terminal error of the herbalists was to imitate reductionist science and to try to play a game that operated according to a different set of rules.

Yet a plant is not easily classified as a drug with a specific usage simply because it has "global" properties rather than one specific action. It is well known in pharmacology that drugs may have different and even contradictory reactions in different subjects, but no one has succeeded in scientifically classifying individual reaction responses to drugs to determine who will react paradoxically or adversely, and if so, at what dosage.

From the point of view of efficacy, it cannot be stated that isolating the alkaloids from plants creates an advantage in clinical potency of the medication. In Japan, for example, it has been demonstrated in clinical trials that using a traditionally prepared formula containing the herb ephedra is more effective than its "active principle," the alkaloid ephedrine. The daily dosage of ephedrine for relief of cough is 75 mg., but in a decoction containing only 3 gm. of Ephedra Combination (*Ma Huang Tang*), with only 20 mg. of ephedrine, a stronger relieving effect is obtained, despite the presence of licorice in the formula functioning to decrease the plasma levels of ephedrine. It seems that the scientific quest for an "active principle" in plants has neglected the buffering and nutritive properties of herbs (and also numerous "subactive" principles as well) that act synergistically with the harsher "active" ones that individually shock physiological systems into responding with an alarm reaction.

Investigations into the use of essential oils for the treatment of infections in France have shown that there is no definitive relationship between so-called active principles and destroying or controlling *in vivo* microorganism populations. Phenolic components such as thymol, eugenol and carvacrol found in essential oils have microbicidal properties identified since the late 1800's. The properties of an essential oil, however, appear to be much more complex than simply being the carrier of an active principle.

Oil of thyme, which contains 40 percent geraniol, is effective in treating staphylococcus *in vitro*, but oil of geranium, containing 80 percent geraniol, was found to have no effect. Oil of geranium is much more effective than oil of thyme in treating streptococcus, even though they both have high concentrations of the same "active principle". In destroying the bacteria *E. coli*, *Enterococcus*, *Pseudomonas* and *Klebsiella*, the effect of Chinese oil of cinnamon, which contains no eugenol, was found to be almost identical to oil of cinnamon from Ceylon (Sri Lanka), which contains a high percentage of eugenol. Oil of thyme was found to be equally effective with these microbes whether it was the type of thyme that contained thymol or carvacrol. In some cases, essential oils that were fortified with extra "active principle" actually had weaker microbicidal properties. It appears that the global properties of a botanical species are primary and more than the sum of their components.

In this cybernetic age, we understand the need to specialize information-handling systems; yet our biological sciences still operate from obsolete principles based on the influence of Pasteur and Lavoisier and the dominance of reductionist thinking. This type of thinking results in the concept of diseases as individual autonomous entities, and the idea that the entire value of a plant can be "reduced" to an active principle. We persist in making causal and sequential connections in observing phenomena and ignore important correspondences.

By our education we tend to think in terms of cause-effect logic in order to be methodical or scientific. Yet this mode of cognition is only one half of understanding and it is the half that forces us to isolate a unit of information from its natural matrix. We might say that this mode of perception produces *in vitro* data. If we want to understand our subject *in vivo,* we must think in terms of the whole system functioning interactively. Thinking in terms of whole systems has been out of fashion academically since the age of Descartes and Newton. That is why many traditional models of cognition have a quaint and archaic tone. They seldom appear in academia except as arcane curiosities, but are still found in "quasi-sciences" or "proto-sciences" such as astrology, numerology and the *I Ching*.

Carl Jung found it essential to understand these traditional intuitive models for ascertaining the full scope of human psychological experience. He coined the word "synchronicity" to describe the principle of understanding systematic correspondences. Joseph Needham, the eminent Chinese scholar, used the term "correlative thinking" to describe the mode of thought pervading Chinese science.

Quantum physics resulted from observing the behavior of subatomic particles, a process that Newtonian physics could not perceive. Yet qualitative analysis of chemical components, even at the molecular level, is inadequate to describe the behavior of whole organisms. The purpose of a health-related science should be to correlate data that lead to logical and effective therapeutic action.

It is important today to develop scientific system models, and to study the traditional ones to define and develop whole-system models for a science of healing. Not only is the set of rules in reductionist systems different from the traditional whole-system models of herbalism, the rules of conventional scientific thought are inimical to the development of herbalism's full range of power and efficacy, which can only be achieved in the context of whole-system models. This is the way herbalism has been understood and developed traditionally, as we shall see, and this is the direction in which it is possible to create a new and powerful nonlinear whole-system science for the future.

Defining a Whole-System Model

Disease naming today is based on a specific set of symptoms, attributable to a single cause and affecting a specific anatomical structure. This method is seldom disputed by natural healing practitioners, although they function in a completely different context than attempting to "conquer" disease. Chinese medicine, especially its popular Americanized form, "T.C.M.," is perhaps the most visible example of a nosology based on the properties of herbs and observable symptoms and signs in the context of a whole-system model. Patients are not simply diagnosed with a stomach ulcer. Rather, they might have "damp phlegm," a "Liver-qi" disturbance, "Stomach heat" and so on. Once diagnosed, they would be given appropriate substances to dry up phlegm, cool heat and so forth.

The use of units such as the Chinese five phases of Wood, Fire, Earth, Metal and Water, rather than being merely quaint, are very practical because familiar items with the greatest variety of associations are the most useful for correlative thinking in a system model. On the one hand, a system of correspondences must have an abundance of familiar associations; on the other hand, except that they should be recognizable, there is no conclusive argument for any particular choice of symbols for correspondences or for any particular number of them.

Categorization has become an important area of study among linguists, anthropologists and psychologists. From the viewpoint of cognitive science, categorizing perceptions is a key factor. A classification can seem quite bizarre outside its proper context. For example, a conventionally-trained dermatologist would be annoyed and confused by a Chinese herbalist's diagnosis of a case of atopic dermatitis being described as a "wind-heat" type of pathology. The philosophical question that emerges is whether any form of classification reflects intrinsic properties of the external world, or if all forms of classification are properties of the mind and the collective bias of shared perceptions of people who share a common language and culture.

It doesn't matter how many ways one chooses to cut the pie. It can be cut into yin and yang of Chinese philosophy, or into three as in Ayurveda. It can be divided into four elements such as the Socratic humors, six like the *I Ching*, seven as in the Law of Octaves. Traditional Chinese Medicine divides diagnosis into eight entities or parameters, the Enneagram consists of nine divisions. Twelve is a common divisor, best known in astrology, seven is found throughout Biblical numerology. The end result is the same. Whole-system thinking strives to collate a wealth of associations and phenomena that Dewey-Decimal-System thought places in different parts of the building.

A whole-system model assumes that all units in a system are a function of the whole, and that all units in the system affect all other components of the system. This means that a whole-system model is useful for depicting situations in which many different factors are at work simultaneously and for characterizing how the different factors interact with each other. For this reason it is not so concerned with cause-effect within the system, but with correspondences among different phenomena.

In self-organizing, self-regulating living systems, the operative term for the phenomenon of physiological self-regulation is homeostasis. Although the body's internal environment is maintained in what appears to be a relatively constant condition, it is not static or unchanging. It exists as a dynamic steady state in which the input and output of materials are balanced either by physiologic mechanisms or by compensating mechanisms. A whole-system model gives us a dynamic picture in which many diverse phenomena can be tracked according to their interactions with one another.

THE TERRAIN AND WHOLE-SYSTEM MODELS

"It is much more important to know what sort of patient
has a disease, than what sort of disease a patient has."

—C.H. Parry (1755-1822)

THE TERRAIN CONCEPT

In France, where the concept of the "terrain" originated, and where it still influences educated thought, serious practitioners of phytotherapy have solved the problem of creating appropriate system models in several ways. We will examine two in some detail, which will allow serious practitioners to build on their own knowledge and experience and develop new insights from another context.

The terrain concept is essentially a description of the condition and nature of the body fluids considered as a whole system and as a fundamental representation of a physiological or pathological function. Its decline as a scientific model paralleled the ascendancy of the "doctrine of specificity," in which diseases are considered to have an autonomous existence and a single cause. The concept of biological individuality is inherent in the concept of the terrain, but not in the notion that perceives a disease as "attacked," as an autonomous entity, with scant attention paid to the individuality of the "host."

Implicit in the idea of the terrain, likewise, is that even if we assume a specific external disease pathogen, an individual living organism's response is so complex that there is no predictable outcome of the disease or its treatment.

The doctrine of specificity still rules most contemporary habits of thought with regard to disease and therapeutics. A contemporary example is how AIDS is defined as the presence of the HIV virus. With this definition, of course, there is a 100% correlation between the disease and the presence of the virus. Thus according to the model of specificity, even though the reality of the situation is vastly more complex, we have a disease name (AIDS), a "causative" micro-organism (HIV), and therapeutics designed to destroy the micro-organism. During the mid to late 1800's, it appeared to many scientists that a disease could have a single cause. *Cholera vibrio* was found in cholera cases and typhoid bacillus in typhoid fever. Diseases like scurvy or beri-beri could be reversed by ingesting a single nutrient.

A result of this preoccupation with microbes as the cause of disease is a situation in which a patient suffering gastrointestinal discomfort, followed by malaise, stiffness and eventually joint pain can be diagnosed as having Salmonella, Lyme's disease, Reiter's syndrome, influenza or fatigue syndrome. These conditions are differentiated based on which microorganism is found, or, in the case of Lyme's, is assumed to be there. The therapeutic strategy is to attempt to destroy this microbe, which may or may not be there, and which is only assumed to be the cause.

The advocates of the doctrine of the terrain, the most famous of whom were Antoine Béchamp and the more famous Claude Bernard, proposed that factors regulating the cellular environment played a primary role in the health of the organism, as opposed to external factors. Furthermore, they espoused the view that the microbes living in the body's fluids were the result of the medium in which they were cultivated, rather than the creators of their own culture medium. This vastly more complex view did not become popular among those involved in creating the reductionist model, nor among those standardizing diagnostic systems and treatment protocols. Nor did it sit well with those who preferred a more militaristic view where disease is conquered by destroying these invisible causative agents.

The traditional concept of the terrain is used in pathology as a global description of pathological states, as in "cancer terrain," and in therapeutics as a description of a designated responder to a certain substance. For example, a patient for whom hawthorn might be prescribed could be referred to as having a "hawthorn terrain," although this usage would be less common, since a terrain is more often described as a characterization of the individual's unique physiological balance. Constitutional types and diatheses, or inherited pathological tendencies, can also be described generically as a type of terrain; an allergic diathesis can be described as an "allergic terrain," for example.

Thus the term "terrain" itself has diverse and subjective usages. As a metaphor, it refers to an environment, like soil, in which things grow and can be cultivated. In this context, the nuance of the word terrain is that it is a "medium" in which there is an ecosystem, a "ferment" of life. (It was called the *milieu interieur,* or "internal medium," by the physiologist Claude Bernard.) In the human body, the term has come to refer specifically to the fluid environment of the cells and the way in which the condition of this medium relates to health and disease. The most common use of the word terrain is in the different nosologies and whole-system models that have been developed for clinical diagnosis and treatment in phytotherapy.

The diagnostic system determines the method of classification of plant substances. The terrain models are by nature system models, meaning that they are nonreductionist. Since they represent a type of nosology that is functional-individualistic, disease names from the conventional nosology are not used. Typologies are an intrinsic feature of a terrain model. We can say, for example, that an individual has a pathology that is sympathotonic – meaning that there is hyperactivity of the sympathetic nervous system – and we can call this a sympathotonic terrain. Perhaps this individual is a sympathotonic type and tends toward this type of condition, and perhaps not. Within the framework of the five phases model, the same individual might be perceived as "Wood yang replete," which requires drainage of the repletion of "Wood" by means of "Wood yang" plant substances. Borrowing from traditional Chinese medicine, we might likewise say that a patient has a "damp-heat terrain," or a "yin vacuous terrain."

This concept addresses the main weakness of the classical herbals in which a plant is indicated for a symptom or disease. The classical herbals will tell us that "X" herb is good for a cough, or that "Y" herb is good for rheumatism. It is no wonder that phytotherapy became haphazard and lost so much of its power and position in the therapeutic world. If we are told that coltsfoot is good for a cough, we are seldom told if it is good for a wet cough or a dry cough. Nor are we told if it should be used for a robust or asthenic constitution, or for a cough that is worse at night, a cough with a fever, a cough with perspiration, a cough accompanied by frequent or infrequent urination, or by nausea and vomiting. In many cases the herbals are written by authors whose chief expertise is in the historical lore of herbs, and who are not experienced herbal practitioners with developed diagnostic skills. Some modern herbals claim to be "scientific" (meaning reductionistic), because they are based on data accumulated in reference to one or more "active principles" contained in various plants. In some cases controlled clinical trials are cited. One of the weaknesses of controlled clinical trials is the lack of consideration of biological individuality, the fact that different types of people respond differently when ingesting the same substance.

Most therapeutic plant substances do not qualify as pharmaceuticals for several reasons. The potency of the first plant-derived pharmaceuticals was based on the fact that the "active principle" was isolated from all of the natural buffers present in the whole plant. These alkaloids were fast acting in part because of the shock presented to the system by their toxicity. Complex plant substances often have multiple properties, a notion not congenial to the dogma of specificity. To understand how deeply the doctrine of specificity has penetrated our collective psyche, we have only to recall the discovery that a common pain drug, aspirin, could also be used prophylactically for heart attacks. A drug with two properties was instantly front-page news nationwide. That a single plant substance could be used for headaches, coughs, diarrhea, skin problems and externally to speed up wound healing was beyond belief. For this and other reasons, phytotherapy does not benefit by imitating the prevailing mindset in medical thought. It is unfortunate that the doctrine of specificity has created habits of thought, even among natural healing practitioners, that are inimical to a deeper understanding of using plant substances to rectify health problems.

The way in which we interpret plant properties is rooted in how we perceive and classify pathological phenomena. In other words, how we diagnose determines how we treat. We could say that the plant rosemary has intrinsic properties, but we need a language to describe its properties and how it will interact with human physiology. For a given nosology, the plant is described according to elements of that nosology. We can say that rosemary is sympatholytic and parasympathomimetic, indicating that it calms the sympathetic branch and fortifies the parasympathetic branch of the autonomic nervous system. It could thus be prescribed beneficially for a patient with vagal insufficiency or a sympathotonic terrain. We could also say that rosemary is Wood-yin, meaning that it is strengthening to systems and structures associated with the Wood phase in a patient who has a Wood-yin terrain. We can say that rosemary is ruled by the sun, or that it is a nervine. We can assign it properties according to the Socratic model of fire, earth, air, or water; or Ayurvedic properties according to vata, pitta or kapha. We can select any software or language we like. But rosemary is still just rosemary – more than the sum of its parts and pieces.

Choosing a model to describe the activity of rosemary, or any other potentially therapeutic substance, is an individual matter, one that depends on the practitioner's background and the patient's needs.

The superiority of using the first paradigm detailed in this book, the neuroendocrine model, is in its familiarity for practitioners who have had conventional training in a school of medicine, osteopathy or chiropractic. The second paradigm, the five phases of classical Chinese medicine, will naturally be more familiar to practitioners trained in aspects of East Asian healing, including acupuncture or shiatsu.

Many practitioners will find familiar concepts in both approaches and can expand their knowledge by filling in conceptual gaps and studying plant properties according to both paradigms. Above all, we should develop our own models of practice based on insights and short-cuts provided by understanding different models, rather than adopting existing paradigms as though they were holy writ. We can gradually discard artificial classifications as one trades them in for real experience. Systems are tools for guiding perception and intuition, and for developing judgment. As our direct perception is developed by experience, we can discard intermediary concepts. We can then learn to write our own software, and finally, once again, rosemary is just rosemary.

Typologies

The particularities of each person, each terrain, are specific to the individual. Equilibrium is maintained by the functional regulation of constitutional factors. The study of typologies is usually based on an understanding of a person's individual strengths and weaknesses.

Typologies are very important in whole-system models, since a "type" is a basic, definable unit of a whole system, i.e., individuals with their characteristics of personality, temperament and constitutional tendencies. Typologies in general have been a subject of interest and speculation throughout human history. They have always been a part of East Asian medical diagnosis and have been a part of Western medical tradition since Hippocrates. Handwriting analysis, astrology, palmistry, physiognomy, phrenology, Jungian archetypes, the Enneagram, to name a very few, have been developed with an eye toward understanding individual differences.

The *Atlas of Man* by Dr. William H. Sheldon is one well-known scientific attempt to classify morphology and temperament. Modern typologies in the West tend to be based on the endocrine system, the classic glandular types being the adrenal, the thyroid and the pituitary. "Diathesis" is a conventional medical term for a constitutional, pathological susceptibility of different tissues to stimuli. Tendencies toward allergies, biliary dysfunction, gout and diabetes are considered to be disorders typical to a predisposed diathetic type (e.g., "allergic diathesis," "arthritic diathesis," "exudative diathesis," "apoplectic diathesis").

As mentioned before, in East Asian traditional medicine there are various constitutional typing systems for herbal prescription as well as for acupuncture. They are most often based on the five phases: Wood, Fire, Earth, Metal and Water. Korean constitutional acupuncture according to Jhema Yi (1836-1900) describes four types: *tae yang in* (Metal), *su yang in* (Earth), *tae-um in* (Wood) and *so-um-in* (Water). In Japan also, "Fire" types are frequently omitted because they are considered to be either rare or nonexistent and five phase typologies are often comprised of four or eight types.

Freud, Jung and others developed psychological typing systems. The eight character types of Gaston Berger are useful as a model for temperament types according to acupuncture channel classifications (see Y. Requena, *Character and Health*). Much of the research in this book matches the character types of Berger with physiological and pathological tendencies in the framework of the five phases.

Many physicians in France, where the "terrain" concept is very much alive and integrated into cultural ideas of health and medicine, use other models of typology, such as the oligoelement diatheses of Ménétrier and the neuroendocrine model of Lapraz and Duraffourd. Many French practitioners of phytotherapy feel that the five phase model is a more digestible introduction to the concept of terrain, yet the more complex neuroendocrine model appeals to many physicians whose background and personal inclination is toward a more detailed and exhaustive approach.

These two paradigms are not, as stated before, the only two that can be chosen. Ayurveda is useful, as is traditional Chinese medicine. The five phase model is more directly useful to acupuncturists, because it provides a meaningful bridge between acupuncture and internal treatment.

CLASSICAL WHOLE-SYSTEM MODELS
IN PHYTOTHERAPY

The term "terrain" implies the use of a humoral model, since the terrain refers to the physiology and pathology of the body's system of fluids (The word "humor" refers to the body's fluids, which were thought to be the basis of one's psychological profile as well as one's moods; hence the word "humor" later came to mean one's state of mind). To the extent that any of the traditional systems use humoral typologies, they would be considered in the context of this book to incorporate a terrain model.

The oldest of the well-known extant Eastern systems of healing is Ayurveda, and in the West the system of so-called "Socratic humors," the Unani system used in the days of Hippocrates. This model is still used today by several healing systems in various interpretations. Proponents would dispute that these systems are strictly "humoral" models because, in the case of Ayurveda in particular, the concepts of *prana,* energetic channels and vibrational healing with mantras also play an integral, if not fundamental role. Anthroposophical physicians would probably concur with Rudolf Steiner's proposition that the Socratic humors were originally considered to interpenetrate with cosmic forces which are more fundamentally causal in the manifestations of health and disease.

THE DOCTRINE OF SIGNATURES

The doctrine of signatures is a way of thinking that was characteristic of pre-Enlightenment approaches to herbalism. The properties of plants were classified by patterns of growth, by their morphology, or by other "signature" traits. *Anemone hepatica,* having leaves shaped like a liver, was considered to be effective for liver complaints. Dandelion root, with a reddish-brown "liver" color, was also considered to benefit the liver. In East Asian tradition, beans, which are kidney-shaped, were thought to benefit the kidney functions. Plants with long, penetrating roots were thought to strengthen virility, and snakes and eels were attributed similar properties for the same reason. Plants that grow in water – sea algae, watercress and horsetail, for example – were thought to be beneficial for "water" functions. The roots of mandrake and ginseng, both of which have a humanoid form, were attributed magical properties in proportion to their size and actual resemblance to the human form.

As an intuitive guide, signatures are clearly a logic of correspondences and pattern recognition. After the Middle Ages, however, thought processes gradually became more biased toward reductionism and the doctrine of signatures became arcane.

AYURVEDA

Ayurveda is the ancient healing system of the Vedic tradition of India dating back to at least 1500 B.C. Like Chinese philosophy, Ayurveda incorporates a system of five elements or phases. The five elements of Ayurveda – Earth, Water, Fire, Air and Ether – are different from those of Chinese philosophy but fulfill the same purpose in the context of classifying phenomena. Each of these five phases contain all the other four phases, and all five combine and interact to manifest all form in the Universe. Earth represents solidity; Water represents fluidity; Fire represents heat, electricity, vision and consciousness. Air represents gases, wind, movement and sensation, and Ether represents space, empty or filled. The three of these that are most fundamental to the observable manifestations of life are Air, Fire and Water. Air includes both Air and Ether, and Water includes both Water and Earth.

The physiological manifestations of Air are the body's motor and sensory functions. The manifestations of Fire, the heat principle, are the digestive function and the function of the liver, eyes and skin. Water, the cold principle, includes fluids such as saliva, mucus, phlegm, lubricants such as synovial fluid, pleural fluid and cerebrospinal fluid. We can see how all their functions combine in the digestive tract, for example, in that peristalsis is an Air function, secretion of enzymes and digestive juices is a Fire function, and lubrication of mucous membranes a Water function.

Pathology is considered to be the result of a disharmony of Air, Fire and Water, usually when one of them is in excess. There is also the notion of "mala," probably similar to the idea of "evil qi" in Chinese medicine. The constitutional balance of these forces is the basis of individual distinctions based on a humoral typology. The Air type is referred to as "vata," the Fire type as "pitta," and the Water type as "kapha," and subtypes are based on combinations of these fundamental three types. We might then say that these constitutional types represent terrains, or predisposing factors toward certain types of physiological and pathological manifestations.

THE UNANI MEDICAL TRADITION

The influence of Hippocrates, a contemporary of Socrates, on medical thought was at its apex in Greece during the fifth and fourth centuries B.C. The four phases – fire, earth, air and water – and the four accompanying types – choleric, melancholic, sanguine and phlegmatic – are based on the four fundamental humors: yellow bile, black bile, blood and phlegm, respectively. There were systems based on their use, especially from the time of Galen (2nd century A.D.) through to the 15th century. It may have been a variation of a still more ancient way of thought, probably originating before the time of Hippocrates. The Socratic humors have survived as a tradition in conjunction with astrological systems of thought, and more recently in Anthroposophical medicine.

Similar to Ayurveda, the essential idea is that pathology is the result of imbalances in the ratios and functioning of the different fluids. When the combination of the fluids is proper, and when their functions are properly regulated, the organism functions properly.

Constitutional types are based on the predominance of certain fluids. The terms sanguine, phlegmatic, choleric and melancholic still maintain approximate meanings to the original descriptions of personality profiles based on these "humors." For example, Nicholas Culpepper wrote that Sweet balm (*Melissa officinalis*) "driveth away all troublesome care and thoughts out of the mind, arising from melancholy and black choler." As a conspicuous feature of Western tradition, the humors have been adopted as an important feature of numerous types of healing philosophy, especially in Europe. Throughout history, descriptions of the types themselves have maintained remarkable consistency, although how they are used diagnostically and therapeutically has varied considerably.

TRADITIONAL CHINESE MEDICINE

As its name suggests, traditional Chinese medicine, most commonly known as T.C.M., is a modern adaptation of a traditional medical system. Created in post-revolutionary China, it represents an attempt by the Communist government to centralize and standardize many diverse traditional healing practices into a single theoretical structure based in herbal medical theory. Even acupuncture theory was included in this sometimes incongruous framework. The apparent purpose of this system was to be able to train physicians and traditional-style practitioners to provide the lower-cost health care of acupuncture and herbs, rather than exclusively using the more expensive and hazardous technological medicine.

As a system, it also individualized treatment to a greater extent by evaluating patients according to functional pathology rather than by disease names. Thus, a patient with a diagnosis of "kidney-yin vacuity" could be suffering from diabetes mellitus, bronchial asthma, nephritis or several other diseases. A patient with hepatitis might be sub-classified according to different types related to the functions and interactions of the Spleen[1], Stomach and Liver, each of which is categorized functionally as a part of a larger organ system.

AROMATHERAPY AND ITS ENERGETIC COMPONENTS

As we will see later, the use of essential oils has challenged conventional ideas about clinical treatment and microbiology, which has made it necessary to learn to use them according to the appropriate terrain. Essential oils can be classified according to their global properties by their five phase, nervous system and endocrine influences, T.C.M. classifications and so forth. Dr. Pierre Franchomme and Daniel Penoël of France devised a method of taking the "parts," the plant components that were taken apart by reductionism, and "reassembling" them into a whole-system model.

Their work was based in part on the work of Jean Mars, an engineer who explored some of the electrodynamic properties of different essences while researching mechanisms for dispersing aromatics into the air. Inside an aerosol generator, a floating ionized electrode plate that came in contact with essential oils discharged from an ultrasonic soundhead carried a change in potential which was measured as an electric current on an ammeter. It was immediately apparent, and precisely measurable, that different oils had different degrees of positive and negative charge.

Essential oils and isolated molecules with a negative charge are anions and thus electron donors, possessing a higher degree of mobility. The essences and molecules with a positive charge are cations, or electron acceptors, exhibiting a reduced degree of mobility. Their charge was classified as mild (-), medium (–) , or strong (—) in negative charge and in the same way for a positive (+, ++, or +++) charge. Aromatic oils and molecules are negative or positive energy vectors, and have the properties of being electron donors or acceptors just like all molecules in the metabolic chains of living systems.

---

[1]Throughout the text, capitalized terms such as "Liver," or "Heart," refer to the traditional medicine system of correspondences of the "Liver" or "Heart," including the physiological functions, pathological manifestations and channel systems associated with them. Lower case letters in words like "liver" or "heart" refer to the organs themselves.

The compatibility with water or lipoid (fatty) materials of aromatic oils or molecules is referred to as the polarity (hydrophilia) or apolarity (lipophilia) of the substance. By classifying oils and their dominant molecular features according to these two independent parameters, Franchomme and Penoël were able to create a two-dimensional graphic representation of a number of oils, terpenes and functional groups. With this chart they began to make global, systematic observations.

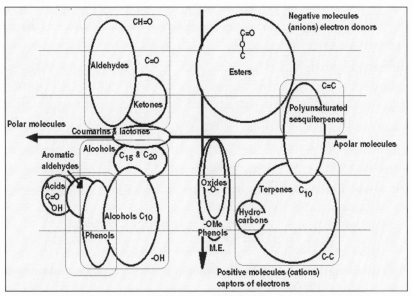

Diagram 1: Oils, terpenes and functional groups[1]

They observed that the oils and molecules that are electron donors have cooling and soothing characteristics, whereas the positively charged electron acceptors are stimulating. Esters and oils rich in esters like lavender and chamomile are cooling, soothing and anti-inflammatory. These are found in the upper right quadrant of the chart. They observed the opposite in the lower left quadrant with the phenols, which are hot and stimulating. They also observed the color spectrum in the chart. In the upper right quadrant is a predominance of blues and greens, such as the factor "chamazulene," found in German chamomile and *Artemisia arborescens;* chamazulene has cooling and antalgic properties. Red oils like oils of cinnamon, clove and thyme that contain phenols like eugenol and thymol are charted in the lower left quadrant.

The two doctors speculated that the four quadrants might also characterize the four Socratic humoral types of the Unani tradition. The upper right quadrant, cool and dry, is like the "melancholic." The hot and dry lower right quadrant would correspond to the "choleric." The upper left, cool and damp, would represent the "phlegmatic" temperament, and the lower left, the "sanguine," which is warm and damp. The most beneficial type of influence for each type would be the diagonal opposite, e.g. warming, drying terpene-rich oils like pine, eucalyptus and terebenthine found in the lower right quadrant would balance the cool, damp, phlegmatic type of the upper left quadrant.

[1]From P. Franchomme and D. Penoël, *L'aromathérapie éxactement* (See Bibliography).

A WHOLE-SYSTEM MODEL OF GEMMOTHERAPY

The "investigative gemmogramme," developed by Dr. Pol Henry of Brussels and his collaborators, is a profile of blood proteins that characterizes the terrain of the patient. According to the theory, each type of pathology reveals itself as a unique profile of several parameters that present themselves as a unique pattern in each patient. Several parameters, including plasma protein electrophoresis, reticulo-endothelial index, levels of haptoglobin, ceruloplasmin, flocculation tests of different globulins and other proteins are measured and correlated.

Based on laboratory research on animals and on clinical research on humans, they have been able to determine the influence of different gemmotherapeutic agents on these various aspects of the protein profile. A given protein fraction can be increased or reduced in a specific manner according to the type of plant buds used. In this way, the overall protein profile can be corrected to a normal terrain. This method represents another way in which data derived by conventional methods can be reorganized to create a whole-system model.

This method for evaluating the effects of gemmae has been used for other types of therapeutic substances. The use of this system established the effectiveness of various gemmae preparations, but did not establish gemmotherapy as a form of therapeutics that is readily distinguishable from other types of phytotherapeutic extracts. Nonetheless several gemmae, such as *Ribes nigrum* and *Juniperus communis,* are very widely used by phytotherapy practitioners.

WHOLE-SYSTEM MODELS COMMONLY USED IN EUROPEAN BOTANICAL THERAPY

Two main systems of botanical therapy are in use in Western Europe: the neuroendocrine model and the five phase model. A third system, less extensively used, is oligotherapy.

The neuroendocrine model has been a familiar model to European physicians since early in the 20th century. Terms such as "sympathomimetic" or "vagotonic" are not exclusively used by practitioners with a phytotherapy or other natural therapeutics orientation. A description such as "sympathotonic," which means a hypertonic sympathetic branch of the autonomic nervous system, has implications for the total physiological picture of the individual. The signs of excessive sympathetic nervous system activity are well established. The distribution of alpha and beta sympathetic receptors throughout the body are likewise well known. The genius of doctors such as Duraffourd and Lapraz is to extend this knowledge into the arena of clinically applied natural medicine.

This work by Duraffourd and Lapraz is based on an extensive knowledge of endocrinology as an interactive model, the anatomy and physiology of the various organ systems and the locations of various hormone and neurotransmitter receptors. By rigorous research into anatomy and physiology and from years of careful clinical observation, it is possible with physical examination to determine the hormonal and neurotransmitter status of the patient's entire system. For example, one can observe that a swollen condition of the left lobe of the liver is from high stress, because of the preponderance of beta-sympathetic receptors in the left lobe. One can palpate a swollen and tender ascending colon and attribute it to a high level of follicle stimulating hormone (FSH), given the high density of FSH receptors in the vicinity. Morphology, personality traits, the sound of the voice and even social attitudes can be clues to the fundamental nature of the patient's terrain.

Based on this physical examination – and often along with the results of laboratory work – the practitioner can select fumitory and lavender for liver drainage, because of the sympatholytic (sympathetic nervous system calming) properties, and also choose chaste tree (*Vitex agnus castus*) because of its FSH-inhibiting properties.

This qualitative evaluation of a patient's condition is familiar to the East Asian-style practitioner. In France, the five phase model is used more by acupuncturists, who already use the framework of Chinese classical medicine. This five phase system was developed to juxtapose with acupuncture treatment using the available and familiar materia medica common to most Western European countries. Through interrogation and physical examination, the practitioner can determine whether a patient with bronchitis is a Metal yin type or an Earth yang type and use Metal yin or Earth yang herbs at the center of the treatment plan.

The system of oligotherapy developed by Ménétrier has been adopted by both camps. The five phase practitioner thinks of the allergic diathesis (Diathesis I) as related to the Wood phase. The neuroendocrine practitioner thinks of Diathesis I as allergic or sympathotonic-hyperthyroid. This oligotherapy system can be used as a single treatment, but more commonly as an adjunct to phytotherapy or nutritional supplements.

THE NEUROENDOCRINE SYSTEM

The link between the nervous system and the endocrine system has been investigated for decades. Hans Selye, the pioneer of stress research, has elucidated the sequence of metabolic events that takes place in the body when there are unfavorable conditions. The "general adaptation syndrome," or stress response, consists of the stages of alarm, defense and exhaustion. The alarm phase – falling temperature, blood sugar instability and depressed nervous function – is followed by a summoning of vital resources in the form of the defense reaction: physiological adaptation that reverses the changes occurring during the alarm phase. The final stage is exhaustion, wherein the adaptive strength is spent and time is required to replenish vital resources or degeneration results. In response to alarm signals, ACTH is secreted, raising the blood levels of corticoid hormones.

Eventually, the role of the hypothalamus as a link between the central nervous system and the endocrine system was uncovered. The pituitary gland (hypophysis), which secretes ACTH, is anatomically a part of the hypothalamus, but is thought of as physiologically separate. This is the primary interface between "neuro" and "endocrine." The hypothalamus is the master adaptation center in the brain and secretes many substances that induce hormone secretion by the pituitary.

In addition to its functions of thermoregulation, regulation of appetite, gastric secretions, sympathetic functions and emotional expression, the hypothalamus controls hypophyseal (pituitary) function by means of numerous releasing and inhibiting factors that govern the secretion of pituitary hormones. This linkage involves the nervous system in endocrine function so that hormone secretions throughout the entire endocrine system will respond to nerve input. Some of these releasing factors include corticotropin releasing hormone (CRH), follicle stimulating releasing hormone (FSH-RH), luteinizing releasing hormone (LH-RH) and thyrotropin releasing hormone (TRH). There are numerous others as well.

The use of the neuroendocrine system as a model of systemic physiological function is more widely used in Europe than in America, where the model has been more pharmacologically-based, and where the emerging paradigm is molecular biology. As an academic tradition, the focus on the nervous and glandular systems as an index for overall physiological function is in the tradition of Walter B. Cannon (who coined the term "homeostasis"), Pavlov and Speranski. The science of typologies according to physical and behavior types that correspond to individual pathology has been a subject of serious scientific interest in the recent history of conventional medical thought. In addition to the classification system of W.H. Sheldon, which combines observations of morphology corresponding to temperament, other classifications were developed by Ernst Kretschmer, Carl Jung, H.J. Eysenck and R.B. Cattel, who belong to a school of thought from earlier in this century that endeavored to develop reliable psychological and emotional profiles corresponding to somatic pathology. Books describing observations of the emotional and psychological profiles typical of arthritics and diabetics attempted to bring scientific insight into an understanding of the pathological process as a multi-level complex of factors related to the full spectrum of human experience.

The depression associated with jaundice and liver dysfunction is well-known, and the psychological characteristics of patients with high levels of serum cortisol or amphetamines has been amply documented. It follows that people with naturally high levels of sympathetic neurotransmitters, such as norepinephrine, or thyroid hormones, or even more obvious, sex hormones like testosterone, will exhibit character, personality and behavioral characteristics in accordance with known physiological responses.

THE FOUR NERVOUS SYSTEM TYPES

The neuroendocrine system is the principal conventionally recognized coordinating system of the body. In both the nervous system and the hormone system there are pairs of antagonists. The activity of the two divisions of the autonomic nervous system provides an index by which we can classify physiological activity according to a more individualized profile of metabolic function. The autonomic nervous system regulates the activity of visceral organs, smooth muscle, cardiac muscle and glands. Its divisions are the sympathetic (orthosympathetic, thoracolumbar) and the parasympathetic (craniosacral).

The sympathetic nervous system has catabolic functions, discharging impulses to vascular smooth muscle in the skin and to the heart, accelerating heart rate and raising blood pressure. The parasympathetic division conserves body resources and has anabolic functions that process materials for use by the cells. It promotes normal digestion, storage of fuel resources and restrains activity of the cardiac and respiratory systems. It also promotes evacuation of the colon and bladder.

Table 1

EFFECTS OF AUTONOMIC STIMULATION		
ORGAN OR COMPONENT AFFECTED	PARASYMPATHETIC EFFECTS	SYMPATHETIC EFFECTS
IRIS	Pupil size decreases (contracts)	Pupil size increases (dilates)
LACRIMAL GLAND	Secretion	Excessive secretion
SALIVARY GLANDS	Secretion of watery saliva in abundance	Scant secretion of viscous saliva
RESPIRATORY SYSTEM Bronchial muscles Blood vessels	Contracts Constricts	Dilates Dilates
HEART Stroke volume Stroke rate Cardiac output	Decreases Decreases Decreases	Increases Increases Increases
SYSTEMIC BLOOD VESSELS**	Dilate	Constrict
PANCREAS (exocrine & endocrine)	Stimulates secretion	Inhibits secretion
STOMACH Motility and tone Sphincters Secretion	Increases * Relaxes * Stimulates	Decreases Contracts * Inhibits
INTESTINES Motility and tone Sphincters Secretion	Increases Relaxes Stimulates	Decreases Contracts * Inhibits (?)
LIVER	Glycogenesis Increased bile secretion	Glycogenolysis Decreased bile secretion
GALLBLADDER AND DUCTS	Contracts	Relaxes
BLADDER sphincter detrusor	Relaxes Contracts	Contracts Relaxes
SWEAT GLANDS	Generalized secretion	Slight, localized secretion
* Usually, but not always ** There are some sympathetic cholinergic vasodilators		

As we can see from this table, the sympathetic nervous system is generally antagonistic to the parasympathetic nervous system. Based on the chemical mediator released at synapses, the sympathetic and parasympathetic divisions are referred to as the adrenergic and cholinergic divisions respectively. High concentrations of acetylcholine, choline, acetylase and cholinesterase are found at cholinergic nerve endings. Norepinephrine (noradrenalin) is the chemical transmitter at most sympathetic postganglionic nerve endings.

Someone in a state of adrenergia (sympathotonia) has a dry mouth, increased heart rate and blood pressure, increased skeletal muscle tone, decreased digestive activity, hair standing on end because of contracted follicle muscles, enlarged pupils and bronchial dilation resulting in more rapid breathing. Someone in a state of cholinergia will have low blood pressure, lower pulse rate, flushed skin, perspiration, small pupils, shining eyes and an over-active gastrointestinal tract.

A sympathetic dominant type of individual is a classic "type A": rapid heart rate, emotionally driven, with tendencies toward constipation, insomnia, hypertension and hyperactivity. Sympathetic dominant individuals have the following pathological tendencies: high blood pressure, infrequent bowel movements, arrhythmias, angina pectoris, nervous strain, arteriosclerosis, bursitis, dental caries, colitis, cystitis, diabetes, lack of endurance, epilepsy, cold extremities, dry eyes, slow fat metabolism, febrile illness, tension headaches, rapid bone healing, slow tissue healing, irritability, indigestion, nephritis, sensitivity to pain, pneumonia, little sweating, tremors, underweight, emotional sensitivity, cravings for sweets, inability to recall dreams, dry hair, skin and mouth, thin flat chest, thick eyebrows, strong sexual passion, large pupils, strong reaction to noise, thick ropy saliva, soft velvety skin.

A parasympathetic dominant person has very good digestion, tends to have loose stools and diarrhea, poor muscle tone, lethargy, tendency to fall asleep easily, good stamina. They tend to have excessive appetite, allergies, osteoarthritis, asthma, low blood pressure, poor bladder control, dermatoses, diverticulosis, eczema, edema, energy loss after eating sweets, bleeding gums, oily hair, shingles, histamine reactions, obesity, osteoporosis, phlebitis, sexual problems, impotence, excessive hydrochloric acid, a cautious conservative nature, deep cough, ruddy complexion, cravings for fatty or creamy foods, vivid dreams, dislike of exercise, infrequent anger, excessive saliva.

Sometimes a person with parasympathetic insufficiency may appear sympathotonic; a person with sympathetic insufficiency may appear parasympathotonic.

Distinction must be made of pure types from subtypes which are determined by the interrelation of the sympathetic and parasympathetic nervous systems. For example, a subject with vagal insufficiency may be a pure vagal insufficient type or there could be a hyperfunctioning sympathetic nervous system. In the same way, a vagotonic individual could be vagotonic constitutionally due to failure or weakness in the sympathetic nervous system or by reaction to a hypersympathetic condition. One must distinguish the following:

1) Pure vagotonia from vagotonia with reactional sympathotonia or vagotonia due to sympathetic insufficiency.

2) Pure vagal insufficiency from vagal insufficiency with sympathetic insufficiency or vagal insufficiency due to sympathotonia.

3) Pure sympathotonia from sympathotonia due to vagal insufficiency or sympathotonia with reactional vagotonia.

4) Pure sympathetic insufficiency from sympathetic insufficiency due to vagotonia or sympathetic insufficiency with vagal insufficiency.

The listing below gives the tendencies and conditions that correlate with each type.

Sympathotonic type: Impulsive, irritable, anxious, rapid heartbeat with palpitations, vascular spasm, distal trembling, flushing, alternating reddening and pallor. Hypertensive, presents a mucus hyposecretion, dry sticky mouth, but without thirst, oliguria (often with urinary lithiasis), constipation and intestinal atony. Skin dry and cold with reactional sweating, goose flesh. Has a chronic pelvic congestion resulting in hemorrhoids, cystalgias, frequent uterine spasms. Varicose veins are a frequent complaint. One often finds systolic heart murmur, myopia. Tendency to hyperadrenalism, hyperthyroidism or hyperestrogenism due to hyperpituitarism. Skeletal muscles tend to be hypertonic, with shoulder and occipital tightness and dilated pupils.

Vagotonic (parasympathotonic) type: Sunken chest, abdominal swelling, warm clammy extremities, sweats easily, introverted, timid, inhibited. Slow heart rate with frequent extrasystoles, hypotensive, hypermetropic tendency. Mucus hypersecretion: rhinopharyngeal, hypersalivation, chronic bronchitis or asthmatic tendency. Gastritis, colitis with diarrhea, pancreatic insufficiency, tendency to constipation, hypothyroid tendency; vagal crises manifesting in involuntary motor spasms of smooth muscle, vertigo and nausea. Tendency to pelvic congestion, especially the prostate.

Sympathetic insufficiency: Great fatigue, normal heart rhythm, hypotensive with a slight difference in systolic and diastolic. Calm, atonic, never desires to do anything, poor libido. Extremities always warm. Can be subject to waking hallucinations of the type attributed to multiple personalities. Predisposed to circulatory insufficiency: coronary, cerebral, respiratory.

Vagal insufficiency: Vagal insufficiency is synonymous with parasympathetic insufficiency. Soft, flabby musculature with a rapid but hypotonic heart and a small thready pulse. Subject to nightmares, delirium, hyposecretive, subject to constipation. Blood pressure normal or a little higher but there is always a large differential between the systolic and diastolic. Cold extremities, often dry and exhibits a global atonia.

Sympathotonia is treated with sympatholytic (also called adrenergic blocking) agents. Sympathetic insufficiency is treated with sympathomimetic agents. A parasympathomimetic agent such as oil of rosemary can be used to stimulate bile flow, or to relax skeletal muscle tension in cases of sympathotonia.

Vagotonia or parasympathetic hyperactivity is treated with vagolytic (parasympatholytic) agents, or with sympathomimetic agents. Vagotonia is often treated with sympathomimetic agents to balance autonomic nervous activity, even for a temporary effect. An example of this is the use of ephedrine or other types of sympathomimetic agents to treat "reactive vagotonia," as in stress-induced asthma attacks.

As useful as these terms can be, they should not be thought of as opposites. In reality, the activities of the branches of the autonomic nervous system are complementary processes, and as diagnostic labels, they are neither mutually exclusive nor pathological entities.

Table 2

PHYTOTHERAPY FOR THE AUTONOMIC NERVOUS SYSTEM	
SYMPATHOTONIC SUBSTANCES	
Adrenalin-like, vasoconstrictor, blood pressure elevating, dilate pupils, elevate blood sugar.	
Drugs	**Herbs – *Oils***
amphetamines, methylxanthines, ephedrine dopamine	broom, ephedra, digitalis, lily-of-the-valley, milk thistle, centaury, kola, black currant, tea, coffee, *basil*, lemon, pine, savory, sage, thyme, rosemary, hyssop, hypericum*
SYMPATHOLYTIC SUBSTANCES	
Drugs	**Herbs – *Oils***
propranolol, reserpine,	black horehound, woundwort, melilot, rauwolfia, periwinkle, water lily, passionflower, valerian, chaste tree, hawthorn, ergot, peyote, lovage, geranium, lime tree, garlic, verbascum, fumitory, white willow, lavender, opium, lycopus, mistletoe, burnet, shepherd's purse, hops, melissa, lotus, cramp bark, *angelica, marjoram, melissa, cypress, lavender, yarrow, ylang ylang, camomile, mint, coriander, Roman camomile basil, clove, cajeput, oregano, spike lavender, garlic, bitter orange, neroli, rosemary, coriander*
PARASYMPATHOMIMETIC (VAGOTONIC)	
Acetylcholine-like, vagus nerve stimulation, myocardial decontraction, vasodilation, augments bronchial tone, augments peristalsis, constricts pupil, increases salivary, gastric and sweat secretions.	
Drugs	**Herbs – *Oils***
muscarine, pilocarpine	black horehound, gelsemium, marigold, mistletoe, groundsel, vervain, horehound, borage, black elder, orange blossom, red poppy, calendula, foenugreek, chicory, shepherd's purse, fumitory, wood betony, *clove, calamus, lippia, mint, neroli, marjoram, oregano, rosemary*
PARASYMPATHOLYTIC (VAGOLYTIC)	
Drugs	**Herbs – *Oils***
atropine, hyoscyamine, scopolamine	datura, henbane, belladonna, gentian, water lily, horsetail, valerian, coltsfoot, chaste tree, opium, field poppy, black currant, viburnum, centaury, yarrow, agrimony, licorice, *angelica, cypress, lavender, savory, thyme, coriander, yarrow, tarragon, hyssop cajeput, Roman camomile, spike lavender, lovage, basil, German camomile, cumin, serpolet*
*Note: italicized entries indicate essential oils.	

THE ENDOCRINE GLANDS AND ENDOCRINE GLAND TYPES

Glandular types are often related to the nervous system types. The hyperthyroid individual, for example, is more often sympathotonic, but by including the thyroid functions in the description, a wider range of phenomena are incorporated. The glandular typologies simply offer a wider perspective and the ability to evaluate patterns of pathology more deeply. Although there is no "pineal" type, and seldom a mention of a "thymus" type, the "adrenal," "thyroid," and "pituitary" types are used more commonly. Here is a brief review of endocrine function with outline profiles of endocrine types.

The epiphysis (pineal body): It secretes melatonin, serotonin, histamine and norepinephrine. The level of melatonin secretion is influenced by light, being elevated in darkness and lower during the day. Serotonin follows the opposite cycle. Melatonin inhibits gonadotropin secretion, inhibits the thyroid gland and has a hypoglycemiant action. When injected into animals, melatonin induces sleep and inhibits ovulation. The epiphyseal secretion 5-hydroxytryptophol inhibits ovarian hormone secretions as well. Serotonin activates the glomerulo-adrenal, augments the secretion of aldosterone and has a tranquilizing and sexual inhibiting effect. The overall function of the gland appears to be the regulation of biological clocks, that is, circadian rhythms and long-term cycles of maturity such as puberty, menarche, menopause and andropause.

Plants that affect the epiphysis include ergot, peyote, caapi, psilocybe, conocybe, stropharia and panaeolus mushrooms and yohimbé. These are substances that appear to act as serotonin inhibitors.

The hypophysis (pituitary gland): The functioning of the pituitary is abundantly described in texts on physiology. Our concern here is the symptomatology, character and behavior related to the hormone secretions. Seven major hormones are known to be produced in the anterior lobe and two in the posterior lobe.

Anterior lobe:

1. SOMATOTROPIN or "growth hormone" accelerates processes essential to the increase of tissue mass, particularly bone tissue, connective tissue, cartilage and RNA production. Somatotropin increases gastrointestinal absorption of $Ca++$, mobilizes free fatty acids from fat tissue, is hyperglycemiant by inhibiting cellular uptake of glucose and stimulates milk production. Insufficiency or excess of GH results in dwarfism or acromegaly respectively.

2. PROLACTIN (LTH, luteotropin) stimulates and sustains milk production when the mammary glands are under the influence of estrogen and progesterone. Inhibits gonadotropin.

3. ACTH (adrenocorticotropic hormone) increases synthesis of steroid hormones from cholesterol, accelerates protein synthesis, raises blood sugar and muscle glycogen levels, increases stress resistance and mobilizes fat.

4. TSH (thyroid stimulating hormone, thyrotropin) is involved in all phases of thyroid activity including removal of iodide from the blood, conversion of iodide to thyroid hormones and thyroid hormone release from the gland.

5. **MSH** (melanotropin) is responsible for skin pigmentation, is lipolytic and encourages function of the adrenals and the thyroid.

6. **LH** (luteinizing hormone) is called ICSH (interstitial cell stimulating hormone) in males, where it stimulates testosterone in the testes. In females it causes formation of the corpus luteum, matures ovarian follicles and induces ovulation of the mature ovum. It induces hormone secretions of the corpus luteum as well.

7. **FSH** (follicle stimulating hormone) stimulates ovarian follicle growth and oogenesis. In the male FSH controls spermatogenesis. FSH with a small amount of LH stimulates follicle development in the ovary. As the follicle ripens, estrogens are secreted which sensitize the follicle to FSH. The estrogens influence the hypophysis so that FSH secretion is inhibited and LH and prolactin secretion are augmented. LH causes the rupture of the follicle and the release of the ovum and stimulates development of the corpus luteum in the ruptured follicle. Prolactin induces secretion of progesterone in the corpus luteum which inhibits hypophysial secretion of LH and prolactin. LH and prolactin production cease and a new cycle begins.

   FSH and LH appear to affect the involuntary muscles that dilate or constrict blood vessels throughout the body. The heart and intestines also appear to be affected by them. When estrogen secretions decline, as in menopause, there is no inhibition to FSH and LH production. The subsequent increase in FSH/LH climbs to levels at which it is thought that they induce hot flushes. Estrogen is often replaced medically, but increased physical activity can convert fatty tissue into estrogen or prompt the adrenals to release estrogen, which will again inhibit FSH/LH.

Posterior lobe:

1. VASOPRESSIN-**ADH** (antidiuretic hormone) accelerates the rate of water reabsorption by the kidneys. Insufficient ADH results in excessive urine excretion. Secretion of ADH is augmented by dehydration or by increased salt intake. ADH induces vasoconstriction in peripheral arterioles and capillaries. It constricts coronary and pulmonary blood vessels and dilates cerebral and renal vessels. Decreased levels of ADH appear to have a connection with memory loss.

2. OXYTOCIN is important in labor and milk secretion because of its effect on smooth muscle. It induces strong contractions of the uterus and it stimulates the myoepithelial cells of the mammary glands. Oxytocin also dilates coronary arteries and slightly lowers blood pressure. Oxytocin secretion is induced by sexual stimulation, suckling and dilation of the cervix in childbirth.

   In sum, the hypophysis is very strongly affected by stress because of its proximity to the hypothalamus. Indeed, the trophic actions of this gland affect all systems of the body; thus an imbalance of pituitary hormones can result in any number of pathological manifestations. When there is a global hypofunctioning of the hypophysis, however, there is severe weakness with loss of weight and reduction of body temperature, blood pressure and basal metabolism.

The pituitary type

The most prominent physical feature of the pituitary type is the head, and particularly the brow. The brow is often wide and angular with contours that give it complexity and contribute to its size. The body in contrast is slight, thin but usually well-proportioned. Women have soft, delicate skin and small breasts, men have a boyish, youthful appearance. The pituitary type has an intense mental life, tends to be withdrawn, somewhat neurotic and is often obsessed with perfection and detail. The mental life takes on a greater sense of reality than the surrounding physical circumstances. Pituitary types often lack body awareness, refusing to exercise or cultivate physical strength and because of this sometimes develop a stooped posture. Tranquil and unobtrusive, they have excellent memories and excellent capacity for abstract thinking, but are often unable to shut off the brain, which can sometimes lead to problems with insomnia. Exercise can provide relief for this in many cases, especially if the insomnia persists for several nights. Other health complaints include stomach and intestinal problems, frequent colds, allergies, eyesight problems, headaches and blood sugar deviations.

The thyroid and parathyroids

Thyroid secretions include thyroxin (T4, tetraiodothyronine), tri-iodothyronine (T3) and calcitonin (once thought to be a parathyroid secretion). The basic functions of the thyroid are regulation of cellular metabolism, regulating cholesterol metabolism, elimination of toxins, oxygenation of cells and regulation of the calcium-phosphorous ratio. Calcitonin appears to inhibit bone resorption and thus decreases loss of calcium from the bone. The calcium level is also regulated by parathormone (PTH) which is released when b-adrenergic fibers induce its secretion because blood calcium levels are reduced.

Tri-iodothyronine is functionally more important that thyroxine with respect to physiological function. In addition to being produced in the thyroid gland it is also produced by the pituitary gland and the liver. This is an important functional link between the liver (Wood) and the thyroid (Wood). Because of this link, and also because of the burden of detoxification passed on to the thyroid by a hypofunctioning liver, compromised liver function can lead to reduced functional capacity.

If the thyroid function is normal, cholesterol levels stay low and progesterone production is normal. Without adequate thyroid hormones, progesterone production will be abnormally low. Estrogen inhibits thyroid secretions. If the liver function is also impaired, estrogen breakdown and excretion will be impaired resulting in hormone imbalances that, if allowed to persist, can result in different types of pathology.

Thyroid hormones, as with adrenalin, have effects similar to a stimulation of the sympathetic system. They accelerate the heart, promote breakdown of lipids and cholesterol, activate glycogenolysis, stimulate erythropoiesis, potentize the action of somatotropin, stimulate the growth of cartilage and stimulate peristalsis and intestinal mobility.

Thyrocalcitonin is also found in the parathyroids and thymus. At the level of the kidney it opposes the excretion of calcium in the urine. Increased thyroid activity affects the calcium-phosphorus in favor of phosphorus, increasing the need for calcium. Decreased thyroid activity has the opposite effect.

Hyperthyroid symptoms: Tachycardia, sweating, weight loss, tremors, vertigo, irritability, temperamental instability, spasmophilia, hyperalertness, profuse sweating (especially palms and soles), easily overheats. Cholesterol levels are decreased or normal; often deficient in calcium.

Hypothyroid symptoms: Weight gain (especially arms and chest), mental dullness, tinnitus, coarse hair, thick skin, thick tongue, lips, decreased temperature, coldness in the hands and feet with paresthesias, thick, ridged, often brittle nails, elevated cholesterol and calcium, functional uterine bleeding and ovarian cysts, slow-moving, docile, indifferent.

Hyperparathyroid symptoms: Von Recklinghausen's disease: Serum calcium is elevated and serum phosphorus is decreased. Leaching calcium from the bones is associated with excessive PTH production. The result is collapse of bone tissue, cyst formation and fibrosis in the bones. Precipitation of calcium compounds can result in stone formation. High blood calcium levels can cause weakness of skeletal, smooth (intestinal pain) and cardiac (arrhythmia) muscle.

Hypoparathyroid symptoms: Tetany. Deficient PTH keeps blood calcium levels low, leading to muscular rigidity and spasms.

THE THYROID TYPE

The thyroid type has extreme energy swings as well as mood swings. Nervous, irritable and intense, they can suddenly become listless, depressed and lethargic. If the thyroid gland is overworked, the classic hypothyroid symptoms of rapid weight gain, sluggishness and swelling (myxedema) can occur with alarming speed. Sensitive to stimuli, the nervous system is easily aroused to hypervigilance. Eating a high fat diet or consuming sugar does not put on weight. On the contrary, it whips the metabolism into a frenzy and the overconsumption can result in weight loss. The overweight hypothyroid type, however, gets caught in a cycle of craving stimulation as lethargy becomes a feature of daily life.

The thyroid type has fine hair and a sculptured body with sculptured features, long thin neck, chest and abdomen, graceful hands and fingers, long limbs and firm sinewy musculature. Smooth skin that bruises easily and tends to erythemas is typical. Restless and fast-moving, the heart rate is high, often over 75. At the energetic part of the cycle they get by with four or five hours of sleep, but need eight to ten during a low phase of the cycle. Thyroid types have poor concentration, but are able to take in and assimilate large amounts of information as though with an antennae.

Often depressed and dissatisfied with life, the thyroid type is well-read, self-absorbed, excessively mental, nervous and restless for new stimulation from travel and new experiences or from internal stimulation from coffee, sugar or alcohol. Although delicate and sensitive, the thyroid type often has a ravenous sexual intensity. The brain and muscles don't turn off easily and so it sometimes takes time for them to settle down into deep sleep.

The menstrual cycle is shortened as well as the length of the menses. The fast-moving thyroid type has a difficult time gauging and managing his or her energy, whipping vital resources mercilessly until the inevitable crash into fatigue and depression.

Health problems tend to be stress-related. Headaches, ulcers, diarrhea, neck and shoulder pain are common. Nervous and mental disorders, spasmophilia, heart palpitations (MVP) and epilepsy are often found in this type. The thyroid type desperately needs exercise to maintain a steady energy level. Strenuous activity increases the level of the active form of triiodothyronine, which makes more energy available.

THE THYMUS

The thymus is the brain of the immune system and an incubator for lymphocytes, which further develop in the spleen and the lymph nodes. Our immunity depends on the proliferation of lymphocytes. A thymus hormone stimulates the spleen and lymph nodes to produce lymphocytes from their own plasma cells. The thymus sends out both lymphocytes and hormones to the spleen and lymph nodes, as well as new information about adapting to environmental changes. Strengthening the thymus can help with autoimmune disorders such as pernicious anemia, rheumatoid arthritis, MS and rheumatic heart disease. Production of antibodies for these conditions may be a thymus function.

THE PANCREAS AND ISLETS OF LANGERHANS

The alpha cells of the Islets of Langerhans produce glucagon and the beta cells produce insulin. Glucagon is the hyperglycemic factor, increasing blood glucose by accelerating glycogenolysis in the liver. Glucagon is produced throughout the gastrointestinal tract as well as by the salivary glands. It stimulates release of catecholamines and strengthens contractions of the heart.

Insulin is the hypoglycemic factor. It increases uptake of glucose by muscle, liver and fat cells, but also exerts an effect on leukocytes, the pituitary and mammary glands. It converts glucose to glycogen and stimulates fat production from liver carbohydrates. Insulin inhibits thyroid activity, promotes protein synthesis and opposes protein catabolism; it facilitates the penetration of K+ into the cells so that they retain water.

Hypoinsulinism results in diabetes mellitus. Blood sugar levels rise (hyperglycemia) because cells fail to take in glucose and glycogen is not converted. Energy needs are compensated for by lipid metabolism and production of sugar from protein. This results in the wasting of body tissues and lipemia, which can cause a fatty liver. High glucose levels exceed the kidneys' capacity to reabsorb it, resulting in glucose in the urine. This loss of glucose creates an osmotic diuresis resulting in polyuria and necessitating the inevitable increase of water intake (polydipsia) that prevents dehydration. Increased food intake is also a result of excessive glucose loss.

Hyperinsulinism (hypoglycemia) is a decline in blood sugar levels which leads to the release of adrenalin and sympathetic nervous system activity. The principal organ affected is the brain. Symptoms include disturbances in locomotion, trembling, anxiety, confusion, loss of muscle tone, fatigue, hunger, respiratory disturbances, depression of reflexes and lowered body temperature.

THE PANCREAS TYPE

This type tends toward an endomorphic build. A great lover of food, the appearance may include big wet lips, often with a jutting lower lip, prominent jowls and a somewhat wet, pasty appearance. The bearing is calm, somewhat imposing, and often the voice is powerful, resonating throughout the voluminous trunk. The neck is thick but loose-skinned, which often results in folds when the body's fat accumulation becomes excessive. Amiable and sociable, this type's body awareness is so strong that there is a tendency to "hold court" and enjoy his own presence immensely and ensure that others do the same. This same intense body awareness magnifies the body's cravings to the level of a fixation on food, drink and physical comfort in general. Often hypogenital, his sexuality is less genital and more idiosyncratic. In this area, the imagination plays a much more important role than body awareness, although he craves touching. The skin is soft and luxuriant, the face is sometimes ruddy and sometimes pale. The temperament is cynical, complacent, slow to be aroused emotionally, but is usually in touch with his emotions because of the feelings being amplified. The midsection is often wider than the shoulders, with relatively thin arms and legs. The fingers and toes are short and stubby and the gums often are prominent and cover more of the exposed tooth area than usual.

Health problems tend to be related to overeating as well as to problems of blood sugar regulation. The liver, kidneys and large intestine tend to get overloaded. The liver and large intestine can become swollen, the latter even grossly distended. The digestion is good and thorough, but stimulation of it is a source of comfort. Obesity is a problem with this type and can shorten the life span. Gout, hypothyroidism, hypertension and arteriosclerosis are other frequently encountered problems with the pancreas type.

THE ADRENALS

The stress glands are associated with the catch phrase "fight or flight," referring to the catecholamines adrenalin and noradrenalin secreted by the medulla. The adrenal cortex secretes steroid and androgenic hormones. The medulla is composed of cells of ectodermal origin and is surrounded by the cortex of mesodermal origin. Secretion of medullar hormones is controlled by direct connection to the sympathetic nervous system. Catecholamine secretion can also be induced by hypoglycemia. The cortex responds to several kinds of stimuli: decreased blood sodium levels, somatotropin, ACTH secretion, angiotensin II secretion or hemorrhage. Steroid hormones are divided into the glucocorticoids (cortisone, cortisol), anti-inflammatory corticoids, which raise glucose levels in the blood and tend to inhibit the body's defensive reactions, and the mineralocorticoids (aldosterone, DOC) or proinflammatory corticoids which bond sodium and excrete potassium.

Adrenalin comprises about 80 percent of the medullar secretions, but is not a neurotransmitter like noradrenalin. Adrenalin strengthens heart contractions and diminishes glomerular filtration of the kidneys. Adrenalin increases the heart rate and stroke volume from b-adrenergic innervation, increases arterial tension by elevating peripheral resistance and induces vasoconstriction of vessels in the intestines, liver, pancreas, the muscles and the skin. Adrenalin causes bronchodilation, decrease in intestinal tone, contraction of sphincters, contraction of the gravid uterus, relaxation of the nongravid uterus, contraction of the spleen; it increases gastric, bronchial and sweat secretions, inhibits pancreatic secretions, stimulates glycogenolysis thus elevating blood sugar, increases blood potassium level and increases cellular respiration, stimulating thermogenesis.

CORTICAL HORMONES

Aldosterone and mineralocorticoids cause reabsorption of sodium by the renal tubules. They increase potassium and hydrogen+ excretion. They cause retention of sodium at the level of the intestine and in the sweat and saliva. The secretion of aldosterone depends partly on ACTH, and the renin-angiotensin system of the kidney. Renin is secreted when there is hypotension from shock, hemorrhage, hypovolemia, sodium depletion and also from sympathetic stimulation. Under stress more steroids are released. Steroid hormones in general lower the quantity of immune antibodies needed to reject foreign tissue as well as to fight infection. The action of mineralocorticoids is inhibited by progesterone and testosterone.

Cortisol and glucocorticoids are called glucocorticoids because of their hyperglycemiant action. They promote protein synthesis in the liver, but promote catabolism by inhibition of amino acids in the muscles. They favor reabsorption of sodium and the excretion of potassium.

ADRENAL SEXUAL STEROIDS

In both men and women the adrenals secrete androgens like DHEA and relatively few estrogens, but some of the androgens are chemically converted to estrogens in the blood circulation. Their secretion is not under the control of the pituitary gonadotropins LH or FSH, but from ACTH. Their function is to provide hormone precursors to the sexual organs and to supply anabolic androgens when they are deficient. They participate more actively in the body's physiology during puberty, change of life (menopause or andropause) and during the general adaptation syndrome (sustained stress).

HYPERFUNCTION OF THE ADRENAL CORTEX

Mineralocorticoids: Hyperaldosteronism (Conn's disease), characterized by high blood sodium and hypertension. Polyuria and polydipsia.

Glucocorticoids: Excessive production (cortisol) results in moon face, fat accumulation in the abdomen, hypertension, osteomalacia, sluggish calcium absorption and secretion, hyperglycemia, tachycardia with hypertrophy of the left heart, seborrhea and psychological hyperexcitability (Cushing's syndrome).

Hypofunction of the adrenal cortex (Addison's disease): Fatigue, elevation of potassium and depression of sodium in the blood, anemia, muscular weakness, hypoglycemia, impotence or frigidity, hypothermia, anorexia, hypotension, constipation and gastric achlorhydria. One of the most specific signs of this malady is melanoderma, dark brown pigmentation of the skin, especially in the palms of the hands, lips and gums.

Adrenogenital syndrome: Hypersecretion of cortical androgens causes masculinization of the female (Stein-Leventhal Syndrome).

THE ADRENAL TYPE

Solid and durable, the adrenal type is the physical powerhouse of the glandular types. With abundant stamina and strongly built, this type bristles with vitality and almost never suffers from fatigue. The head is square with a low forehead and low hairline, the hair is thick and coarse, often curly, and the body is often covered with thick hair. The nose is wide and the lips well-developed; the teeth are large and the jaw heavy and often protruding. The skin is thick, dry and warm, the neck is short and thick and the ear lobes are large, long and thick. The chest is broad and the female has large, well-developed breasts. The lungs and heart are large, giving the adrenal type an excellent oxygen supply to the cells. The muscles are well-developed and have excellent tone. Smooth muscle tone results in excellent peristalsis and bowel tone. The skeletal muscles are large with exceptional endurance and strength. This is an "action" type of individual who thrives on competition and challenge.

An abundance of ACTH and ADH with an abundant supply of endorphins give adrenal types an insensitivity to pain and a feeling of invincibility. Love of competition and challenge makes them doers. Preoccupied with their influence on others, their lives are plunged headlong into accomplishing their goals, spending relatively little time in self-reflection and in self-restoration. The sexual nature is strong, simple and direct. They are fond of using salt and alcohol to stimulate the adrenals, getting away with a high level of dietary abuse compared to other types. Health problems are mostly chronic degenerative problems or athletic injuries. Hypertension, kidney problems, heart problems, low back pain, osteoporosis, bone and arthritic problems are typical of this type later on in life.

THE GONADS

It is one of the obvious facts of life that the diversity of secretion of sexual organ substances results in two major classes of primary and secondary sexual and psychosocial characteristics. The extreme changes in appearance and behavior induced by such hormones as somatotropin and thyroxin are profound and obvious but also show up most clearly when there is related pathology. The differences induced by normal values of masculinizing and feminizing hormones are no less profound. We are concerned primarily with testosterone, estrogen and progesterone. Sex hormones not only influence sexual appetite, but also fat distribution on the body, protein metabolism and numerous secondary sexual characteristics. The secretion of testosterone and progesterone are induced by LH (ICSH) from the hypophysis and estrogen secretion is induced by FSH.

Testosterone: It is responsible for the sex drive of both men and women. The brain also has testosterone receptors and enzymes for its conversion to estrogen. Testosterone helps build bone tissue and increases metabolic rate. In addition to sex drive, aggressiveness, combativity, thickness of vocal cords, the size of the sexual organs, thickened facial and body hair, muscular development and ossification of the long bones are also dependent on testosterone. Testosterone levels peak in the male in the early 20's and decrease until age 40 when the levels drop more gradually (andropause).

Estrogens: The ovary is where most estrogens are produced. Testosterone is their immediate precursor. Nature has, as the biologist Rostand put it, "divided the species economically." Estrogen is regulated in the hypothalamus by FSH-RH and LH-RH, which control secretion of FSH and LH respectively. Estrogen stimulates growth and maturation of the reproductive system and reproductive capacity of the female. It increases all metabolic activities of the uterus – vascularization, water-electrolyte balance and cell division. During adolescence, estrogen stimulates breast development and controls fat and hair distribution and enlargement of the pelvis.

Estrogens increase fat metabolism turnover, decrease the level of blood lipids, elevate serum calcium and phosphorus levels and diminish hypersecretion of sebaceous glands in the skin induced by testosterone. Estrogen levels are elevated 48 hours prior to onset of menses causing accumulation of blood along with water retention in the uterus region, increased secretion of mucus by the cervical glands and proliferation of the endometrium and vaginal mucosa.

Progesterone is produced by the corpus luteum in the ovaries after ovulation. It induces mucus secretion in the endometrium, which has been prepared by estrogen to precede implantation of the ovum, and it relaxes the uterus. If pregnancy occurs, prolonged secretion of progesterone is essential. Progesterone also stimulates growth of the breasts and inhibits the release of oxytocin from the pituitary gland. Progesterone elevates body temperature and causes the temperature shift at ovulation. It has a beneficial effect on almost all premenstrual syndrome symptoms, such as headaches, sugar cravings, breast pain, mood swings, acne and edema. It also reduces breast and ovarian cysts. Excessive estrogen or insufficient progesterone results in many symptoms and syndromes familiar to female patients and caregivers alike. The balance between estrogen and progesterone is thrown off by caffeine consumption or by impaired liver function.

Estrogens, progesterone and androgens are conjugated and excreted in the bile. They are then hydrolyzed by intestinal bacteria and returned to the liver by the portal vein. Congestion of the bile duct system can result in the accumulation of abnormal levels of estrogen. Progesterone and androgens are also broken down in this fashion, and to a lesser extent in the kidneys and uterus.

It is not known if symptoms related to high estrogen are because of a failure in the process of breaking them down or if it is related to an imbalance of estrogen and progesterone. PMS symptoms have been alleviated by therapeutic use of progesterone and high progesterone symptoms sometimes occur when estrogen levels drop too suddenly after ovulation. The two in combination appear to stimulate sex drive. Women who have high amounts of female hormones are often more sexually responsive when both increase after ovulation.

Hyperfolliculine symptoms: Estrogen binds water, so excess amounts can cause water retention. Edema, swelling, headaches, epigastric, back or abdominal pain, nausea and vomiting can also occur. Excess estrogen can cause thickening of the uterine lining and heavier bleeding. "Endogenous" estrogen is converted from androstenedione in the body fat, so excess weight can be a cause of hyperfolliculine symptoms. Blood clots and fibroid tumors are also linked to high estrogen levels. Estrogen also makes a woman's skin smooth.

Hypofolliculine symptoms: Hot flushes are the most common symptoms. Insufficient vaginal lubrication, deficient calcium and anosmia are also associated with low estrogen.

Hyperluteal symptoms: When progesterone is in excess, women suffer fatigue, depression, hypoglycemia with sugar cravings and ravenous hunger. Sometimes the body temperature is elevated. Resistance drops, however, making the woman more susceptible to infection or allergies. Acne sometimes breaks out and bladder pressure and constipation with gas can occur. Libido in many cases is exaggerated.

Hypoluteal symptoms: Mood swings, uterine cramping and many hyperfolliculine PMS symptoms occur.

THE GONADAL TYPE

The contrast is sharp between the sexes for obvious reasons.

Male: Possessed with an indomitable will and tremendous pride, it is difficult to compromise with this type. Intense and self-reliant, he lacks the ability to lay back and relax. Always the strategist, he moves forward with indefatigable force and has a taste for vengeance. Sexually strong, he is ruled by the desire for conquest as well as by passion. He enjoys challenges of all kinds and loves to demonstrate physical prowess. He is not overly verbose, is even secretive and can be insanely jealous and possessive. This is a warrior type of man who is not overly self-reflective, but decisive. This type has a rock-hard jaw, thick hard bones, powerful muscles and hardly any fat on his body.

Female: She has a small head, thick eyelashes, a pear-shaped body with small breasts but large buttocks and thighs and smooth creamy skin which is very sensitive. She sleeps well, and retains water easily so must exercise for that as well as for weight control. She is prone to breast lumps, pelvic congestion and urinary tract infections. Also secretive, she sometimes has a mysterious demeanor. Her emotions are deep and sexual desires are strong and passionate.

Table 3

PHYTOTHERAPY FOR THE ENDOCRINE SYSTEM

PINEAL

Stimulation of pineal function: Indole alkaloid-containing substances: peyote, psilocybe, stropharia & panaeolus mushrooms, *clary sage, jasmine, lavender, sandalwood, myrrh, frankincense, ylang ylang*

PITUITARY

Strengthen pituitary function: elecampane, eleutherococcus, laminaria, licorice, black walnut, *sage, savory, mugwort, sassafras*

Inhibit pituitary function: pasque flower, chaste tree (particularly FSH), stoneseed, *marjoram*

Oxytocic: lady's mantle, woundwort, goldenseal, motherwort, snakeroot, vervain, honeysuckle, elecampane, fennel, shepherd's purse; *clove, cajeput, cinnamon*

Antioxytocic: pasque flower, lovage, white willow, cramp bark

Stimulate prolactin secretion: galega, vervain, fennel, black elder, *anise, fennel*

Inhibit prolactin secretion: periwinkle, sage, scarlet pimpernel, clary sage, sage

Gonadotropin stimulants: mugwort (FSH & LH), sage (FSH), elecampane (FSH & LH) wild oat (LH), sarsaparilla (LH), *anise (FSH), caraway (FSH), sassafras (LH)*

Gonadotropin inhibitors: stoneseed, white willow, hops

Growth hormone: elecampane, sage, eleutherococcus, laminaria, *sage, sarsaparilla, savory, Canadian fleabane*

THYROID

Strengthen thyroid function: laminaria, bladderwrack, wild oat, horseradish, *garlic, onion*

Inhibit thyroid function: brassicas (cabbage, turnip, etc.), lycopus, white hellebore (veratrum album), shepherd's purse, *cumin, fennel*

THE PANCREAS AND ISLETS OF LANGERHANS

Normalize blood sugar regulation (hyperglycemiant, hypoglycemiant): agrimony, artichoke, bilberry, black walnut, burdock, eleutherococcus, foenugreek, geranium, goat's rue, horsetail, lady's mantle, maize, nettle, periwinkle, wild oat, *lemon, eucalyptus, ginseng, juniper, geranium*

ADRENALS

Medulla: sympathomimetic herbs stimulate medulla

Herbs to stimulate cortex: licorice, black currant, periwinkle, cypress, valerian

Essential oils to stimulate cortex: *sage, savory, rosemary, pine, black spruce (picea), sandalwood, thyme, cinnamon* (zeylanicum)

Herbs with steroid-like effect: black currant, licorice

GONADS

Estrogenic: black cohosh, hops, ivy, white willow, lovage, scarlet pimpernel, *sage, clary sage, cajeput, angelica, anise, caraway, coriander, cumin, cypress, fennel*

Estrogen antagonists: pasque flower, chaste tree, *cumin*

Luteotropic: sarsaparilla, lady's mantle, blessed thistle, yarrow, licorice

Aphrodisiac: sea holly, wild oat, licorice, sarsaparilla, Chinese ginseng, *jasmine, cinnamon, clove, ginger, mint, pine, rosemary, sandalwood, savory, thyme*

Anaphrodisiac: chaste tree, marjoram, white willow, *melissa, ylang ylang*

Thermoregulation in the autonomic nervous system: stoneseed, witch hazel, yarrow, melilot, passionflower, *melissa*

SUMMARY

Regulation of the terrain with regard to the neuroendocrine system treats global pathological and constitutional tendencies perceived as nervous system and glandular functions. For example, a diabetic patient who is underweight and asthenic might require herbs for the stimulation of gonadal function. For remineralization and for blood sugar regulation, we could select foenugreek, wild oat and horsetail. The hyperthyroid, sympathotonic diabetic, on the other hand, would be treated with oils to regulate blood sugar, such as *juniper*[1] or *geranium, cumin* for thyroid regulation and a sympatholytic agent, such as *lavender*.

The possibilities of combination depend on the practitioner's familiarity with physiological processes from observing these interrelationships between the glands and the nervous system. The conventionally trained practitioner must strive to view the pathological process of the individual in a unified fashion. The diabetic with a urinary tract infection may respond more favorably to urinary antiseptics that have an influence on blood sugar regulation, i.e., on the "diabetic terrain." These would be, for example, oils of *juniper, sage* or *eucalyptus*. On the other hand, a urinary infection in a patient who is asthmatic may respond more favorably to oils of *pine, rosemary* and *thyme*. The section on therapeutic principles and examples is organized to assist practitioners in taking a global overview of the patient's pathology.

THE FIVE PHASES[2]

Practitioners of traditional Chinese medicine will be familiar with the correspondences presented here and will recognize most aspects of these interpretations of Chinese traditions[3]. The following theoretical explanation, as well as the herb profiles in the next section, are a compendium of how doctors who practice acupuncture, but who have no access to Chinese herbs or to Chinese herb theory, have applied East Asian classical ideas to the practice of phytotherapy using the indigenous materia medica.

THE FIVE PHASES AS A SYSTEM OF CORRESPONDENCES

To illustrate the dynamic aspect of the five phases, let us examine two interactive five-phase "cycles": the generative, or "creative" cycle and the mutually restraining, or "destructive" cycle.

---

[1]Throughout the text, italicized botanical names refer to essential oils, to distinguish them from whole plants or plant components.

[2]The earlier term, "five elements," is in fact a misnomer. The term "elements" is defined as something immutable, a building block of matter. The Chinese character popularly rendered as "element" is closer to being an antonym. Variously translated as "to go," "to effect," or "to carry out," professional translators who have grappled with the philosophical issues of denoting the appropriate nuance and range of meaning have suggested that the term "five phases" is more precise.

[3]There are differences in how terms such as "Liver yin," or "Earth vacuity" are interpreted in different traditions. Japanese interpretations and schools of thought in five phase theory are different in many fundamental ways from how five phase theory is taught in England or the U.S. Much of the French approach to five phase theory originates from the Vietnamese tradition. The way these principles and classical ideas are interpreted and extrapolated here are based on how the practice of acupuncture has developed in France, along with entrenched biases about how herbs and their functions should be adapted to medical practice.

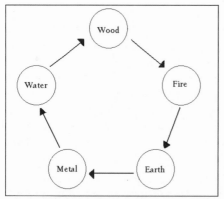 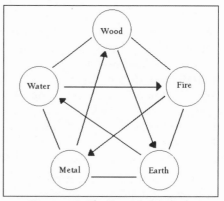

Diagram 2: The Generative Cycle   Diagram 3: The Restraining Cycle

The diagram on the left illustrates that Wood creates Fire; Wood as fuel allows us this image. Fire burns into ash. Volcanic soil is often cited as an image of Fire becoming Earth. Earth produces Metal, and Metal produces Water. Underground water sources are said to be found where there are mineral veins and ore deposits. Wood absorbs Water from the soil and the cycle begins again.

The restraining cycle, portrayed in the diagram on the right, presents its images with greater clarity. Wood[4] (roots) anchor the soil to prevent erosion, Fire melts Metal, Earth absorbs Water, Metal cuts Wood and Water extinguishes Fire.

We can see how this is applied in botanical medicine first by observing that each flavor associated with one of the five phases nourishes its organ and corresponding channel as explained in the Chinese classic known as the *Su Wen*. Sour nourishes the Liver, bitter nourishes the Heart, sweet nourishes the Spleen (and Pancreas), pungent the Lungs and salty the Kidneys. Extremes of these flavors are known to be detrimental to these organs. Excessive salt is implicated in renal hypertension, and excessive sugar in diabetes. A number of alkaloids, which are bitter, can damage the circulation, most notably caffeine. Hot, spicy foods can quickly aggravate asthma or chronic sinusitis. These correlations between flavors and organs are not static ones, however. We can observe their dynamic in the two inter-relative cycles. In the generative cycle, Wood is said to be the "mother" of Fire and conversely Fire is called the "son" of Wood, and, in sequence, Fire is the mother of Earth, and so forth.

Five phase systems have played an important role in the history of East Asian thought. Each phase correlates diverse phenomena that have a common function or essence. These correspondences can be used to create recognizable patterns out of the multitude of observations and perceptions that occur in our experience, and thus feed our judgment and intuition.

---

[5]The five phases – Wood, Fire, Earth, Metal, Water – are capitalized to clarify their identity as a conceptual entity associated with the five phases.

ESSENCES OF EACH OF THE FIVE PHASES

WOOD

To grasp the essence of Wood, think of the elasticity of stalk fibers in the living plant, rather than boards in the lumberyard. The essence of Wood is adaptability, based on pliant, limber, lithe strength. The nature of Wood is organization and persistence. In human physiology, the liver's functions are numerous. It is considered to be the "General" of the organs, that is, it gives orders. The organ of patience and decisiveness, it is an organ of digestion, being particularly involved with fat metabolism. As an endocrine organ, it is associated with hormone regulation, particularly with respect to female hormone cycles. It is identified with venous blood, in that it stores venous blood during sleep and it detoxifies venous blood at the end of the circulation cycle. The muscles and tendons are the primary means of motion for the venous blood from the body's periphery.

Signs of Wood pathology include tightness and tension in the muscles and tendons, restlessness, impatience, anger, migraine headaches, allergic syndromes, biliousness, nausea, a bluish or greenish pallor, bulging veins at the temples and hemorrhoids and other types of varicose veins. In plant classifications, herbs with a sour flavor or herbs that appear in the spring (the classic "spring tonic" herbs) might be classified as Wood depending on their traits and on how they can be used therapeutically.

The liver is a true organ of detoxification. At the end of the circulation cycle, it receives the oldest, darkest, most toxic venous blood. The liver also has close nervous system and thyroid associations. When the liver is unable to handle its toxic load, connective tissue, especially tendons and myofascia, compensate for it. Muscle spasms are an almost universal symptom of poisoning. Chronic autotoxicity creates some degree of chronic tendinomuscular rigidity, or body armor. The liver manufactures part of the T3 supply of the thyroid.

In the tradition of Chinese medicine (and also according to Hippocrates), the Liver is strongly associated with emotions in general. It also helps to make the body's qi and fluid.

FIRE

The essence of Fire is "flaring," that is, rapid centrifugal expansion, engendered by agitation that generates heat. This is the most dynamic of the five phases – energetic activity at its peak. In humans, the most obvious features of being alive are heartbeat and pulse. Correspondences include joy, laughter, running, summertime and verbosity. The Heart is the "monarch" of the organs, the center of activity served by all the other energetic functions.

As well, Fire includes arterial blood circulation. This is the exploding or flaring from the heart that carries vitality and nourishment to all the cells of the body; this is the body's most physically dynamic process.

Nitroglycerin and PETN (pentaerythritol tetranitrate, an explosive used in armor-piercing bombs during World War II) are substances actually in used as drugs to treat angina pectoris and the loss of memory and mental function common after cardiac bypass surgery. This use of explosives to expand a contracted heart graphically illustrates the energetic principle of Fire and corroborates the metaphoric understanding of the Chinese idea of Heart as Fire.

EARTH

The essence of Earth is nourishing and moistening, its nurturance enveloping its charge as a mother's arms envelope an infant. It is soft and moist and supports growth that results in thickening and accumulation. The physiological systems associated with Earth are the digestive and lymphatic systems. Typical Earth pathologies effect digestive, exudative and immune system disorders. The Earth type tends to be corpulent or asthenic and have a great deal or very little stamina, is often slow and easygoing and inclined to be lazy. Blood sugar is usually unstable and needing something to eat can be a minor crisis. Often there is an addiction to sweets and to gustatory stimuli in general. Earth yang types are carefree and good-humored and have a ruddy complexion. Earth yin types tend to worry and have a sallow appearance. Earth types hate humidity and tend to become sluggish in a humid environment. Common ailments are gastritis, ulcers, pancreatitis, hiatus hernia, obesity and poor muscle tone.

The Spleen is synonymous with the lymph system and the upper digestive tract. It is the enzyme headquarters of the body. Digestion takes place not only in the gut, but peripherally throughout the body in the form of macrophage (literally, "big eater") activity, and in the antigen-antibody reaction. Many of the enzymes used in the digestive tract are found outside the gut participating in these functions.

Like Mother Earth, the Spleen or lymph system is the nourishing and protecting mechanism for the cells that live in the tissue fluid. It is moistening, nourishing, digestive, soft and warm. The direction of Earth is the center. The Spleen is truly the center of activity, the actual location of the terrain. It feeds the cells and carries away their waste products and permeates all systems of the body to a depth that no other system can.

METAL

Whereas the essence of Earth is moistening and nourishing, the essence of Metal is drying and tempering. It has superior electrical conducting properties. In East Asian medicine, Metal includes the Lungs, the Large Intestine and the skin. The Large Intestine has the function of hardening and drying the dregs of food in the alimentary canal through mechanical compression and the absorption of water through the intestinal tissues. The lungs eliminate a substantial amount of water in exhaled air as does the skin through perspiration. Metal pathology includes asthma, bronchitis, emphysema, colitis, sinusitis and skin problems.

Through the inhalation of atmospheric oxygen, the lungs provide negatively charged ions to the cells. The skin contains the acupuncture channels, the currents which are fundamental to the distribution of ions throughout the system according to classical acupuncture theory. Metal needles are considered to be especially efficient for correcting functional problems by their conductive properties, which improve conductivity in the skin.

WATER

The essence of Water is cooling and settling. It precipitates and absorbs minerals and electrolytes and maintains salinity and alkalinity to purify and refine the internal milieu. The main Water organs, the Kidneys, are not primarily organs of waste elimination. Their function is to manage pH levels and simultaneously to regulate mineral metabolism. Included in the Water classification are the adrenal glands, the sexual organs, the bones and teeth. Water pathology includes nephritis, renal edema, Addison's disease, impotence, lumbago, osteoarthritis, spinal cord problems, osteoporosis and kidney stones.

Among the range of associations included in the Water tropism are the bones and teeth. (The Spleen is actually the organ system associated with the body's fluids.) The Kidney precipitates minerals for these solid structures. The Kidney is considered to be the root of the body's intrinsic makeup rather than a filter or an organ of waste removal. For example, the skeletal system is the body's actual physical foundation. The Kidney is the reservoir of the genetic makeup and the sexual essence of the body. East Asian medicine teaches that the Kidney is the root of the body's yang and yin. Its main physiological role is to maintain the integrity of the relationship between the ocean-like compartment of the intercellular environment and the intracellular environment.

CYCLES OF THE FIVE PHASES

The rules of logic in the five phase structure are based on mutual engenderment and mutual restraint. The term "cycle," like the word "element," also implies a false idea. The "elements" are dynamic rather than static, as pointed out before, and the "cycles" are simultaneous and not sequential. In other words, we tend to think of Wood generating Fire and then Fire generating Earth, and so on, when we should construct our mental model with Wood generating Fire while Fire generates Earth while Water is generating Wood in a simultaneous activity. Likewise, Water restrains Fire as Metal restrains Wood, and so forth.

The mutual restraint cycle has more obvious associations for those who observe physiological phenomena. These rules of five phase activity are used more frequently and literally in acupuncture treatment strategy, although historically there have been many practitioners who have devised systems of phytotherapy as well as acupuncture by expanding the application of traditional five phase teachings. Below are some examples of how the five phases are manifested in physiological function.

Wood creates Fire: The liver produces 60 percent of the body heat, which is also produced by muscle contractions. Muscles also store glycogen which is converted to sugar by adrenal hormones (Water creating Wood). The heart (Fire) is itself a muscle (Wood) and muscles are necessary for venous circulation (Wood) which connects to the heart (Fire) and becomes the arterial system (Fire). If Wood becomes Fire too easily, blood pressure is elevated and the Fire of the Liver Fire "rises," resulting in irascibility, bloodshot eyes, shouting, tears and other explosive emotions. If Wood does not engender enough Fire, the personality is not expansive, there are few words, muscles are tight, emotional expression is repressed, ambition and purpose are lost and there are palpitations and insomnia.

Wood restrains Earth: Liver and Gallbladder function regulate digestion by emulsifying fats and oils.

Fire creates Earth: Arterial blood (Fire) is distributed to the interstitial fluid of the cells (Earth) where nutrient exchange takes place. Red
blood cells are recycled in the spleen. If Fire becomes Earth too easily,
thought accelerates in the Spleen resulting in confusion and frustration,
which can have an adverse effect on the digestive organs. If Fire does not
warm Earth, the result is abdominal distension, diarrhea, edema and cold
extremities.

Fire restrains Metal: The heart rate (Fire) determines the speed of respiration (Metal) and perspiration (Metal).

Earth creates Metal: Earth moistens and nourishes the body and creates membranes (Metal) that secrete fluids and dry excess. When Earth is
unable to create sufficient Metal, there is fluid production in the form of
mucus, serous fluid or edema. If Earth is unable to moisten sufficiently,
liquid is discharged as in diarrhea, anorexia, shortness of breath and non-
productive cough with thick sputum.

Earth restrains Water: Fluid discharge creates a burden for the kidneys. Edema is an example of this.

Metal creates Water: The drying influence of Metal (Lung, Large
Intestine, skin) regulates fluid in the system and begins the process of precipitation and separation completed by the Kidneys. The perspiration conducted by the skin, the exhalation of moisture performed by the Lungs and
the regulation of abdominal fluid levels accomplished by the Large Intestine are all functions that separate usable from unusable fluid, which the
Kidney then manages. If Metal becomes Water too easily, the subject
becomes physically hyperactive and driven to physical performance. If
Metal does not become Water, there is weak adrenal function, loss of will
power, scant urine and hardening of the body.

Metal restrains Wood: Large Intestine function assists Liver function
in detoxification and conjugation of hormone substances excreted in the
bile. Enzymes in the lung convert angiotensinogen produced by the liver
into angiotensin.

Water creates Wood: Adrenal secretions trigger the conversion of
glycogen from the Liver into sugar in the blood. Bones support the musculature of the body. If the Water is insufficient, there is demineralization
which causes muscle cramps, coldness, vertigo. Water becoming Wood too
easily causes an accumulation of hormones in the blood and the subject
becomes willful and domineering.

Water restrains Fire: Kidney function regulates arterial tone and the
adrenals secrete heart regulating factors such as adrenalin.

As a system of correspondences, these relationships can help us understand why numerous herbs have been used as digestive "bitters," or why
salty foods can affect blood pressure. In general, we classify herbs according to the phase where they have the greatest influence on the corresponding organ system, but we also anticipate secondary effects according to
these five phase relationships. Seldom do we see a plant substance that has

a single five phases tropism, just as we seldom see an individual who represents a pure five phase or neuroendocrine type. Often we see that plants have secondary characteristics simply because the complex personality of its characteristics defies a singular description. As we will see in the section on flavors, it is important to understand the engendering cycle relationships to understand some of the indications of herbs.

One difficulty with understanding the interconnections within a whole-system model is that within the system, it is possible to logically "deduce" anything. On the other hand, sometimes more complex situations occur. For example, a vacuity of Wood can result in a vacuity of Fire. Fire is then unable to restrain Metal, which causes Metal to hyperfunction, and in turn reinforces the vacuity of Wood. This is a way of organizing experience that is more often used in acupuncture than in phytotherapy. It depends more on organizing personal observations than on the formalities of logic.

We can use these principles to make our own observations and systematize our own experience. If we combine systems and interchange them as freely as our experience with them grows, we become experience-centered, rather than theory-centered. Theories are not precious jewels, but rather software for specific kinds of tasks. We need to learn to generate them effortlessly in order to keep up with their rapid obsolescence.

FLAVORS AND THE FIVE PHASES

"When the liver suffers constraint, one can release it with sweet food."

"If the heart is excessively loose [cardiac insufficiency], one can retract it with sour."

"If the spleen suffers from dampness, one can dry it with bitter."

"If the lung suffers from reflux of qi, one can drain it with bitter."

"If the kidney suffers dryness, one can moisten it with spicy flavor which opens the orifices, attracts fluids and circulates the qi."

Su Wen, Chapter 22

THE FIVE FLAVORS AND THEIR INFLUENCE

We can extrapolate from these traditional explanations to develop a useful perspective on allopathic diagnoses, for example:

— Excessive spiciness destroys wood (spasmophilia).

— Excessive saltiness destroys fire (arteriosclerosis, HBP).

— Excessive sour destroys earth (collagen disease).

— Excessive bitter destroys metal (dry skin, lung damage).

— Excessive sweet destroys water (arthroses, dental caries).

Reading books is only one way to learn about herbs and their properties. The oral tradition of herbs required the learner to obtain direct experience with plant substances and patients as the primary learning method. As much as possible, it is beneficial for students of phytotherapy to acquaint themselves with plants through direct experience, in order to activate intelligence at levels other than those that can be evoked by intellectual understanding.

We can understand much about plants from our intuitive process without much training. Would the starving lost hiker be tempted to eat a plant like jimson weed, with its delicate, purplish-white trumpet-shaped flower, and its black-tinged leaves with a coarsely-toothed margin? However, a deep, intuitive understanding of plant properties requires training and practice. Our esthetic sense and personal experience is the starting point. Anyone who has experienced sinus drainage from eating *wasabi* (Japanese horseradish) or experienced bronchial drainage from eating very hot curry, has had the experience that leads to the intuitive understanding of how spicy-warm herbs can be used therapeutically.

SOUR-COOLING

Sour-cooling herbs neutralize heat repletion in the Liver (also known as "Liver Fire"). They are sympatholytic, antithyroid and antiestrogenic. They respond to the Liver's tendency to distribute and disperse. Dispersing the yang of the Liver in effect disperses the Heart yang. The effect is sympatholytic with secondary parasympathomimetic and hypoglycemic effects. Several examples of sour-cooling herbs that act directly on the Liver and the Gallbladder are pulsatilla, witch hazel and nettle. Hawthorn calms the yang of the Heart. Agrimony, nettle and oil of lemon have a purgative action by promoting bile secretion.

SOUR-WARMING

These herbs have the effect of astringing Liver yin repletion (fatty liver), and by stimulating the bile ducts and the Liver yang. The result is an increase in sympathetic activity. They are hepatotonic and stimulate the liver's immunity functions. They promote thermogenesis, stimulate the thyroid and decrease venous pressure, especially in the portal circulation. Angelica, milk thistle and oak are examples of sour-warming herbs.

BITTER-WARMING

The function of bitterness is to harden. Bitter-warm compresses the Heart yin and supplements the Heart yang. Thus it is sympathomimetic and exerts a cardiotonic effect: accelerates rate, reinforces heart contractions, accelerates propagation, diminishes excitability and augments tone. This effect of stimulation of the heart (which is Fire) also affects the pituitary gland and its sphere of influence.

The bitter-warming influence dries excess moisture of the Spleen (Earth) which results in the Spleen (Earth) yang being supplemented. This is another way of describing their use as aperitifs. Appetite is stimulated by drying the phlegm that accumulates in the upper digestive tract as well as by stimulating digestive secretions. They are glandular stimulants (with the exception of insulin secretion) that can relieve hypoglycemia. Lymphocyte production, a Spleen (Earth) function, is also increased, thereby enhancing immunity. Bitter-warm herbs that particularly influence the Heart (Fire) are adonis, digitalis and Peruvian bark (cinchona – which contains quinine). Bitter-warm herbs that particularly influence the Earth phase are cinchona, chamomile, centaury, yellow gentian, barberry, hops and foenugreek.

BITTER-COOLING

In contrast to bitter-warming herbs, the effects of bitter-cooling are sympatholytic, heart-regulating and tranquilizing. They are also febrifugal, emetic and purgative. Herbs affecting Heart yin are hawthorn, black hellebore, oil of bitter orange, rauwolfia and valerian. Herbs affecting earth are arnica, fumitory and oil of birch.

SWEET-COOLING

These influences are harmonizing and moderating. Sweet-cooling herbs are emollients, laxatives, diuretics and moistening agents that are used in cases of pathologically excessive heat or dryness. Sweet-cooling herbs disperse heat repletion in the Spleen (Earth), diminishing the yang of the Spleen. They supplement the yin of the Spleen increasing the secretion of saliva, perspiration and tears through their parasympathomimetic action. They also stimulate insulin secretion. Sweet-cooling herbs include burdock, calendula and European linden (lime tree).

SWEET-WARMING

Sweet-warming herbs supplement and regulate. They supplement the Spleen yang. They have vagolytic effects; they stimulate the corpus luteum and elevate blood sugar. Sweet-warming herbs have a sudorific effect and warm the Lung in cases of chill.

Excess sweet destroys the Liver and Kidney yin and creates a sympathotonic Kidney and Liver yang hyperadrenal state, with adrenalin-like and cortisol-like bone and teeth catabolism: "Eating excessive sweet grieves the bones and causes loss of hair." Sweet-warming herbs include anise, cinnamon, coriander, melissa and sage. Mallow and coltsfoot also warm the lungs.

PUNGENT-COOLING

Pungent-cooling herbs are parasympathomimetic. They dissipate pathological heat in the lungs and are sudorific. Pungent-cooling herbs moisten the Kidney (Water) and soften and open the pores to attract fluids to the periphery. When there is heat in the Lung with a yellowish-green or bloody discharge, these herbs can have a soothing effect. When the Kidney yang is encumbered by a repletion of heat and dryness, from anuria or urine retention from repletion (stones) or heat (pyelonephritis), there is oliguria because undischarged urine impedes flow. Pungent-cooling herbs include bryonia, white horehound, senna and oil of sandalwood.

PUNGENT-WARMING

Pungent-warming herbs dissipate. They dry excessive moisture by dissolving phlegm and allowing it to drain. We can treat stomach ulcers with such substances as ginger or cayenne is because of this property of dissolving irritating mucoid plaque adhering to mucous membranes. In cases of chill, they have a sudorific effect and warm any pathological cooling of the Lung. Pungent-warming herbs nourish the Kidney yang, an adrenalin-like function, and they assist the Kidney when they become excessively cold (oliguria, proteinuria, glomerulonephritis). Pungent-warm herbs include eucalyptus, pine, juniper, ginger, nettle and sassafras.

SALTY-COOLING

Salty-cooling herbs promote the repletion of Kidney yin. This promotes elimination and prevents any backup in the kidneys that could result in pathology such as stone formation. Bearberry, barberry and heather are salty-cold herbs.

SALTY-WARMING

Like salty-cooling herbs, salty-warming herbs are purgative and diuretic but their role is to "harden" the Kidney yang. They stimulate the secretion of the adrenal medulla and cortex and especially androgen (sex and growth hormones) secretion. Chickweed, hyssop, honeysuckle, horsetail, laminaria, goldenrod and broom are salty-warming herbs.

CONSTITUTIONAL TYPES AND PATHOLOGY

The Center for Disease Control in Atlanta informs us that that 75 percent of deaths by disease are due to five primary causes. Interestingly, we can correlate each of these causes with a distinct phase:

1) cardiac and cerebral vascular accidents (Fire)
2) obstructive pulmonary disease, e.g. emphysema (Metal)
3) chronic liver disease and cirrhosis (Wood)
4) malignant neoplasms (Water)
5) diabetes (Earth)

(These five are followed by suicide, AIDS and infectious diseases.)

Each of the constitutional profiles are divided into two types, yang and yin.

WOOD CONSTITUTIONS

THE WOOD YANG CONSTITUTION

The Wood-yang type is a choleric-enthusiast. Such an individual likes to be in charge mainly because he or she does not like to go unnoticed. Authoritarian, but not coercive, the Wood yang type likes to assume the position as leader either to gain distinction, or simply because of impetuosity and irrepressibility. Cordial, exuberant, the life of the party and perhaps a bit hot-tempered, Wood yang is optimistic but anxious, always in a rush because always afraid of being late. The Wood-yang type is impulsive, deciding to do something and vigorously pursuing it. However, Wood yang can get involved in too many things, and be unable to follow through on everything initiated.

They often have a square build, short legs, thick hard-to-cut nails, a square jaw and sometimes a stern, austere demeanor. They are night owls and are sometimes slow to get started in the morning.

In childhood and adolescence, they are rarely sick except for the occasional fever. They possess tremendous drive, stamina and organizational ability. The Liver is sometimes referred to as the General of the organs and the Wood type often possesses a military bearing. Very outward in emotionally, they are easily moved to tears by sentiment as well as by stress. Their emotional outbursts blow over quickly as a rule and seldom do they hold a grudge or attempt to prolong a conflict. Anxiety attacks and insomnia are common in this type, and matters that do not resolve quickly are most stressful for them, since they are impetuous and decisive individuals.

Typical Wood yang disorders are high blood pressure, calf cramps, gastric spasms, sudden onset pains, varicose veins, phlebitis, stomach ulcers, constipation, hemorrhoids, gum problems, gout, rheumatic pains, anxiety neurosis, seasonal allergies, biliary dyskinesia, hyperfolliculine dysmenorrhea, hyperthyroidism, chronic muscle spasms, ophthalmic migraines, genital herpes, shingles, myopia, keratitis and blepharospasms.

THE WOOD YIN CONSTITUTION

The Wood-yin type is the nervous temperament: emotional, inactive, anxious, indecisive and timid with a repertoire of nervous gestures that classically include nail-biting. Possessing great intelligence and imagination, they have the need to embellish reality, to add to the truth, and could be criticized for being subjective. Craving attention, they will use various seductive means to get it. They need frequent change, excitement and diversion, and often escape into dreams and unreality. Moody, temperamental, inhibited and timid, they also have a flair for performance. They are sometimes irritable, and they may sometimes become suddenly tearful. Because of their excessively rational nature they store or deny these feelings and their outbursts may thus appear for no apparent reason. Their emotions can be stored as an excessively rigid musculature that may release as emotional outbursts or as nervous tics or twitches.

Often they are very attractive with a charismatic mystique, and can be amazing entertainers and performers despite their reclusive inclinations. They tend to have a wiry build that begins to expand in middle age. Very firm and fairly muscular, they have good reflexes but poor flexibility.

As children, they seldom have problems except for gastric crises with headaches, nausea and vomiting. Throughout adulthood they continue to have a digestive sensitivity, but do not usually become seriously ill. They usually do not follow medical advice and seldom seek treatment.

They work irregularly and only on projects that interest them. In the same way, their memory for details which do not interest them is very poor. They have difficulty in organization, but have a strongly original creative power and an urge to innovate and pioneer new territory. They have a powerful mental life that often makes them seem distracted and brooding. In fact, they have so many ideas it may be difficult for them to concentrate enough to focus on work, or to bring ideas into reality. Often they suffer anxiety, which causes them to internalize and refuse to express themselves, rather than to emote. Depression is a problem, because they tend to store anger and implode it, creating a morbid sense of self-criticism. They love escape of all kinds, sleep very deeply with few dreams and love to sleep well into the morning.

Typical health problems are headaches, especially from the back of the neck to the temples, hepatitis, epilepsy, myopia, allergic rhinitis, dermatitis, hypoglycemia, polymenorrhea, frigidity, estrogen deficiency from hepatic origin, impotence due to testosterone insufficiency of hepatic origin and various neuropathies.

WOOD PATHOLOGY

THE LIVER

It is particularly true of Wood pathology that it affects almost everyone at one time or another and is not confined to Wood constitutional types. Because the Liver overlaps so many other systems, including the circulatory system, the digestive system, the endocrine system and the musculoskeletal system, there is scarcely an individual who does not manifest some chronic Wood pathology. The way the pathology manifests depends on the constitutional type. One person may develop arteriosclerosis where another person may develop fatty degeneration of the liver, another constitutional type may develop renal calculi, but all are due to a common origin in a liver dysfunction, usually impaired fat digestion or detoxification.

PHYSIOLOGICAL MANIFESTATIONS

Toxicity: Tendinomuscular spasms and irritation of the nervous system are typical symptoms of chronic dysfunction of Wood. There is inflexibility, rigidity and spasticity whether it is rigidity of tendons, muscles, a spastic colon or seizure disorders. Restlessness, tics and insomnia all indicate irritation of the Liver.

Fat metabolism: Varicose veins, neoplasms, especially fibroid tumors and crystallization of waste products such as lactic acid and uric acid are often noted in the Liver Wood pathology. Bile, which is secreted by the liver, emulsifies fat globules, neutralizing fatty acids and resulting in a substance that is emulsified, i.e., water-soluble, and thus easily absorbed and utilized. Bile is also an intestinal lubricant. When there is insufficiency, the resulting accumulation of mucoid plaque can exacerbate or create conditions leading to endogenous toxicity.

BEHAVIORAL MANIFESTATIONS

Normal liver function results in behavior that is patient, calm and in control. When liver function is abnormal, the result is generically referred to as anger. In Chinese medicine, anger is sometimes referred to literally as "rebellious Liver Fire." The Japanese word for anger, *kanshaku*, means liver spasm.

The hallmark of negative Liver behavioral manifestation is inflexibility. There is a tendency to be nervous, impatient, restless in mood and movements and with an overall bossiness, the classic choleric temperament of a General. Shouting and clenching, which are also associated with Wood, are images of anger. Morning fatigue, or difficulty in rousing oneself is typical. In the evening, on the other hand, there is a tirelessness or euphoria that can lead to insomnia.

A common Liver symptom is subcostal distress, a tightness that is found bilaterally under the ribs. This area is referred to anatomically as the "hypochondrium," an indication that there has been some recognition in our own tradition that the region is related to the Liver as seat of the emotions. Someone with symptoms believed to be of emotional origin is referred to as a "hypochondriac."

WOOD YANG PATHOLOGY

Symptoms of heat repletion and hyperactivity in the Liver system include seasonal allergies (hay fever), varicose veins, hemorrhoids, biliary dyskinesia, cholecystitis, hepatobiliary constipation, hepatomegaly of liver abscesses, hyperfolliculinism with dysmenorrhea, amenorrhea or metrorrhagia (fibroma), allergic conjunctivitis, myopia, anguish, nervous anguish, hyperthyroidism, hyperparathyroidism, spasmophilia, spastic colon, migrating arthralgias, gout, ophthalmic migraines, epilepsy, genital herpes, keratitis and blepharospasms.

WOOD YIN PATHOLOGY

Coldness or vacuity of the Liver can result in any of the following pathologies: estrogen insufficiency of hepatic origin (polymenorrhea, frigidity), myopia, cirrhosis, chronic hepatomegaly, melancholia, gallstones, uterine fibroma, chronic hepatitis, liver cancer, hepatic coma, myelitis, fibrositis and muscular rheumatism.

FIRE CONSTITUTIONS

THE FIRE YANG CONSTITUTION

The Fire yang temperament is idealistic and extremely volatile, with violent swings between joy and dejection, ecstasy and despair. Extroverted and quick to embrace an idea or cause, Fire yang feels destined for noble causes and difficult challenges. He or she is inspired, acts intuitively and can pursue aims to the point of fanaticism, always willing to surpass and transcend their own efforts.

The two Fire yang types are intellectual and emotional. The intellectual Fire type is not often heavy, sometimes even tall and slender; the face has a prominent luster or sheen. A large head with a small body is often observed.

The intellectual Fire types are people with uncommon information-handling skill and phenomenal memories, especially in mathematics or computer science. Extremely inventive, they almost never have a conventional outlook on life, yet enjoy great emotional stability. Disciplined, quick with the facts and eager to insist on their point of view with a rapid-fire, dazzling display of supporting evidence, this type loves information and ideas. The intellectual Fire type is more rare than the typical passionate Fire type and may suffer from manic depression and mental disorders involving aphasia and confusion, but when healthy often obtains distinction in his or her field of endeavor.

The emotional Fire type is passionate in the stereotypical way of having an "artist's temperament." Many actors are Fire yang types, possessing a proud demeanor, and easily inspired by the enthusiasm of others, preferring to be led rather than to lead. When inspired, they will work tirelessly and sacrifice themselves for a cause, especially a noble cause capable of arousing strong sentiment in themselves and others. Often they become devoted to an ideal or cause, but they seldom become a leader unless they embody the cause or unless the role of leadership involves martyrdom. They like movement, are athletic and often enjoy athletics for the sake of surpassing themselves. Long distance running, tennis, handball and other sports requiring fast reflexes are well suited to this type. The emotional Fire type will climb the mountain "because it is there." They possess an excellent memory for data and often have a superior intelligence, but the intellect is subordinate to passion, giving them the enormous zeal necessary for working to the point of exhaustion.

The typical Fire yang type is often attractive with long, lean muscles, somewhat delicate, a reddish cast to the face, a rigid frame but with good posture and a smooth, flowing movement. They have wide shoulders and narrow, almost non-existent hips, a wide, prominent forehead and a penetrating gaze. They have a proud bearing, a strongly developed sense of honor and a rebellious nature. Having a very excitable sexual nature, they frequently fall in love with love beyond all rational considerations.

Health problems are typically cardiovascular. As children they suffer extremely high fevers and may even have convulsions. They typically get at least one attack of scarlatina, scarlet fever or rheumatic fever, which not infrequently leaves a defect resulting in mitral valve prolapse or stenosis. They have difficulty sleeping and often wet the bed.

As adults, there are often problems with cardiac rhythm, coffee addiction, alcohol abuse, arterial problems, angina pectoris, myocardial infarction, cerebral hemorrhage, arterial hypertension, enteritis and Crohn's disease. Other frequently observed problems include anxiety disorders, manic depressive and bipolar depressive disorders, hysterical amnesia, ovaritis, impotence (narcissistic) and hyperpituitarism.

THE FIRE YIN CONSTITUTION

The Fire yin temperament is sentimental. Emotional, introverted, hypersensitive, the sentimental type is often troubled by unfortunate events that seem to cling to them easily due to a pessimistic, defeatist attitude. Inclined to be uneasy and concerned for others as well as themselves, they are susceptible to sudden mood changes. They are idealists who remain steadfast in their aspirations and never renounce what they believe to be true and right. They are able to wait years to fulfill their hopes and dreams.

Romantic by nature, Fire yin individuals often feel misunderstood early in life because they believe no one can understand the depth and sensitivity of their feelings. At an early age, they learn or decide not to trust others, and sometimes armor themselves to hide their emotional fragility. They are great lovers of beauty – natural and man-made – and have free-flowing artistic temperaments. They are never happier than when intoxicating their senses with beautiful sights, sounds, smells or journeys into romance or trips to foreign lands.

The restless mind of the Fire type needs very little sleep. The Fire type can be quite articulate and often has the exceptional intellectual qualities of a creative genius despite lapses of memory. The heart organ itself tends to be weak.

FIRE PATHOLOGY

> "We know the truth, not only by reason, but
> also by the heart."
>
> —Blaise Pascal

THE HEART

In the Chinese medical tradition, the Heart is the organ that is the dwelling place of the *shen*. In his numerous French-language publications, Nguyen Van Nghi, the Vietnamese acupuncturist who was instrumental in shaping the practice and profession of acupuncture in modern France, defined *shen* as the vital spirit, or mental energy. It is the cohesive force of psychosomatic unity of the organism. According to Needham, the *shen* is the force that governs instinct and emotion and is at the root of the body's metabolism. This represents a strong conceptual link to the thyroid gland, which is the main regulator of the basal metabolism. Many heart syndromes and most symptoms of Heart fire repletion would be described as thyroid-related in the context of conventional medicine in the West.

Psychic processes, especially emotions, resonate throughout the body. This resonance not only has a component of psychic experience, but also an outward motor expression and an internal visceral manifestation. Since cessation of the function of the heart and the arterial circulation results in almost instant termination of life, the heart system, the fire of the vital process, is one of the most important organs of internal visceral expression. The force that supplies life to all cells and all physiological functions is the force that binds psyche and soma into a unity.

For this reason, the Heart has an intimate relationship with the emotional life, and has become a symbol of individual expression and intuitive knowledge. Some things we know in our minds, and some things we know in our Hearts. In other contexts, the Chinese character for *shen* has also been translated as God, or Divine force. This adds the implication that the concept of *shen* may be viewed as similar to the Hebrew concept of *nefesh* (popularly translated as soul), or *atman* in the Hindu tradition or the Holy Spirit of the Christian tradition. The *shen* can be thought of, then, as that which is individual in a person, but also universal, which resides in the Heart of human beings and is an integrative force in human consciousness.

As explained earlier, the essence of Fire is flaring or rapid centrifugal expansion. The most obvious manifestation of this is the blood vessels that emanate from the heart. These arteries comprise a reservoir of blood pressure that plays an important role in regulating the flow of blood throughout the arterial system and in maintaining arterial tone. They assist the heart in propelling blood through the entire body.

The pathology of the Fire system, like most Fire manifestations, is conspicuous. Even if gross physiological signs are not manifest, the anxiety level of the patient is difficult to overlook.

Physiological manifestations

The heart, the thyroid gland, the pituitary gland, the tongue, the arteries and the small intestine are the main sites of pathology of the Fire system. The thyroid is often classified as part of the Wood phase, but it is important to remember that the heart, the thyroid gland and the tongue all spring from common embryological tissue and are considered to maintain a functional relationship throughout life. In fact, hyperthyroidism results in tachycardia and high anxiety states, both of which are associated with the Heart even though they may be hepatic in origin. Those who suffer from angina pectoris commonly report that their tongue feels as if it is being pulled out during an attack.

The Fire organ that is most difficult to describe is the Small Intestine. According to East Asian medicine, the Small Intestine is the organ that produces blood, therefore it is the origin of the blood, a primary manifestation of Fire. This description contradicts Western physiology. However, researchers in both Japan and Russia have reported that in normal, healthy individuals, erythrocytes (red blood cells) are formed in the small intestine. These researchers claim that the conventionally accepted research, which is responsible for the belief that blood is produced in the bone marrow, was conducted with people who were already in a pathological state, or on fasting test animals.

Behavioral manifestations

The emotion associated with the Heart is joy; however, other manifestations of this are giddiness, nervous laughter, the desire to be outrageous, humorous, perhaps even to the point of hysteria. High anxiety states are associated with the Heart system. Other behavioral manifestations include loss of consciousness and loss of memory, signs of a lack of circulation to the head and a lack of oxygen in the brain.

Fire yang pathology

Ulcers on the tongue, left-sided cardiac insufficiency, arrhythmias, arterial hypertension, endocarditis, myocarditis, pericarditis in a bacterial or fungal terrain, arteriosclerosis, cerebral hemorrhage, hemiplegia with aphasia, high fevers, sexual overexcitation, manic-depression, mania, hysteria.

Fire yin pathology

Mitral valve prolapse, hypotension, syncope, myocarditis, viral pericarditis, cardiac insufficienc (global and right-sided), tachysystole, fibrillation, cerebral circulatory insufficiency, cerebral anoxia, intestinal malabsorption, cancer of the small intestine, extreme timidity and inhibition, manic-depressive states, amnesia.

The Earth Constitutions

The earth yang constitution

The Earth yang temperament is sanguine. The sanguine type loves verbal sparring, but without malevolence. A braggart and a joker by nature, the Earth yang loves word games, puns and banter. They dramatize everything and sometimes act precipitately with excessive optimism. They are diplomats and opportunists who adapt themselves to all circumstances.

They love to facilitate reconciliation between people in dispute, and will devote much time to pleasure in general and to society life.

An august presence, Earth yang dominates with the sheer strength of their presence. They have a prominent abdomen, a large, square pelvis and short, round arms and legs, with white, thin, elastic skin. Above all else they love to sleep and to eat. Their thick-set constitution tends toward obesity, the classic "viscerotonic" constitutional type described by the physiologist Sheldon. A great lover of sweets, they are capable of consuming enormous amounts of food, their efficient guts maintaining considerable bulk on their frames with relative ease. The build of the Japanese sumo wrestler is a classic Earth yang constitutional type. In Japan, diabetes mellitus is sometimes referred to as the "sumo disease," so common is it among these wrestlers who train for years on a bulk-producing diet.

Earth yang is cheerful, gregarious and carefree and does not care to dwell on unpleasant aspects of life. However, they have a well-developed sense of reality and do not spend their lives hiding from difficulties and unpleasantness. They can be blunt and outspoken and somewhat insensitive to the feelings of others.

Earth yang has a narrow forehead, large lips, a resonant and powerful voice (many opera singers are Earth yang types) and a dramatic manner of self-expression, filled with wit and self-effacement (although we know they do not believe it). They dislike heat and humidity and have a tendency to perspire freely and profusely. Earth yang has a tendency to become flushed and is in general "moist," often suffering from stiffness and aching in the shoulders that can easily become headaches. The blood pressure can become elevated and often there will be hypertension, skin disorders, constipation, obesity and digestive disorders such as ulcers, pancreatitis, colitis with chronic diarrhea, and hiatus hernia.

The Earth yin constitution

The Earth-yin type is amorphous, living a life of heedless but excessive concern. They are content to sleep and lounge about and are inclined to sloth. They prefer to let things manage themselves, but nevertheless can become overwrought even about trifles. This excess of concern substitutes for an emotional life in someone who is essentially emotionally detached. Earth yin types prefer to hear about the feelings of others before recounting their own. Conciliatory and accommodating, they do not intervene in events but stay in the background. They are skillful in weighing the pros and cons of a situation, and at grasping the subtleties of ideas and words. They are not so much intellectuals but rather they fix on mental activity and seek to have a meaning, explanation or answer for everything to soothe their anxiety. This tendency takes precedence over whether or not they have the skill or talent for intellectual pursuits. A worrier by nature, Earth yin tends to be a cynic and to habitually look for flaws and inconsistencies.

With a hypersensitive digestion, they often have food sensitivities and an inability to digest many different foods. Their facial expression sometimes resembles a sneer or smirk as if they had a bad taste in the mouth. They may be skin and bones, or carry a fair amount of weight, usually "water weight," and they have a prominent, bony pelvis. There is a certain boniness to the hands and joints, which gives the appearance of awkwardness of movement. The lips are often large and the nipples are large, even in Earth yang women whose breasts are not large. In a weaker type, the lips are sometimes quite thin.

Obsessed with detail, Earth yin is usually quick to learn and does well in occupations that require careful thought and attention to detail. Very sensitive to sugar, he or she often craves sweets and the feeling of being "spaced-out" that they provide, relieving overconcentration. They like to nap during the day, and dislike exercise even though it benefits them greatly by restoring body sensitivity and a heightened awareness of external reality. They have poor muscle tone, or the opposite, a hypertonic condition. As a patient, the Earth yin is easy to recognize, because they must have an explanation for everything and because they are quick to notice any inconsistencies in explanations or arguments. Earth yin types are also extremely self-critical and can easily be ensnared by a tendency toward fixed ideas. They are prone to jealousy and think that everyone else has life better than theirs. They envy those who do not make such severe demands on themselves and are able to take life a little easier. There is a tendency to hypoglycemia and often the worst bouts of depression or self-criticism follow dietary excess or other indulgences.

EARTH PATHOLOGY

PHYSIOLOGICAL MANIFESTATIONS

The organ for Earth is the Spleen, considered as a unit with the pancreas, the stomach and the lymph system. Between the two circulations of fluid, the yang circulation being the blood circulation and the yin circulation being the lymphatic system, the spleen itself, along with the systemic lymph node aggregations of the body, comprises a type of "liver" for the lymph circulation. Of course the lymph system is the physical location of the immune system, so the concept of Spleen links digestive function, blood sugar regulation and immunity. The fact that the spleen and pancreas are considered as a unit introduces to us the relationship between blood sugar and allergic sensitivities. Clinically it is noteworthy that allergic susceptibilities are high when blood sugar is low. Hence, the first important manifestation of Earth pathology is poor immunity such as low white cell count or lymphatic stagnation. In addition, we may find various digestive problems, blood sugar instability and problems with lactation and the abnormal function of the smooth muscle, which includes all the viscera and entrails of the abdomen. Smooth muscle prolapses of either digestive organs or even the uterus are considered to be problems of insufficiency of Earth.

BEHAVIORAL MANIFESTATIONS

The emotion associated with Earth is obsession. Overconcentration or excessive thought is said to be damaging to digestive function and immunity. Thus, in our own culture, the overwrought, busy executive with stomach ulcers is a symbol of modern civilization. In addition, the high anxiety of the Heart, associated with Fire, is passed on to damage the Spleen. It is illustrative that many of the traditional East Asian formulas for improving digestion are referred to as Heart-sedating formulas. They are used essentially to clear stagnation and tension from the upper digestive tract and to promote normal peristalsis. Obsession, mania and single-minded behavior all fall into the category of Earth. Yet when the Earth phase is strong, there is great presence of mind, a centeredness or ability to be powerful in the present moment. Another negative manifestation of the Earth system is the exact opposite of over-concentration. Being "spaced out" is a common vernacular for a lack of mental focus and clarity. Excessive study and mental activity of any kind that is overconcentrated is considered damaging to the Spleen.

EARTH YANG PATHOLOGY

Typical pathologies include aphthous ulcers, buccal membrane abscesses, gastritis, stomach ulcers, pancreatitis (chronic or hemorrhagic), diabetes and hypoglycemia, obesity, hyperestrogenic menorrhagia or metrorrhagia, mania.

EARTH YIN PATHOLOGY

Typical pathologies include lymphomas, anorexia, malabsorption, coeliac malady, parasites, hyperglycemia, uterine prolapse, rectal prolapse, gastroptosis, gastric cancer, pancreatic cancer, intestinal cancer, diabetes insipidus, infectious mononucleosis, leukopenia, various types of splenomegaly and obsessional syndromes.

METAL CONSTITUTIONS

THE METAL YANG CONSTITUTION

The Metal yang temperament is phlegmatic: methodical, precise, efficient. These people are even-tempered and generally impassive; they criticize more with humor than with outbursts, are objective in making observations, are rarely angered and analyze without emotion. They resolve problems dispassionately, just as one would solve a mathematical equation. This is not to say that they are devoid of emotions, rather that their emotions are filtered through a rational process. The Earth yin type, another great stoic, differs in that the intellectual life is a substitute emotional life, rather than an emotional life rationalized. Thus the Metal yang type gives the appearance of stability, which is comforting to those whose lives flap in the currents of change. This type is capable of working in a plodding, systematic fashion and winning, like the proverbial tortoise in a race with the hare.

Relative to physique, Metal yang has a large nose with thick skin around the nostrils, clear eyes, wide shoulders and an athletic frame. The eyebrows are thick and the musculature is well-toned. The Metal yang is, in fact, a good athlete because of love of movement, the feeling of the body's energy in motion. They also have the temperament to concentrate, pushing feelings aside to succeed in athletic pursuits. They have a good memory, and a capable mind for abstract work as well as precise work such as in law. The Metal yang type has a generally even temperament and does not get upset about anything, but when upset, seems to know exactly why. The skin is dense; emotionally and temperamentally they are somewhat thick-skinned as well. They can be arrogant about rationalizing other people's feelings, because they lack empathy and are condescending to those who indulge in emotion for emotion's sake. Generally, Metal yang is likable and well-liked, possessing a charisma that makes it easy for others to forgive shortcomings, and a pungent wit that is difficult to resist.

There is usually a physiological weakness of the lungs, sinuses or large intestine. If there is constipation, it is more often of the spastic variety, whereas the Metal yin type usually suffers from the flaccid type. Metal yang generally ages gracefully and is often robust and physically active into advanced years.

THE METAL YIN CONSTITUTION

The Metal-yin type is melancholic, loving solitude, liking to organize life in advance and not liking improvisation. Conservative and mistrustful, interactions with Metal yin types can be difficult since they practice the politics of inertia. They also tend to be convinced they are right and are more than willing to debate and split hairs to prove it, but their manner of being with others is characterized by the fact that they are almost insufferably nice. They tend to be claustrophobic and sometimes their way of being nice is to develop refined manners, as Emerson put it, "to keep fools at a distance." Interactions with other people can be fatiguing to Metal yin types and they often economize energy by being somewhat clannish.

The Metal yin constitution is easily tired by many situations. Such persons are often exhausted by evening and require considerable sleep. They lack concentration, are easily discouraged, and tend to be inward-looking. They like sweets and highly seasoned foods and are prone to dental caries. They catch colds easily and colds quickly move to the lungs; in childhood they often suffer from asthma. They are also prone to hypothyroidism and thyroid tumors; the lymph nodes swell easily and skin problems such as acne, eczema and psoriasis often appear. The tendons and ligaments are hypotonic which often results in tightness and spasms.

Metal yin has a bent posture, a thin frame and is not well muscled. The face is thin with a thin chin, almost gaunt with aquiline features, a thin nose and nostrils, sometimes with lots of nasal hair and a prominent Adam's apple in males. Men often have a deep voice and speak in a monotone. The face frequently has a basset hound expression. The arms and legs are long and thin with fine bones and almost no hips. The skin is dry and flaky and very sensitive to temperature changes and other stimuli; pimples will leave pock marks in the skin, especially in the cheeks. The hair is fine and wispy and thins from the front fairly early. The body is often covered with a fine wooly hair, especially on the back at the shoulders and lumbar region. The colon is often sluggish and the resulting bloat can give a bulging or swollen appearance to the lower abdomen. Constipation can be a problem with bowels that at least tend toward sluggishness and flatulence. There is a tendency to have swollen nodes in the neck, armpits, groin or all three, which is typical of what is called a thymicolymphatic constitution.

They are very sensitive to other people's feelings and thoughts and for this reason seem to have a psychic ability. Often they take blame on themselves for social interactions or communications that do not go well and can carry around a pathological level of guilt about nearly everything, even being alive. They have a well-developed ability to know how others are thinking, feeling and reacting. By nature they are philanthropic and in their advanced years are often revered as wise and sagacious.

METAL PATHOLOGY

PHYSIOLOGICAL MANIFESTATIONS

The Metal system includes the Lungs, the Large Intestine and the skin. As noted earlier, the Lungs, Large Intestine and skin all eliminate moisture and have a drying effect on the body. Thus the Lung type tends to catch colds easily and these colds tend to move to the Lungs very rapidly. Because the Metal system also includes the mucous membranes of the body, mucous membrane disorders, particularly allergic problems and digestive problems, are typical of Metal. But the most common pathology is of the Lungs, the Large Intestine and the skin itself. This interrelation between these three organs may be one reason why diverticulitis and emphysema are often concurrent diseases. It also explains why dermatosis often clears when constipation is relieved. Lymph nodes swelling up easily can also be a sign of Metal pathology, showing that the drying capacity of the body is weak enough that wetness can accumulate in the form of lymphatic congestion.

BEHAVIORAL MANIFESTATIONS

The emotion associated with Metal is sadness and the patient with Metal pathology, if not possessed of a sad demeanor, may exhibit a whining or melancholy attitude toward life. In fact, tuberculosis was once referred to as the "illness of sad passion." People with Metal pathology often have great difficulty seeing the positive side to anything that happens in their lives. In treatment, this makes it is important to show them that there are silver linings accompanying many of the dark clouds. Metal types being dry by nature often like things that are moistening: mucus-forming foods like fruits and dairy products. They also tend to like highly seasoned foods, which induce mucous membrane secretions.

METAL YANG PATHOLOGY

Metal yang patterns include bronchial problems and pneumopathies, bacterial pleurisy, chronic bronchitis, constipation, anal fistulas and fissures, dysentery syndromes, cystitis from E. coli bacillus, pyodermatitis, cutaneous abscesses and chronic sinusitis.

METAL YIN PATHOLOGY

Metal yin patterns include influenza, colds – both viral and parasitic – bronchial and lung disorders, pulmonary abscesses, emphysema, sarcoidosis, chronic laryngitis, tracheitis, sinusitis, chronic rhinitis, anosmia, tuberculosis, lung cancer, atonic constipation, colitis, malabsorption colic, colon cancer, psoriasis, eczema, hyperhidrosis, depressive states and diverticulitis.

WATER CONSTITUTIONS

The Water constitution, as mentioned before, is either exceptionally strong or exceptionally weak. The strong type has spectacular endurance and stamina. Fearless, they are driven by ambition and excel in all areas of achievement with the exception of the intellectual. They have tremendous vitality and are physically warm, able to endure harsh physical circumstances and suffering no apparent ill effects from alcohol or dietary abuse. The weak Water constitution, on the other hand, is hypersensitive and is easily chilled. Low resistance and susceptibility make it necessary to scrupulously cultivate health habits that might seem severe to most people.

THE WATER YANG CONSTITUTION

The Water-yang temperament is passionate. These people are emotional but hide their feelings. They are highly demanding of themselves and others. Possessing a natural authority and the temperament of a commander, they feel predestined to noble causes, to adventures and to difficult enterprises. They strive to attain the highest distinction and will make whatever sacrifices necessary to this end. Often they believe they are objects of envy or jealousy to others, and rightly so, for who wouldn't covet such supreme self-confidence?

The Water yang has noble features, Greek god-like, with a Roman nose, prominent brow, a solid jaw, a well-sculpted chin and large ears with thick lobes. The skull is thick and all the bones are dense and hard, to be broken only by the most severe death-dealing trauma. In males, the beard is thick and the hair is dense. When there is body hair it is also dense and abundant. The vocal cords are thick, giving a deep voice, husky in women and sometimes raspy. In terms of health they represent the ideal, but are often abusive to their magnificent constitution simply because they feel no pain.

They have an ability to get things done with seemingly little effort, almost as if by magic. The will is indomitable and they want to dominate and control other people, though usually they are easily led by an individual of strong intellect, because this is often the Water yang's weakest attribute. They have great courage and spirit of endeavor, but sometimes rush in where angels, or lesser mortals, fear to tread.

The Water yang type often seeks to hide the lack of intellectual strength, sometimes going to great pains to develop their vocabulary or seek academic credentials, but this deficiency is their secret shame. It often leads them to be emotionally or socially aloof, so as not to let their secret become inadvertently known. They seek a position of authority and know that it is essential to have strong mental competence to lead others. This type is well suited to athletics, police work and work involving danger and adventure like rescue work, firefighting, exploring and the like.

THE WATER YIN CONSTITUTION

In sharp contrast to the Water yang type, the Water yin type is sentimental, timid, dependent, fearful and easily discouraged. Often they are defeated before they start because they believe they will never succeed. They cultivate their interior life and often keep a private journal. They lack zest for life and seek to compensate for their vulnerability by attaining clarity of consciousness through meditation and other types of spirituality.

Thin, sensitive to cold, their resistance is low so that they catch any epidemic that comes around. There is a certain frailty or delicacy to them, and their sexual nature is not strong. If there is weight gain, it is usually fluid. The voice is soft, feminine, weak; stamina is poor. For one reason or another, they often need to be taken care of by others. The fingers and toes are long, the feet are small and thin. The eyes are wet and sometimes puffy around the lids. The head is small, the chin narrow, the neck long and thin.

The knees are weak and there is a tendency to tremble. Arthritic and urinary tract complaints are not uncommon. The lower back is weak and susceptible to injury, urination is frequent, the skin is clammy and there is sometimes a brownish or greyish tinge to the skin.

By nature the Water yin type is very vulnerable, so they must live a life of quiet seclusion. They have a pathological fixation on cleanliness and a mortal fear of germs. They are fastidious about diet and practice dietary and health management practices that most people would consider severe.

These limitations and a strongly internal nature can actually drive an individual to great achievements, but it does not come easily to the Water yin type, for their stamina to accomplish things is limited. They do not naturally have good coordination and are easily surprised or alarmed by stimuli that would not concern others. Sometimes they can reach a higher spot on the mountain by developing their strength and will, and by careful persistence and wise management of their energy resources.

WATER PATHOLOGY

PHYSIOLOGICAL MANIFESTATIONS

Mineral metabolism is the primary function of Water. When fluids are not charged with electrolytes, they are unable to pass through membranes and can thus stagnate. Stagnation or toxicity in the genitourinary system results in hampered function and congestion of these organs, and can also affect other parts of the body. For example, if there is stagnant fluid around the inner ear, loss of balance or tinnitus can result. This is a common Water pathology. The kidneys are not primarily organs of waste elimination, as is commonly assumed. Their main function is to regulate the pH of the blood and the body's fluids. The kidneys receive fresh arterial blood directly from the heart, unlike the liver, which receives venous blood through the portal circulation at the end of the cycle. It is the role of the adrenals to help maintain normal alkalinity.

The normal pH of both the lymph and the blood is 7.2 to 7.3. When the adrenals are strained, there is a temporary state of excitation, sexual stimulation and well-being, which is one reason why people abuse such substances as coffee, sugar, alcohol and stimulating drugs. When any substance threatens this normal state of alkalinity, it is the role of the kidneys to find minerals to maintain the proper ion exchange so that oxygen can be carried by blood. If minerals are not readily available in the blood, then the connective tissue will be used to obtain them, but in most cases the minerals that are obtained are either magnesium taken from the muscles, which can become hard and stiff, or from the bones and teeth, which can become soft.

BEHAVIORAL MANIFESTATIONS

The Kidney types manifest extreme opposites. People with a strong Kidney function have personalities that can be calm and relaxed or dynamic and overwhelming. Charisma and internal strength allow these people to accomplish a great deal if their likewise overwhelming passions do not dissipate their energies. People with Kidney vacuity or Water pathology, on the other hand, tend to be afraid or apprehensive. They are unable to have an impact on people or events.

WATER YANG PATHOLOGY

Water yang pathologies include renal hypertension, urinary calculi, kidney infections, bladder infections, hematuria, urinary retention in the bladder, nephroangiosclerosis, anemia, anuria, glomerulonephritis, pheochromocytoma, septicemia, over-exertion (hyperadrenalism) and paranoia.

WATER YIN PATHOLOGY

Water yin pathologies include suppurative otitis, deafness, difficulty in hearing, articular rheumatism, Sjögren's syndrome, hypotension, vertigo, enuresis, chronic urinary tract infections, oxalic or phosphatic urinary calculi, nephrocalcinosis, chronic glomerulonephritis, renal insufficiency, diabetes insipidus, renal amylosis, impotence, frigidity, adrenal insufficiency (Addison's disease), global senescence, Paget's disease, osteoporosis, Parkinsonism, ataxia, dental caries, pathological calcification, prostatitis and tinnitus.

Tables 4a-e: The Flavors

SOUR FLAVOR	
FUNCTIONS: Sour nourishes the liver – evacuation	
SOUR-WARMING	**SOUR-COOLING**
Disperses repletion of Liver yin, clears hepatic congestion, stimulates the Liver, diminishes venous pressure, stimulates thyroid and thermogenesis.	Opposes Liver heat repletion.
NEUROENDOCRINE PROFILE	
Sympathomimetic, vagolytic.	Sympatholytic, antithyroidean, antiestrogenic, hypoglycemiant, parasympathomimetic, purgative.
HERBS	
milk thistle, oak, plantain	eyebright, goldenseal, grapevine, horse chestnut, nettle, witch hazel
ESSENTIAL OILS	
lemon, cypress	*cypress, lemon, rosemary*

BITTER FLAVOR	
FUNCTIONS: Bitter nourishes the heart – elimination, vomiting	
BITTER-WARMING	**BITTER-COOLING**
Compresses the Heart yin, supplements Heart yang, dries dampness of the Spleen, clears excessive phlegm in digestive tract.	Disperses Fire of the Heart; febrifuge, emetic, purgative.
NEUROENDOCRINE PROFILE	
Sympathomimetic, cardiotonic, antihyperglycemiant, adrenalin-like (kidney yang).	Sympatholytic, cardiomoderator, tranquilizer.
HERBS	
cinchona, digitalis, foenugreek, lily-of-the-valley, milk thistle	artichoke, hawthorn, hellebore, poppy, rauwolfia, valerian
ESSENTIAL OILS	
hyssop, lavender, niaouli, rosemary, thyme	*bitter orange*

SWEET FLAVOR

FUNCTIONS: Sweet nourishes the Spleen – dispersing

SWEET-WARMING	SWEET-COOLING
Supplements Spleen yang, stimulates pituitary and corpus luteum.	Emollient, laxative, harmonizing, moisturizing (saliva, sweat, tears).

NEUROENDOCRINE PROFILE

Hyperglycemiant, sympathomimetic, adrenalin-like, cortisol-like bone catabolism.	Hypoglycemiant (stimulates insulin secretion), diuretic, parasympathiomimetic.

HERBS

fennel, licorice, sweet balm	ash, burdock, hawthorn, sarsaparilla

ESSENTIAL OILS

anise, caraway, cinnamon, lemon, sage, sandalwood, thuja	*juniper, lemon, sandalwood*

SPICY FLAVOR

FUNCTIONS: Spicy nourishes the Lung – sudorific

SPICY-WARMING	SPICY-COOLING
Warms the Lung, dries and disperses dampness, increases Lung yang; moistens the Lung if affected by dryness.	Disperses heat in the Lung by diaphoresis.

NEUROENDOCRINE PROFILE

Vagolytic, sudorific, adrenalin-like.	Antilithiatic, adrenolytic, sympatholytic, hypotensive.

HERBS

dandelion, mugwort, nettle, oak, sassafras, horehound, horse chestnut	black radish, eyebright, rhubarb

ESSENTIAL OILS

caraway, eucalyptus, ginger, niaouli, peppermint, savory	*eucalyptus, niaouli*

SALTY FLAVOR

FUNCTIONS: Salty nourishes the Kidney– purging

SALTY-WARMING	SALTY-COOLING
Supplements Kidney yang, laxative, diuretic, evacuant, purgative,	Moistening.

NEUROENDOCRINE PROFILE

Salidiuretic, azoturic, eliminates phosphates and oxalates, cortisol, cardiotonic, sympathomimetic, stimulates adrenal cortex and medulla.	Sympatholytic, uricosuric, azoturic, salidiuretic, hypoglylcemiant, inhibits adrenal cortex and medulla, parasympathomimetic.

HERBS

black elder, bladderwrack, cornsilk, elder, horsetail, laminaria	ash, bearberry, black currant, harpagophytum, meadowsweet

ESSENTIAL OILS

hyssop, sandalwood	*thuja*

Table 5

WOOD REPLETION	
CONSTITUTION Wood yang **CHARACTER** Choleric enthusiast **NEUROENDOCRINE PROFILE** Sympathotonic, hyperthyroid, hypoparathyroid, hyperestrogenic, allergic terrain **PHYTOTHERAPEUTIC ACTIONS** Depurative, astringent, cholagogic, choleretic, hypotensive, sedative, tranquilizing, sympatholytic, antithyroidian, antiestrogenic **BITTER-COOLING PLANTS (HERB, *OIL*)** artichoke, black horehound, celandine, dandelion, eyebright, goldenseal, hepatica, horse chestnut, meadowsweet, mistletoe, white willow, witch hazel, *bitter orange, marjoram, melissa* **SOUR-COOLING PLANTS (HERB, *OIL*)** eyebright, fumitory, goldenrod, grapevine, horse chestnut, horsetail, lady's mantle, melilot, mouse ear, nettle, plantain, stoneseed, yarrow *cypress, lemon, rosemary* **SWEET-COOLING PLANTS (HERB, *OIL*)** black horehound, cabbage, chaste tree, melilot, mugwort, passionflower, turnip, stoneseed, water lily, *lemon, melissa* **SPICY-COOLING PLANTS (HERB, *OIL*)** black cohosh, black horehound, black radish, cabbage, eyebright, horse chestnut, turnip, pasque flower, valerian, water lily, *terebenthine*	**PATHOLOGY AND SYMPTOMATOLOGY** muscular tightness pain in the middle of head or behind the eyes bloodshot eyes thermophobia abdominal spasms dry mouth or bitter taste in mouth nausea, vomiting of bile alternating constipation and diarrhea excessive chatter migrating pains circulation problems in legs varicose veins pain in ribs and/or flanks dyspnea, heaving anger, aggressiveness irritability, agitation, anxiety, insomnia vertigo, dizziness, tinnitus angina pectoris chest oppression and pain hemoptysis stomach pain, vomiting bile coagulated menstrual blood pelvic congestion and pain bleeding between menses oliguria and dysuria hemiplegia restlessness in the limbs reddish tinge to the skin insomnia, restless shallow sleep

Table 6

WOOD VACUITY	
CONSTITUTION Wood yin **CHARACTER** Nervous, moody **NEUROENDOCRINE PROFILE** Sympathetic insufficiency, vagotonia, thyroid inhibition, hypofolliculine, hypogenital (genital overexcitation) **PHYTOTHERAPEUTIC ACTIONS** Hepatic immunity stimulant, diuretic, sympathomimetic, coagulant, thyroid stimulant, visual acuity - augmentation, optic nerve strengthener **BITTER-WARMING PLANTS (HERB, *OIL*)** barberry root, centaury, elecampane, germander, hops, milk thistle *ginseng, lavender, mugwort* **SOUR-COOLING PLANTS (HERB, *OIL*)** angelica, black currant, cabbage, plantain, *cypress, lemon* **SWEET-WARMING PLANTS (HERB, *OIL*)** cabbage, germander, ginseng, hepatica, hops, plantain, tarragon *celery seed, cypress, lemon* **SALTY-WARMING PLANTS (HERB, *OIL*)** black currant, hepatica, *celery seed* **SPICY-WARMING PLANTS (HERB, *OIL*)** angelica, elecampane, *lavender, mugwort*	**PATHOLOGY AND SYMPTOMATOLOGY** chills easily weakness of vision, loss of acuity pallor, bluish facial tone chest pain liver pain hepatomegaly vertigo, dizziness dark circles under the eyes skin color tinged blue-green depression dread, feelings of insecurity indecisive, lack of confidence and initiative fear of humiliation, fear of taking action insomnia from worry permanent headache anxiety, anguish, inhibition cramping in the four limbs atonic constipation diarrhea with colorless stool aqueous vomit abundant clear urine abundant menses frigidity or impotence hernias, hemorrhoids hemiplegia dyspnea and cough with glairy mucus

Table 7

FIRE REPLETION	

CONSTITUTION
Fire yang
 	
CHARACTER
Idealistic, volatile, extroverted
 	
NEUROENDOCRINE PROFILE
Sympathotonic, hyperpituitary,
   dopaminergic central hypertonic,
   hyperadrenal
 	
PHYTOTHERAPEUTIC ACTIONS
Antihemorrhagic, antisclerotic,
   sympatholytic, febrifugal,
   calming to the adrenal medulla
 	
SOUR-COOLING PLANTS (HERB, *OIL*)
ash, black currant, chaste tree,
goldenseal, grapevine, hawthorn, horse
chestnut, melilot, stoneseed, periwinkle,
witch hazel, yarrow, *rosemary*
 	
BITTER-COOLING PLANTS (HERB, *OIL*)
ash, birch, black horehound,
convallaria, goldenseal, hawthorn,
horehound, horse chestnut, mistletoe,
meadowsweet, passionflower,
periwinkle, rauwolfia, witch hazel
bitter orange, eucalyptus, lavender,
marjoram
 	
SWEET-COOLING PLANTS (HERB, *OIL*)
ash, black horehound, borage,
chaste tree, hawthorn
 	
SPICY-COOLING PLANTS (HERB, *OIL*)
black horehound, horse chestnut,
water lily, valerian
 	
SALTY-COOLING PLANTS (HERB, *OIL*)
black currant, borage
	PATHOLOGY AND SYMPTOMATOLOGY
	thermophobia
	sensation of heat in the chest
	hypertonic muscles
	dyspnea, labored respiration
	intense agitation
	hemoptysis
	sensation of heat in front of the ears
	insomnia, anguish
	thirst and polydipsia
	mouth dry and bitter
	fever
	ulcerations of the mouth and tongue
	delirious speech
	reddish skin color
	dryness of the skin
	agitation
	absence of sweat
	excessive enthusiasm
	colic pains
	excessive decisiveness
	diarrhea with yellow stool
	irritability and aggressiveness
	hematuria
	painful urination
	precordial pain (neurogenic)
	accelerated heart rate
	tingling in upper limbs
	headaches
	angina pectoris, arterial hypertension
	cracked lips
	excessive or absent sweat
	vertigo, fainting
	thirst, oliguria (dark urine)
	oppression and heat in chest
	skin lesions on the palms
	rapid heartbeat, palpitations
	slurring words, poor pronounciation
	hysterical laughter, sometimes
	   with sudden weeping
	chattering
	fainting, loss of consciousness
	vomiting blood
	memory loss
	epistaxis
	sexual preoccupation, satyriasis,
	   nymphomania
	extravagance, aggressiveness

Table 8

FIRE VACUITY

CONSTITUTION	PATHOLOGY AND SYMPTOMATOLOGY
Fire yin	chills easily
	cold skin
CHARACTER	perspires freely, nightsweats
Sentimental, emotional, introverted, hypersensitive	absence of thirst
	tears, abscesses on eyelids
	melancholia
NEUROENDOCRINE PROFILE	fullness in the chest
Sympathetic insufficiency, hypoadrenal, hypogonadal, hypopituitarism, insufficient cerebral circulation, dopaminergic central hypotonia, vagotonia (upper and middle warmers)	weak respiration
	heart murmurs
	weak digestion
	dyspepsia
	diarrhea
	yellow stool
PHYTOTHERAPEUTIC ACTIONS	coldness of chest and abdomen
Sympathotonic, cardiotonic, adrenal and sexual function strengthening, pituitary gland activating	abdominal pains
	pain in the chest
	pains in bladder and genitals
	urinary incontinence
BITTER-WARMING PLANTS (HERB, *OIL*)	frequent (clear) urination
barberry, convallaria,* digitalis,* elecampane, milk thistle, motherwort, oleander,* strophanthus*	depression, apathy, remorse
	hollow feeling in the chest
	severe asthenia, fatigue
lavender (* toxic)	cold limbs
	arterial hypotension
SOUR-WARMING PLANTS (HERB, *OIL*)	vertigo
angelica, black currant, milk thistle, motherwort	diffuse chronic headache
	tinnitus
	oppression of the heart
SWEET-WARMING PLANTS (HERB, *OIL*)	impotence or frigidity
elecampane, *rosemary, sage*	sexual weakness
	radiating passivity between the shoulder blades
SPICY-WARMING PLANTS (HERB, *OIL*)	joylessness
angelica, elecampane, *rosemary*	dyspnea
	fear of the dark
SALTY-WARMING PLANTS (HERB, *OIL*)	nausea and vomiting
black currant (buds), chickweed	spontaneous sweats
	fainting
	loss of memory
	loss of sperm
	timidity
	confusion

Table 9

EARTH REPLETION	
CONSTITUTION Earth yang **CHARACTER** Sanguine, cheerful, gregarious, carefree **NEUROENDOCRINE PROFILE** Vagal insufficiency, hypergonadic, 　hypoinsulinism (hyperglycemic) **PHYTOTHERAPEUTIC ACTIONS** Sedative, anti-inflammatory, vagus 　nerve stimulant, blood sugar reducing, 　damp heat dispersing **SOUR-COOLING PLANTS (HERB, _OIL_)** agrimony, ash, bilberry, lady's mantle, stoneseed, vervain, _cypress, lemon_ **BITTER-COOLING PLANTS (HERB, _OIL_)** ash, birch, calendula, fumitory, meadowsweet, _eucalyptus, melissa_ **SWEET-COOLING PLANTS (HERB, _OIL_)** ash, bilberry, burdock, calendula, goat's rue (galega), maize, orange blossom, stoneseed, _juniper, melissa_ **SPICY-COOLING PLANTS (HERB, _OIL_)** arnica, birch, goat's rue, _juniper_ **SALTY-COOLING PLANTS (HERB, _OIL_)** fumitory, maize, meadowsweet	**PATHOLOGY AND SYMPTOMATOLOGY** thermophobia sensation of heat in stomach 　and upper body dry lips and mouth pain at root of tongue pimples around lips gum and tongue irritations excessive eating bad breath postprandial nausea or vomiting vomiting tooth pain constipation or diarrhea cervical lymphadenitis acute intestinal pain sore throat and tonsillitis headaches from digestion or 　high blood pressure yellow sclera great thirst polydipsia heart pains dyspepsia overeating jaundice belching abdominal distention oliguria with dark urine hiccough whole body pain, arthralgia esophageal reflux purpura (petechia) dyspnea from thoracic oppression rapid, incoherent speech pain in the big toe obstinate obesity abscesses and pimples on body yellowish skin tone dark urine, oliguria frequent singing facial neuralgia excessive joy, giddiness, gaiety excessive mental and sexual excitation

Table 10

EARTH VACUITY	
CONSTITUTION Earth yin **CHARACTER** Amorphous, emotionally detached, detail-oriented **NEUROENDOCRINE PROFILE** Parasympathomimetic, immune deficient, hyper-insulin, hypothyroid, hypopituitary **PHYTOTHERAPEUTIC ACTIONS** Lymphatic constitutional, eupeptic, aperitif, digestion and absorption enhancing, nourishing, Earth and Metal strengthening **SOUR-WARMING PLANTS (HERB, *OIL*)** angelica, black currant, black walnut, eyebright, oak, plantain, vervain, *cypress* **BITTER-WARMING PLANTS (HERB, *OIL*)** barberry, belladonna, black walnut, blessed thistle, calendula, centaury, colchicum, elecampane, foenugreek, fumitory, gentian, germander, hops, hypericum, mouse ear, mugwort, vervain, yellow dock, *chamomile, eucalyptus, geranium, hyssop, lavender, savory, terebenthine, thyme* **SWEET-WARMING PLANTS (HERB, *OIL*)** belladonna, bladderwrack, blue mallow, calendula, elecampane, fennel, gentian, horsetail, laminaria, licorice, plantain, vervain, *anise, caraway, cinnamon, coriander, cypress, geranium, lemon, melissa, sage, thuja* **SWEET-WARMING PLANTS (HERB, *OIL*)** angelica, elecampane, horseradish, mugwort, oak, thyme, yellow dock *caraway, coriander, eucalyptus, ginger* **SALTY-WARMING PLANTS (HERB, *OIL*)** bladderwrack, black currant, fumitory, horsetail, laminaria, maize, yellow dock, *hyssop*	**PATHOLOGY AND SYMPTOMATOLOGY** chills easily sensation of cold in the limbs craving for warm liquids damp, moist, pinkish lips leg pains, heaviness hypersalivation frequent yawning nausea, aqueous vomitus belching, esophageal reflux anorexia depression abdominal distention, gas fullness in the chest weakness or atrophy in legs intermittent fever craves isolation, misanthropic boredom with anxiety fatigue, sensation of body heaviness insomnia from excessive worry flabby tongue profuse sweating distention and borborygmus sharp epigastric pain jaundice pasty yellow stool diarrhea with undigested food polyuria with clear urine generalized edema leukorrhea heaviness of the pelvis stomach or rectum prolapse sensation of cold in the knees thinness, wasting yellow, sallow skin tone large or frequent sighs obsessions, inflexibility loss of taste for food

Table 11

METAL REPLETION	

CONSTITUTION
Metal yang
 	
CHARACTER
Phlegmatic, even-tempered,
    methodical, precise, efficient
 	
NEUROENDOCRINE PROFILE
Vagal insufficiency
 	
PHYTOTHERAPEUTIC ACTIONS
Emollient, sedative, febrifugal,
    expectorant, antidiarrheal, antiseptic
 	
SOUR-COOLING PLANTS (HERB, *OIL*)
agrimony, ash, periwinkle, *lemon*
 	
BITTER-COOLING PLANTS (HERB, *OIL*)
ash, horehound, opium, periwinkle,
rhubarb, *eucalyptus, niaouli, savory,*
thyme
 	
SWEET-COOLING PLANTS (HERB, *OIL*)
borage, burdock, lungwort,
marshmallow, senna, *lemon, ylang ylang*
 	
SPICY-COOLING PLANTS (HERB, *OIL*)
horehound, rhubarb, senna,
eucalyptus, niaouli, terebenthine
	PATHOLOGY AND SYMPTOMATOLOGY
	thermophobia
	dry lips and mouth
	bad breath
	thirst
	yellow sclera
	inability to recline
	cervical adenitis
	tonsillitis
	epistaxis
	pain in teeth
	arterial hypertension
	intestinal colic aggravated by pressure
	dry skin
	tenesmus
	rectal prolapse, anal fissures
	constipation with dry stool
	diarrhea with pus and blood
	melena
	dry dermatosis
	pyodermatitis
	irritable, aggressive
	sensation of heat all over body
	hot palms
	dry mouth, absence of saliva
	dry sore throat or nose
	yellow, thick nasal discharge
	thoracic pain
	shoulder and back pain
	sensation of energy rising
	dyspnea
	dry cough, or cough with dry,
	    yellow expectoration
	phlegm accumulation in throat
	constipation
	cough with chills
	fever with chills
	nightsweats
	oliguria with dark urine
	agitation, aggressiveness, excitability

Table 12

METAL VACUITY	

CONSTITUTION
Metal yin
 	
CHARACTER
Melancholic, conservative,
  easily fatigued
 	
NEUROENDOCRINE PROFILE
Parasympathomimetic, hypothyroid,
  hypogonad, hyperparathyroid,
  immune deficiency (thymus
  hypofunction)
 	
PHYTOTHERAPEUTIC ACTIONS
Immune stimulant, emollient, adrenal
  and gonadal strengthening (esp. luteal
  function), expectorant, antiseptic
 	
SOUR-WARMING PLANTS (HERB, OIL)
angelica, black walnut, oak, *myrtle*
 	
BITTER-WARMING PLANTS (HERB, OIL)
belladonna,* black walnut,
blessed thistle, centaury, elecampane,
foenugreek, gentian, germander,
hypericum, mugwort, violet, wild oat,
yellow dock, *eucalyptus, hyssop,*
lavender niaouli, oregano, pine, sage,
savory, terebenthine, thyme
(* toxic)
 	
SWEET-WARMING PLANTS (HERB, OIL)
belladonna,* blue mallow, coltsfoot,
groundsel (senecio), laminaria, licorice,
plantain, violet, wild oat, *cinnamon,*
cypress, fennel, rosemary, sage (* toxic)
 	
SPICY-WARMING PLANTS (HERB, OIL)
angelica, dandelion, datura,*
elecampane, eyebright, henbane,*
horseradish, mugwort, nettle, oak,
sarsaparilla, violet, yellow dock,
cajeput, eucalyptus, ginger, myrtle,
niaouli, peppermint, pine, sassafras,
terebenthine (* toxic)
	PATHOLOGY AND SYMPTOMATOLOGY
	chills and trembling
	cold limbs
	cold sensation in the teeth
	frequent yawning
	clear nasal discharge
	severe asthenia, prostration
	chest oppression
	intestinal distention and gas
	dyspepsia
	borborygmus
	abdominal pain
	depression, sadness, insomnia
	atonic constipation
	aqueous stool
	rectal prolapse
	anal pruritus
	polyuria with clear urine
	boredom
	discouragement
	fever and shivering
	evening fever
	cold sweats, nightsweats
	hypersalivation
	cold sensation in teeth and gums
	pain in shoulders and back
	cough with abundant clear
	  expectoration
	hoarse voice
	nausea, vomiting
	postprandial diarrhea
	oligomenorrhea, amenorrhea
	paralysis of upper limbs
	dry skin
	weight loss, wasting
	difficulty speaking, weak voice

Table 13

WATER REPLETION

CONSTITUTION	PATHOLOGY AND SYMPTOMATOLOGY
Water yang	thermophobia
	yellow sclera
CHARACTER	excessive tears
Passionate, self-confident	sharp sensations in the eyes
	fever with shivering
NEUROENDOCRINE PROFILE	headache in nuchal region
Sympathotonia, dopamine excess	sensation of intense internal heat
(central hypertonia), global	abuse of authority
hyperadrenalism, hypercorticism	abundant reddish or yellowish
(glucocorticoid or mineral corticoid)	urine with strong odor
	pelvic pain
PHYTOTHERAPEUTIC ACTIONS	priapism
Hypotensive, sympatholytic,	cutaneous abscesses
antisclerotic, uricosuric, salidiuretic	hemorrhoids
azoturic, astringent, emollient,	pain in the entire back
parasympathomimetic	lumbar pain
	irritability, authoritarian
BITTER-COOLING PLANTS (HERB, *OIL*)	convulsions
ash, birch, black currant, dandelion,	delirium
goldenrod, horehound, meadowsweet,	agitation, extravagant behavior
periwinkle, valerian, white willow	abuse of authority
	fever
SWEET-COOLING PLANTS (HERB, *OIL*)	dry mouth without thirst
ash, bilberry, black elder, borage,	lumbalgia
horsetail, melilot, passionflower,	blepharospasms
sarsaparilla, water lily, *juniper,*	dizziness and vertigo
sandalwood, ylang ylang	heat in the palms and soles
	arterial hypertension
SPICY-COOLING PLANTS (HERB, *OIL*)	edema of the eyelids
horehound, valerian, water lily	constipation
eucalyptus, sandalwood, terebenthine	difficult urination
	infrequent urination, urine red
	or dark yellow
SALTY-COOLING PLANTS (HERB, *OIL*)	generalized contractures
ash, barberry, bearberry, bilberry,	continuous sexual excitement,
heather, melilot, rest harrow, *thuja*	erotic dreams
SOUR-COOLING PLANTS (HERB, *OIL*)	
ash, barberry, bearberry, bilberry,	
heather, melilot, rest harrow, *thuja*	

Table 14

WATER VACUITY	

CONSTITUTION
Water yin
 	
CHARACTER
Hypersensitive, sentimental, timid
 	
NEUROENDOCRINE PROFILE
Sympathetic insufficiency, global
  hypoadrenalism, hypogonadism,
  cerebrospinal hypotonia
 	
PHYTOTHERAPEUTIC ACTIONS
Immune strengthening, adrenal and
  sexual organ strengthening,
  azoturic, spasmolytic, tonic,
  parasympatholytic, salidiuretic
 	
BITTER-WARMING PLANTS (HERB, _OIL_)
bearberry, black walnut, chickweed,
convallaria,* elecampane, mistletoe,
mouse ear, solidago, yarrow
eucalyptus, geranium, hyssop,
lavender, pine, sage, thyme (* toxic)
 	
SWEET-WARMING PLANTS (HERB, _OIL_)
bladderwrack, black currant, dog rose,
heather, horsetail, laminaria, licorice,
lonicera, lovage, madder, nettle,
celery seed, fennel, geranium, lemon,
rosemary, sandalwood, sage, thuja
 	
SPICY-WARMING PLANTS (HERB, _OIL_)
birch, elecampane, henbane,* madder,
cajeput, eucalyptus, ginger, juniper,
myrtle, niaouli, pine, rosemary,
sandalwood, sassafras,* savory,
terebenthine, thyme (* toxic)
 	
SALTY-WARMING PLANTS (HERB, _OIL_)
bladderwrack, black elder, black currant,
chickweed, laminaria, lonicera, nettle,
maize, sea holly, solidago, _celery seed,_
hyssop
	PATHOLOGY AND SYMPTOMATOLOGY
	cold intolerance
	extreme chill ("to the bone")
	cold in the limbs, feet are
	  completely cold
	asthenia
	clear nasal discharge
	epistaxis
	acute and chronic pulmonary
	  afflictions from cold
	abundant clear urine
	frequent urination
	incontinence
	nocturnal enuresis
	impotence, spermatorrhea
	sharp pain in intestines, groin
	  or lumbar area
	facial edema
	depression
	feeble psyche
	hypersomnia
	confusion
	sharp headache pain, especially
	  at the vertex
	tinnitus, difficulty hearing
	weakness, fainting
	excessive sweating with no
	  physical effort, or at night
	dyspnea with any physical exertion
	depression and misanthropy
	diarrhea in the morning
	frequent abundant urination
	generalized edema and edema
	  around eyes
	weakness of spinal column
	chronic lumbalgia
	ataxia
	deep pain in the bones
	extreme timidity
	inhibition
	lack of initiative and will

Oligotherapy

In the early 20th century,. J.U. Sutter, M.D. began treating patients with an oil-based concoction containing manganese and copper. This product was often used with dramatic success in cases of asthma and eczema. Dr. Sutter was not able to determine how to select the patients appropriate for this therapy, but when it was effective, the cure was rapid and thorough.

Jacques Ménétrier, probably the principal pioneer of oligotherapy, attempted to solve the problem of how the therapeutic use of trace elements could result in such dramatic beneficial results in some cases, with no perceptible change in others. To solve this problem, he grouped patients according to hereditary background, disease predispositions and morphological and psychological traits. He eventually developed a system of typologies, termed diatheses, to correlate different groups of oligoelements, or oligoelement compounds.

Ménétrier proposed that the patient's diathesis (i.e. "terrain") was the primary orientation of treatment, not the symptoms. Each trace element was specific to a diathesis, not to the symptoms. Furthermore, he proposed that the action of trace elements is regulatory and normalizing rather than destructive to microbes or suppressive to symptoms.

Ménétrier named the five diatheses the "allergic," the "hyposthenic," the "dystonic," the "anergic," and the "maladapted." The similarity of Ménétrier's diatheses to the five phases fundamental constitutional types is remarkable. Ménétrier himself was actually the first to point out the similarities between the diatheses and the five phases. Late in his life he actually attempted a scientific investigation of acupuncture points and the channel system. He even suggested that, like oligoelements, acupuncture seemed to be catalytic in its effects.

The correlations between Diathesis I (the allergic) and Wood include allergic problems of the respiratory system, the energetic, nervous, irritable temperament and the predisposition to migraine headaches. Diathesis II (the hyposthenic) is related to sadness and to respiratory problems such as chronic bronchitis, tuberculosis and colitis, which can be categorized as Metal. Diathesis III (the dystonic) corresponds to fire: arterial problems, heart disease and anxiety are common to both. Diathesis IV (the anergic) corresponds to fear, depression, thoughts of suicide, and indications of low adrenal cortex activity, which can be classified as Water. Pathological conditions associated with Diathesis V (the "dysadaptation" diathesis) include digestive disorders such as gastric distension and colic, ulcers, diabetic syndromes and hypogenital conditions, which correspond to the Earth phase.

The appearance of any of these diathetic patterns can be an indication for botanical medications belonging to the corresponding five phases classification. The oligoelement associated with each diathesis can often be used as a fundamental or constitutional treatment for patients who clearly exhibit a specific corresponding pattern according to the five phases. For example, the patient who is a Fire yang or yin type can usually benefit from intermittent use of MANGANESE-COBALT (MN-CO)[1], the oligoelement corresponding to Diathesis III.

---

[1] The abbreviations used here for the trace elements are also used in the therapeutic index along with the abbreviations for trace elements listed in the "Plant Profiles" section.)

DIATHESIS I

The allergic diathesis (MANGANESE, MN) is a terrain more typical of adolescents and young adults. As this type of terrain devolves, or as the subject ages, the terrain tends toward the dystonic diathesis (MANGANESE-COBALT, MN-CO). Most pathology for this type is acute and not serious. This diathesis is energetic, optimistic, nervous, irritable (sympathotonic-hyperthyroid), but very adaptable. This type has difficulty getting started in the morning and sometimes is a night owl. He or she suffers from excessive muscular tension. Pathology of the allergic type includes all types of allergies: allergic rhinitis, asthma, eczema, urticaria, muscle aches, nerve pains, migraine headaches, biliary sluggishness and stasis, hemorrhoids, dysmenorrhea, hypermenorrhea, nervous digestive and intestinal upsets, and mild cardiopathies such as tachycardia and precordalgia. Manganese is used along with sulphur to treat some of the hepatic tendencies, with iodine added for thyroid imbalances. The allergic diathesis is a Wood type, according to the five phase classification.

DIATHESIS II

The hyposthenic diathesis (MANGANESE-COPPER, MN-CU) was also called the "arthrotuberculous" diathesis by Ménétrier. The temperament of the hyposthenic individual is calm and deliberate. Their emotions are not easily aroused and they generally view life with pessimism. Fatigued easily, and having difficulty with concentrating, they require a great deal of rest on a regular basis. The hyposthenic type has an ovoid face with fine, sometimes fragile skin. The body is round and larger at the pelvis, and can accumulate weight easily in this area. Children of this type are sometimes developmentally slow. There is a sensitivity of the respiratory and digestive mucosa to irritation and infection. Colds are frequent, rectocolitis is a typical somatic compensation for emotional stress in this type. Bronchial asthma, arthritis, inflammatory rheumatism, ligament laxity, flaccid constipation and enuresis are all typical "paratubercular" manifestations of this hypotonic constitution. In contrast to the more hypertonic Diathesis I, the hyposthenic diathesis is hypothyroid, hypoadrenal and hypogenital. SULPHUR (S), IODINE (I) and PHOSPHORUS (P) can supplement the activity of MANGANESE-COPPER (MN-CU). This type is classified as Metal in the five phases model.

DIATHESIS III

The dystonic diathesis (MANGANESE-COBALT, MN-CO), also called the neuroarthritic diathesis, manifests latent tendencies to neurovegetative and circulatory pathology in middle age. In youth, this type often manifests more tendencies to the allergic diathesis. Nervous and emotional, the dystonic individual frequently suffers anxiety. Often there will be warm, moist, reddish skin and firm muscle tone, and large-boned types can gain considerable weight. In childhood they often have high fevers even with convulsions. Typical pathologies include heart and circulatory disorders such as functional hypertension, mitral valve prolapse, loss of memory, cardiac asthma, edema of the lower limbs, epigastric problems, stomach ulcers, muscle cramps, degenerative arthritis, mental disturbances and paresthesias. SULPHUR (S), IODINE (I) and MAGNESIUM (MG) can supplement the activity of MANGANESE-COBALT (MN-CO) for this type. In the five phases system, the dystonic diathesis is classified as Fire.

Diathesis IV

The anergic diathesis (COPPER-GOLD-SILVER, CU-AU-AG) has a severe lack of physical, emotional or psychological resilience. The weakness and sensitivity of this type are reminiscent of the Water yin constitution of the five phases. An anergic terrain can also be caused by numerous types of strains on the system such as prolonged drug treatment or drug abuse, major accidents, surgery and emotional shocks that require a prolonged recovery period. The anergic person has low vitality and must eat well, rest and in general pursue a very cautious lifestyle. They need to rest frequently, becoming overexcited and exhausted by too much stimulation, mental or physical. The anergic patient is tired of life and tired by it, is indecisive, lacks spirit and enthusiasm, has poor concentration, poor libido, and suffers from irregular sleep. Morphologically, this type has a malnourished, wasted appearance, a greyish skin that is cold and dry.

Typical pathologies include tuberculosis, viral hepatitis, leukemia, lymphadenitis, chronic and recurrent viral infections, fatigue syndrome, articular rheumatisms, cancers, osteoporosis, depression with suicidal tendencies and frequent kidney and urinary tract infections.

The treatment of this diathesis has been supplemented with numerous other trace elements. Originally this diathesis was treated with LITHIUM (LI) and MAGNESIUM (MG). It is also treated with COBALT (CO), PHOSPHORUS (P) and ZINC-NICKEL-COBALT (ZN-NI-CO). It is important to treat the anergic diathesis as soon as possible, especially since the patient may require prolonged therapy.

Diathesis V

The maladapted diathesis is treated with ZINC-COPPER (ZN-CU) and ZINC-NICKEL-COBALT (ZN-NI-CO). This type suffers from cyclic weakness, with periods of exhaustion often accompanied by hunger. Usually during these periods there is also mental dysfunction such as depression, memory problems and poor mental concentration. It is associated with dysfunction of different endocrine axes. When it is associated with the pituitary-pancreatic axis, there is a prediabetic terrain, treated with ZINC-NICKEL-COBALT (ZN-NI-CO). When it is a dysfunction of the pituitary-genital axis, it is treated with ZINC-COPPER (ZN-CU). Dysfunction of the pituitary-genital axis manifests as symptoms of dysmenorrhea, abnormal ovarian function, cryptorchidism, retarded sexual development, impotence, frigidity and prostate disorders, among others. This diathesis is often considered to be a transformation or variation of one of the other diatheses, usually the allergic diathesis, but also the hyposthenic. Treatment in these cases involves the use of the trace elements associated with the other diatheses.

PART TWO:
PLANT PROFILES

Five Phase Listings

The plants profiled in this section are categorized according to five phase classification. The key words assist in gaining familiarity with the materia medica of European phytotherapy. Most plants in this listing are used primarily in the form of extracts: tinctures, suspensions, water extracts, or as teas in the bulk form. Some indications are based on references that can be found in the bibliography, but most of the indications are based on the observations of clinicians who use either the five phase model, the neuroendocrine model, or Ménétrier's diathetic model. They may also be indications based on traditional use.

HERBS FOR WOOD YANG PATHOLOGIES

WOOD YANG PROFILES – QUICK REFERENCE

ARTICHOKE	choleretic hypocholesterol
BLACK COHOSH	antispasmodic analgesic hypotensive
BLACK RADISH	cholagogue digestive spasms
CELANDINE	jaundice stomach pain
DANDELION	cholagogue hypocholesterol diuretic
EYEBRIGHT	eye secretions
GOLDENSEAL	hemostatic, pelvic vasoconstrictor
GRAPEVINE	varicose veins hemorrhages menopausal complaints
HORSE CHESTNUT	menopause prostate congestion hemorrhoids
LADY'S MANTLE	oxytocic sedative menopause
MISTLETOE	hypertension tachycardia convulsions
PASQUE FLOWER	PMS headache allergies
PLANTAIN	eye secretions allergies
STONESEED	menopause mastosis
WITCH HAZEL	menstrual problems menopausal problems hemorrhoids

ARTICHOKE *Cynara scolymus*

ACTIONS: Hepatoprotective, choleretic, cholagogue, diuretic, hypoglycemiant.

CONSTITUENTS: Flavonoid derivatives of luteolol, cynarin, provitamin A, tannins, orthodihydroxyphenolic acids, bitter principles, polyphenolic derivatives, aliphatic acids and alcohols, mineral salts (zinc, nickel, cobalt, manganese and selenium). Enzymes including ascorbinases, catalases, oxydases, peroxydases and cynarases.

FAMILY: Compositae.

FLAVORS: Bitter-cooling, sour-warming.

FIVE PHASE CATEGORIES: Wood yang, Fire yang.

PRINCIPAL INDICATIONS ACCORDING TO TERRAIN:

1) WOOD — Viral hepatitis, ascites; protects the liver cells; choleretic (stimulates the production of bile); cholagogue (stimulates the flow of bile into the duodenum); enhances digestion; has an antilithiatic function, is hypocholesterolemic and has an antitumor action.

2) FIRE — Slows metabolism, calms thyroid function; arteriosclerosis; hypercholesterolemia; arterial hypertension; azotemia (excess of urea or other nitrogenous substances in the blood); arthritis; calculi; obesity; diabetes (hypoglycemiant); protects the kidney and liver cells.

Artichoke was cultivated by Italian horticulturists as far back as the 15th century. By the 18th century, it was popular all over Europe and commonly used for treating jaundice. Since the advent of the 20th century, doctors in France have used it as a choleretic for digestive problems. Its diuretic properties have made it useful for problems with renal elimination as well. The edible portion has the same activity as the leaves, but is not as strong. Artichoke is used primarily as a digestive medication. It is non-toxic and has no known side effects. It can be useful in any type of terrain for symptoms related to liver congestion.

The artichoke extract used in Europe is taken from the leaves of the plant. The artichoke itself is a member of the Compositae family and is the largest thistle. It has a bitter, cooling property and drains heat repletion in the liver and drains the bile ducts. It is a general stimulant to hepatic cells and can be used to facilitate regeneration of the liver as well as to protect liver cells.

BLACK COHOSH *Cimicifuga racemosa*

ACTIONS: Antispasmodic (musculotrope and neurotrope), sedative, sympatholytic, vagolytic, LH antagonist.

CONSTITUENTS: Cimicifugin, bitter principle racemosin, triterpenes, 27-deoxyacteine, resins, wax, starch, fat, gum, sugars.

FAMILY: Ranunculaceae.

FLAVOR: Pungent-cooling.

FIVE PHASE CATEGORY: Wood yang.

PRINCIPAL INDICATIONS ACCORDING TO TERRAIN:

1) WOOD — Migraine headaches, opthalmic headaches, cluster headaches, hypertension, vertigo, Menière's syndrome, neuralgia, spasmophilia, menstrual cramps, menopausal complaints including depression, anxiety, hot flushes, vaginal dryness and atrophy, genital herpes, asthma, pertussis (whooping cough), anxiety, panic attacks.

Black cohosh is primarily indicated for neurological symptoms related to the Liver. It is a powerful antispasmodic and sedative. Its primary efect is to inhibit gonatropins. Although it contains some estrogen-like substances, it can be helpful in relieving symptoms for patients with high estrogen levels, particularly if the cause of the excess estrogen is depleted liver function. It is used in several preparations and in standardized form in some European countries for relief of menopausal symptoms in lieu of hormone therapy.

Its sedative properties are effective for anxiety, nervous spasms, muscular spasms, respiratory spasms including asthma and cough, even pertussis and tuberculosis. Because it relieves tension in the shoulders and occiput along the Gallbladder channel, it is used for several different types of headaches. It should be used carefully in the case of a true migraine, because it can easily induce vomiting. A high dose can induce vomiting even in a less sensitive patient. The most typical clinical applications are for menstrual cramps, headaches, anxiety and vertigo. It is also commonly used for facial neuralgia and rheumatic pain.

Black cohosh is strictly contraindicated during pregnancy.

BLACK RADISH *Raphanus sativus niger*

ACTIONS: Cholagogue.

CONSTITUENTS: Senevol, glucoraphenine, zinc, nickel, cobalt and sulphur.

FAMILY: Cruciferae.

FLAVOR: Pungent-cooling.

FIVE PHASE CATEGORY: Wood yang.

PRINCIPAL INDICATIONS ACCORDING TO TERRAIN:

   1) WOOD — Disperses Wood; biliary dyskinesia; alternating constipation and diarrhea; arthritis and rheumatism; allergic asthma; allergic rhinitis; whooping cough. Like most of the Wood herbs, it can be used effectively in most terrains, since liver dysfunction is such a frequent occurrence.

   Black radish is a powerful cholagogue. Traditionally, it is the juice of the root that is used. A familiar garden plant, there are numerous varieties; the white and black varieties are sometimes referred to as Spanish radish. It is an excellent remedy for stones and gravel. The juice has been used in the treatment of gallstones and as an aid in preventing their formation. It is best known for its effectiveness in discharging bile from an engorged gallbladder, though it is equally useful as an antispasmodic for the lungs. It can be a powerful sedative for coughs and is used effectively for treating asthma in Wood yin and Wood yang constitutions. It also has antiallergic properties against urticaria.

   Black radish is an excellent medication for an arthritic or allergic constitution (of the diatheses according to Ménétrier).

CELANDINE *Chelidonium majus*

ACTIONS: Antispasmodic, hypotensive, purgative, choleretic.

CONSTITUENTS: Chelidonine (an alkaloid with opium-like characteristics), chelerythrine, methoxychelidonine, oxychelidonine, sanguinarine, berberine, fumarine, other alkaloids, a saponin, essential oil, pigment, enzymes and acids.

FIVE PHASE CATEGORIES: Wood yang, Earth yang.

FAMILY: Papaveraceae.

FLAVORS: Bitter-cooling, pungent-cooling.

PRINCIPAL INDICATIONS ACCORDING TO TERRAIN:

1) WOOD — Biliary dyskinesia (biliary calculi), icterus from retention, stomach pain, duodenal ulcer, hypertension, cardiovascular problems, arteritis, allergic asthma.

2) EARTH — Splenomegaly, edema, indigestion.

3) METAL — Ringworm (externally), tetters, tuberculosis, skin cancers.

Historically, the juice of celandine has been used to sharpen the sight and for cleansing the eyeball of mucus deposits and films. Externally, it is applied to spreading ulcers, ringworm, malignant swellings and skin tuberculosis. The milky juice can irritate healthy skin.

The whole plant, especially the leaves and root, is used to relax smooth muscles and to treat cases of biliary dyskinesia, biliary calculi with icterus from retention, gastric pain and duodenal ulcers. It is also prescribed for cardiovascular problems such as arteriosclerosis, coronary pathology, hypertension and arteriopathy. Traditional usage includes treatment of eczema and scrofulous disease, where it is reputedly effective in cases of cancer. Modern usage is primarily as a hypotensive, antispasmodic and for bile duct congestion including jaundice.

DANDELION *Taraxacum dens leonis*

ACTIONS: Cholagogue, laxative, diuretic (azoturic).

CONSTITUENTS: Inulin, choline, vitamins A and E (nearly six times more vitamin A than carrots), taraxacin, taraxercerin, silica, potassium, magnesium, manganese, calcium, vitamin B-complex, riboflavin, vitamin C, tannin, lactupicrin.

FAMILY: Compositae.

FLAVORS: Bitter-cooling, pungent-cooling.

FIVE PHASE CATEGORIES: Wood yang, Metal yin, Water yang.

PRINCIPAL INDICATIONS ACCORDING TO TERRAIN:

1) WOOD — Biliary dyskinesia, vesicular calculi, constipation, obesity, cellulitis, urea, gout, hypercholesterolemia, varices, acne, herpes, eczema.

2) METAL — Acne, chronic rheumatism.

3) WATER — Excess of uric acid, urinary calculi, urea, renal insufficiency.

Dandelion is indicated in various states of congestion of the liver and the pancreas, such as hypercholesterolemia, excess of urea, gout, biliary lithiases (calculi), urinary lithiases, constipation, obesity, cellulitis, the first stages of mastitis, varices and other cutaneous afflictions such as acne and herpes (cold or heat of the liver). Used in medicine in all parts of the world, it is mentioned in Arabian medicine of the 10th and 11th centuries and has been cultivated in India for centuries as a remedy for liver complaints. Throughout England and Western Europe, it is taken as a spring tonic, and the leaves are commonly consumed as food. An extract of the root is used in Japan as a general constitution-strengthening agent. In East Asian medicine, the root and the entire herb of the species *Taraxacum mongolicum* are used. It is described as entering the Liver and Stomach channels, and is administered in a formula to treat acute appendicitis and for hepatitis. It is given as a detoxifying agent and anti-inflammatory agent for a number of acute illnesses, such as bronchitis and tonsillitis, as well as various suppurative infections. As an eyewash, it is used for acute conjunctivitis. *Taraxacum mongolicum* also contains taraxacin, which is found in the *Taraxacum dens leonis*.

EYEBRIGHT *Euphrasia officinalis*

ACTIONS: Anti-inflammatory, analgesic, astringent.

CONSTITUENTS: Essential oil, tannins, the glycoside aucubin, aucuboside, glucosides, resin, bitter principle.

FAMILY: Ranunculaceae.

FLAVORS: Bitter-cooling, pungent-warming and cooling.

FIVE PHASE CATEGORIES: Wood yang, Metal yin, Earth yin.

PRINCIPAL INDICATIONS ACCORDING TO TERRAIN:

    1) WOOD — Rhinitis and asthma, conjunctivitis, herpetic keratitis, blepharitis, styes. Eye problems related to diabetes mellitus. Used for colds accompanied by conjunctivitis.

    2) METAL — Rhinitis, common cold, otitis media and other nose and throat infections, especially pediatric.

The flowering plant has been used from antiquity all over Europe for various types of eye problems. Used externally as a lotion and also internally, it is said to be excellent for general disorders of the eyes. The dried herb is an ingredient in British herbal tobacco, which is smoked for chronic bronchial colds. A medicinal tincture is prepared from the whole plant and spirits of wine, from which a lotion is made with rose water for use in simple inflammation of the eyes. According to Culpepper, eyebright mixed with mace "comforteth the memorie."

Eyebright is used for allergic rhinitis and asthma, conjunctivitis, herpetic keratitis, blepharitis and styes. It is frequently used for treating head colds, sinusitis and rhinitis in children. Applied locally, it is also useful for drying up clear, watery secretions from the nose and eyes.

GOLDENSEAL *Hydrastis canadensis*

ACTIONS: Anti-inflammatory, hemostatic, pelvic vasoconstrictor.

CONSTITUENTS: Alkaloids (berberine, berberastine, tetrahydroberberine, hydrastine, phytosterine), various fatty acids.

FAMILY: Ranunculaceae.

FLAVOR: Bitter-cooling.

FIVE PHASE CATEGORIES: Wood yang, Fire yang.

PRINCIPAL INDICATIONS ACCORDING TO TERRAIN:

1) WOOD — Venous congestion (including hemorrhoids), uterine tonic, conjunctivitis, indigestion, nausea, heartburn related to biliary dyskinesia.

2) FIRE — Inflammation of the mucous membranes, especially intestinal.

Goldenseal has a general supplementing effect on the veins, especially in the pelvic area. Hydrastine is a vasoconstrictor and oxytocic agent. Berberine is anti-inflammatory and its presence is an important factor in the usefulness of the herb in treating dysentery and intestinal parasites.

Goldenseal stimulates bile production and secretion, is strongly antibacterial (staph, strep and E. coli), antifungal, astringent and antiseptic. It is used for such diverse infections as conjunctivitis, vaginal mycosis, pharyngitis and giardia infestation, and was used successfully in the treatment of cholera during an epidemic in Calcutta in the 1960's. Prophylactically, it can be used to protect the intestines from amoebic infestation.

GRAPE VINE *Vitis vinifera*

ACTIONS: Astringent, hemostatic, choleretic, diuretic.

CONSTITUENTS: Tannins, gum inositol, quercitin, quercitrin, oxalic acid, tartaric acid, potassium bitartrate, glucose.

FAMILY: Vitaceae.

FLAVORS: Sour-cooling, bitter-cooling.

FIVE PHASE CATEGORIES: Wood yang, Fire yang.

PRINCIPAL INDICATIONS ACCORDING TO TERRAIN:

1) WOOD — Dysmenorrhea, "liver depression" and other problems of menopause, varicose veins, phlebitis, hypercholesterolemia, gallstones, conjunctivitis.

2) FIRE — Hemorrhage, hypertension, circulation problems of menopause, red blotches on the skin.

Grapevine has anticoagulant properties, but is hemostatic because it reduces hypercoagulability. It is used for dysmenorrhea, hypertension (especially in cases of hypertension where there is blood stasis), thrombophlebitis, hypercholesterolemia and gallstone formation. Grapevine is useful for streptococcus infections and is even helpful for treating hemolytic streptococcus when used synergistically with essential oils (oils of *lavender* and *lemon* are especially useful for this purpose). The gemmae (buds) are used for treating scarlatina, and can prevent circulatory complications of scarlet fever and scarlatina. It can be used to drain the bile ducts and locally as a pelvic decongestant.

HORSE CHESTNUT *Aesculus hippocastanum*

ACTIONS: Astringent, hemostatic, anti-inflammatory, vasoconstrictive.

CONSTITUENTS: Tannins, saponins (aesculus, aescin), aesculic acid, aesculinic acid, flavonoids (esculin, esculetin, rutin), kaempferol, coumarin heterosides, potassium phosphate, salts of magnesium, sodium, iron, manganese, cobalt and iodine, high in starch.

FAMILY: Hippocastanaceae.

FLAVORS: Bitter-cooling and pungent-cooling (nuts);
sour-cooling, bitter-cooling (leaves).

FIVE PHASE CATEGORIES: Wood yang, Earth yin, Fire yang.

PRINCIPAL INDICATIONS ACCORDING TO TERRAIN:

1) WOOD — Varices, hemorrhoids, prostate congestion, varicoceles, edema.

2) FIRE — Hot flushes.

3) EARTH — Prostate congestion, obesity, cellulitis, varices, edema, acrocyanosis (Raynaud's phenomenon).

Traditionally, horse chestnut bark has been used as a tonic, narcotic and febrifuge for intermittent fevers. In the absence of quinine it was recommended for malaria. It was also used in a bath for this purpose. The nuts and leaves have been employed in the treatment of rheumatism, neuralgia and hemorrhoids. It treats Liver blood vacuity, blood stasis, congestion of the prostate, hemorrhoids, varices, varicoceles and hot flushes. It is also prescribed for treatment of edema and cellulitis.

LADY'S MANTLE *Alchemilla vulgaris*

ACTIONS: Tonic, stomachic, astringent, oxytocic, luteotropic.

CONSTITUENTS: Ellagiac acid, tannin, glycoside, traces of salicylic acid.

FAMILY: Rosaceae.

FLAVORS: Sour-cooling.

FIVE PHASE CATEGORIES: Wood yang, Earth yang.

PRINCIPAL INDICATIONS ACCORDING TO TERRAIN:

1) WOOD — Biliary dyskinesia, nervousness, mood swings, insomnia, headaches, arthritis, arteriosclerosis, conjunctivitis, menopausal complaints, menstrual disorders, uterine hemorrhage.

2) EARTH — Diarrhea, obesity, diabetes, leukorrhea, mastodynia, cystic breasts.

Lady's mantle secretes a rose-colored exudate, sacred to alchemists for preparation of an elixir. It is sour-cooling and a powerful agent for calming Liver Fire, which manifests in such symptoms as agitation, insomnia, nervousness, hot flushes and headaches. It is also useful for Liver depression, biliary dyskinesia (nausea and indigestion, especially after fat consumption), subcostal pressure or discomfort and mood swings.

In addition, Lady's mantle is known to stimulate the secretion of luteinizing hormone (LH) and can be useful when necessary for dysmenorrhea and amenorrhea. It is used as an oxytocic agent, and for treatment of leukorrhea (yellow discharge), vulvar pruritus, menorrhagia and metrorrhagia especially in a Wood-yang or Earth-yang terrain (when there is damp obstruction of the Spleen).

In a diabetic terrain, it is used to treat obesity, diarrhea and Liver symptoms. It is a useful agent in the treatment of arthrosis and arteriosclerosis in an Earth-yang or Wood-yang terrain. Externally it is used in the treatment of conjunctivitis.

MISTLETOE *Viscum album*

ACTIONS: Hypotensive, antispasmodic, immune stimulant, diuretic (volumetric and azoturic).

CONSTITUENTS: Mucilage, tannins, organic salts, viscin, resins, sugars.

FAMILY: Loranthaceae.

FLAVORS: Bitter-cooling and bitter-warming.

FIVE PHASE CATEGORIES: Wood yang, Fire yang, Water yin.

PRINCIPAL INDICATIONS ACCORDING TO TERRAIN:

1) WOOD — Neuropsychiatric disorders such as hysteria, convulsions, epilepsy; hypertension, arteriosclerosis, asthma.

2) FIRE — Hypertension, tachycardia, arteriosclerosis, hemorrhagic syndromes, menorrhagia of menopause.

3) WATER — Chronic renal insufficiency, proteinuria.

Mistletoe calms Heart Fire, and is used clinically for hypertension, arteriosclerosis, tachycardia, convulsions, hysteria and epilepsy, and as well to treat hysterical bleeding and for hemorrhage in menopause. It is sympatholytic and parasympathomimetic. European mistletoe is strongly luteotropic and was used by the Celts during the Beltane festival to protect the members of the community from pregnancy following the week's sanctioned sexual license. The custom of kissing women standing under mistletoe during the Christmas season is derived from this tradition. In anthroposophical medicine, a mistletoe extract called "Iscador" is used in the treatment of cancer.

PASQUE FLOWER *Pulsatilla vulgaris*

ACTIONS: Antispasmodic, emmenagogue, sedative, estrogen antagonist, sympatholytic.

CONSTITUENTS: Anemonin (protoanemonin, which rapidly converts to anemonin), saponins, tannin, sterols and a fatty oil.

FAMILY: Ranunculaceae.

FLAVORS: Pungent-cooling, sour-cooling.

FIVE PHASE CATEGORY: Wood yang.

PRINCIPAL INDICATIONS ACCORDING TO TERRAIN:

1) WOOD — Tachycardia, migraines, neuralgia, allergic rhinitis, allergic asthma, colonopathy and colitis, pelvic congestion and pain, anguish, phobia, estrogen antagonist.

One of the best plants to drain repletion of Liver yang, the whole plant is used to treat syndromes of Liver Fire, hyperthyroid symptoms, tachycardia, neuralgia, migraines, bronchial spasms of pertussis, allergic rhinitis and asthma, spasms of colonopathy on the right side, dysmenorrhea, Liver congestion, symptoms of depression with the sudden mood swings of menopause, pain in the pelvic and genital area, hysteria and phobias. It also has diaphoretic and diuretic properties. All parts of the fresh plant are dangerous, causing nausea, vomiting, diarrhea, intestinal spasms, skin inflammation and asphyxiation.

PLANTAIN *Plantago major*

ACTIONS: Astringent, diuretic, sympathomimetic, pituitary stimulant.

CONSTITUENTS: Rich in mucilage, glucides, tannin, mineral salts, potassium, calcium.

FAMILY: Plantaginae.

FLAVOR: Sour-cooling, sweet-cooling, sweet-warming.

FIVE PHASE CATEGORIES: Wood yang, Wood yin, Earth yin, Metal yin.

PRINCIPAL INDICATIONS ACCORDING TO TERRAIN:

1) WOOD — Conjunctivitis, allergic rhinitis, allergic asthma, allergic eye conditions.

2) METAL — Emaciation, retarded development, bronchitis, laryngitis, tuberculosis, constipation, chronic diarrhea, leukorrhea, eczema and acne.

3) EARTH — Strengthens the stomach and upper digestive functions; good for malnutrition, retarded development, nephrotic syndromes.

The healing virtues of plantain have been known from antiquity. A decoction of plantain has long been considered beneficial for disorders of the kidney, and the root powder is often used for complaints of the bowels. Others have recommended the expressed juice for spitting of blood and for hemorrhoids. It has legendary properties for removing toxicity from the bites of dogs, snakes and spiders, and even burns and scalds when used as a poultice. As a decoction, it is recommended as a treatment for intestinal parasites. Culpepper stated that the water is used for "all manner of spreading scabs, tetters, ringworm, shingles, etc." In addition, he used the seeds to treat epilepsy, dropsy, jaundice and to open obstructions of the Liver, Spleen and Kidney.

In Chinese medicine, the seed of *Plantago asiatica* is used as a diuretic to treat ascites and edema and to calm coughs and eliminate phlegm. It is prescribed for weakness of the Lung (depletion of Lung yang), bronchitis, and laryngitis, for example, chronic bronchitis where there is an abundance of watery secretions. Clinically, it is used for inflammations of the kidney or gonorrhea, for their associated low back pain and for eye diseases.

The leaves are used for gonorrhea and for diarrhea resulting from bacterial enteritis and other acute forms of enteritis. The whole plant is used as a styptic and astringent for hemorrhoids and is used on the skin as a vulnerary, a hemostatic and as a poultice for rheumatic pain. Plantain can be used for emaciation and retarded development of infants due to growth hormone and androgen insufficiency. Its mucilaginous quality is useful in constipation and its sour astringent quality is used for chronic diarrhea; however, it is also effective for water retention.

In modern European phytotherapy, it is used as an astringent, expectorant and blood purifier. It is used in Europe primarily for allergic types of rhinitis, allergic asthma and conjunctivitis.

STONESEED *Lithospermum officinale*

ACTIONS: Diuretic, emmenagogue, inhibitor of pituitary gonadotropins (FSH and LH), TSH antagonist.

CONSTITUENTS: Mucilage, pigments, mineral salts, especially those of calcium and silicon.

FAMILY: Boraginaceae.

FLAVORS: Sour-cooling, sweet-cooling.

FIVE PHASE CATEGORIES: Wood yang, Fire yang, Earth yang.

PRINCIPAL INDICATIONS ACCORDING TO TERRAIN:

1) WOOD — Biliary dyskinesia, urinary and biliary calculae, hyper-folliculine dysmenorrhea, mastosis, mastitis, hot flushes, spastic colon.

2) FIRE — Excess pituitary hormone secretion; especially inhibits FSH and LH.

3) EARTH — Hyperfolliculine dysmenorrhea and premenstrual syndrome.

Stoneseed is sour-cooling, which directly cools Liver Fire. The fruit, leaves and flowers are used. Its main indications are for hyperestrogenic dysmenorrhea, Liver depression, mastosis, mastodynia and hot flushes of menopause. A diuretic, it dissolves stones of the biliary tract and urinary tract. It is also indicated for colonopathy from Wood yang origin. It is considered to have cardiotonic properties, antiphlogistic properties, antibacterial and antiviral (influenza virus) properties. In addition, it has proven utility for eczema and also for pruritus of the perineum. In Chinese medicine, it is used externally in an ointment for a wide variety of skin afflictions.

WITCH HAZEL *Hamamelis virginiana*

ACTIONS: Astringent, hemostatic.

CONSTITUENTS: Rich in tannins, especially hamamelitannin, saponins, resinoids (hamamelin), flavonoid pigments.

FAMILY: Saxifragiceae.

FLAVORS: Sour-cooling, bitter-cooling.

FIVE PHASE CATEGORIES: Wood yang, Fire yang.

PRINCIPAL INDICATIONS ACCORDING TO TERRAIN:

1) WOOD — Hemorrhoids, varices, pelvic congestion, painful menstruation, genital hemorrhages, varicoceles, pruritus, urticaria.

2) FIRE — Hot flushes, various types of hemorrhage, hemorrhagic purpura.

A common household remedy, witch hazel has been used for generations for burns, scalds and inflammatory conditions of the skin. It can provide relief for the pain of diarrhea and dysentery when there is excessive mucus elimination. A tea made from the leaves or bark can be taken safely for bleeding in the stomach.

Externally, it can relieve eye inflammations and varicose veins other than hemorrhoids. The native American Indians used it as a poultice for painful swellings and tumors. It can be applied as a mouthwash for bleeding gums and for mouth and throat inflammations.

The bark and leaves treat pelvic congestion, uterine, ovarian or testicular congestion and dysmenorrhea, Liver depression, mood swings during menopause and hot flushes. It is good for varicoceles, metrorrhagia, hemorrhoids, varices and phlebitis due to Liver vacuity, and is the main ingredient of a number of products used for bleeding hemorrhoids.

HERBS FOR WOOD YIN PATHOLOGIES

WOOD YIN PROFILES - QUICK REFERENCE

ANGELICA	nervousness
	cramps
	spasms
	headaches
BARBERRY	subcostal distress
	constipation
	hemorrhoids
ECHINACEA	strengthens Liver
	immunity
	Wood-yin
	Earth-yin
LOVAGE	headache
	edema
	low estrogen
MILK THISTLE	toxic liver
	menorrhagia
	melancholia
MUGWORT	low estrogen
	anemia
	cholagogue
TARRAGON	choleretic

ANGELICA *Angelica archangelica*

ACTIONS: Tonic, eupeptic, carminative, parasympatholytic, sympatholytic, estrogenic.

CONSTITUENTS: Tannins, glucides, angelic acid, valeric acid, wax, an essential oil containing phellandrene, a coumarin (angelicin) and organic acids.

FAMILY: Umbelliferae.

FLAVORS: Spicy warming, sour-warming, sweet-warming.

FIVE PHASE CATEGORIES: Wood yin, Metal yin, Fire yin, Earth yin.

PRINCIPAL INDICATIONS ACCORDING TO TERRAIN:

1) WOOD — Asthenia of hepatic origin, hepatic insufficiency (hemorrhoids, constipation), insufficient immunity of hepatic origin, viral hepatitis, vertigo, syncope, migraine headaches, seasonal allergic asthma, muscular cramps, nerve problems, spasms, estrogenic activity; sedative (action comparable to diazepam); diminishes excess of both the sympathetic and parasympathetic branches of the autonomic nervous system.

2) FIRE — Vertigo, syncope, hypotension, anguish, spasms, nervous excitation and fatigue; calms sympathetic and parasympathetic branches of ANS.

3) EARTH — Anorexia, gastric pain, dyspepsia, poor digestion, exhaustion, emaciation, amenorrhea, dysmenorrhea due to insufficiency of estrogens; insufficient immunity: prevents colds, influenza and epidemics.

4) METAL — Anorexia nervosa, chronic bronchitis, emphysema, anemia, estrogen secretion stimulation.

Highly prized in Europe, angelica commanded a high price for its medicinal qualities and was used as well as a confectionary ingredient in wines and liqueurs including Chartreuse and Benedictine. Culpepper recommended its use in epidemic disease. Legend holds that the Archangel Raphael introduced angelica to mortals to treat the plague, as a snakebite remedy and to prolong life. In the Middle Ages, it was used for protection against witchcraft and the forces of evil.

An important herb in traditional European herbology, the root, herb and seeds have been used as a remedy for colds, coughs, colic, rheumatism and urinary tract disorders. It was considered a useful agent for fevers, acting as a diaphoretic. In Russia it was used as a sedative for hysteria, epilepsy, nervous exhaustion and for gastric hyperacidity and bloating.

Useful in syndromes of Earth yin and Wood yin constitutional types, it is a gentle cardiotonic for cardiac insufficiency and syncope. It improves digestion by stimulating the liver, dilating the biliary passages, and increasing pancreatic secretions. It also elevates blood sugar. It is not recommended during pregnancy. (See Angelica in "Essential Oils")

BARBERRY *Berberis vulgaris*

ACTIONS: Cholagogue.

CONSTITUENTS: Alkaloids (berberine, palmatine, columbamine, berbamine, berberubine, oxyacanthine), chelidonic acid, mucin, glycosides including oxyacanthine; the berries are rich in vitamin C.

FIVE PHASE CATEGORIES: Wood yin, Wood yang, Earth yin, Fire yin, Water yin.

FAMILY: Berberidaceae.

FLAVORS: Bitter-warming (bark), sour-cooling (berries, leaves).

PRINCIPAL INDICATIONS ACCORDING TO TERRAIN:

1) WOOD — Biliary dyskinesia, cholelithiasis, hepatomegaly, atonic dyspepsia, constipation, hemorrhoids, dysmenorrhea, fibroma, varices.

2) FIRE — Strengthen heart contractions, psychasthenia, general fatigue.

3) EARTH — Fatigue, anorexia, scurvy, splenomegaly, malaria, mycotic infections.

4) WATER — Urinary calculi.

As a folk remedy, the common barberry has been used for generations to treat dyspepsia and functional derangement of the liver. The root, bark and berries have been used in jaundice, general debility, biliousness and diarrhea. East Asian medicine uses berberine, a yellow, crystalline, bitter alkaloid, for bacterial dysentery and throat infections. A bitter tonic, it promotes bile flow and activates the lymphatic system. In Ayurvedic medicine it is used with turmeric for gallbladder and liver problems. The Navajo native American tribe used barberry leaves and branches as a treatment for rheumatic stiffness.

The fruits have also been used as a laxative. The root contains up to 8 percent alkaloids and has been used as a hemostatic agent for postpartum uterine bleeding and for kidney stones.

ECHINACEA (PURPLE CONEFLOWER) *Echinacea purpurea*

ACTIONS: Depurative, immune stimulant, febrifuge, hepatostimulant.

CONSTITUENTS: Echinacin, inulin, betaine, phytosterols, fatty acids including oleic, cerotic, linoleic, and palmitic acids.

FAMILY: Compositae.

FLAVORS: Sweet-cooling, sour-warming.

FIVE PHASE CATEGORIES: Wood yin, Earth yin, Fire yang.

PRINCIPAL INDICATIONS ACCORDING TO TERRAIN:

1) WOOD — General detoxifying, liver congestion, hemorrhoids, hot flushes of menopause; to increase general immunity, to speed recovery in acute infections.

2) FIRE — Acute febrile infections, hot flushes and nightsweats of menopause; to speed recovery in acute infections.

In recent years, Europeans have used echinacea as a general immune stimulant, popularly consumed at the acute stage of colds and minor respiratory infections. Native to North America, it was widely used by the Eclectic school in the 19th century for acute febrile infectious diseases including typhoid, meningitis, diphtheria, abscesses and insect and reptile bites.

Echinacea influences the liver by enhancing the liver's detoxifying functions, its thermoregulating function and its connective tissue building function. It elevates the white blood cell count, stimulates lymph drainage and activates T-cell function. It also accelerates the healing process by accelerating granulation.

LOVAGE *Levisticum officinalis*

ACTIONS: Diuretic, choleretic, carminative, antispasmodic, emmenagogue.

CONSTITUENTS: Coumarin, tannin, angelic acid, benzoic acid, malic acid, logulin, resins, gums, starches, sugars, vitamin C, an essential oil containing phthalidin, terpinol, bergaptene, umbelliferone and butylphthalide.

FAMILY: Umbelliferae.

FLAVORS: Sweet-warming, sour-cooling.

FIVE PHASE CATEGORIES: Wood yin, Water yin, Wood yang.

PRINCIPAL INDICATIONS ACCORDING TO TERRAIN:

1) WOOD — Hepatic insufficiency, dyspepsia, migraines, acne, insufficient menstruation.

2) WATER — Edema, oliguria, glomerulonephritis, urinary tract infections, pyelonephritis, cystitis, urinary retention, amenorrhea, menstrual insufficiency, dermatoses, acne on the back, seborrhea, psoriasis.

The root, fruit and leaves of lovage have classically been used in herbal medicine for stomach disorders, fevers, colic and flatulence in children. Culpepper reported that it was useful as eyedrops to take away eye redness. Even today, the juice of the leaves is used for conjunctivitis. Children's complaints figure among its main indications, especially flatulence, but it is useful for adults as a carminative, for headaches and for edema.

Because it absorbs excess moisture in the body, it is prescribed for obesity, edema and sluggish lymph circulation. It is used as an emmenagogue for asthenic women, and strengthens kidney function in the treatment of oliguria of glomerulonephritis, proteinuria, oliguria of cystitis, pyelonephritis and urinary retention in the bladder. It is useful for skin problems related to the Water phase.

MILK THISTLE *Silybum marianum*

ACTIONS: Hepatoprotective, cardiotonic, sympathomimetic.

CONSTITUENTS: The flavonoid silymarin consisting of the flavono-lignins silybin, silychristin and several others, the amines histamine and tyramine, an essential oil and bitter principle.

FAMILY: Compositae.

FLAVOR: Bitter-warming.

FIVE PHASE CATEGORIES: Wood yin, Fire yin.

PRINCIPAL INDICATIONS ACCORDING TO TERRAIN:

1) WOOD — Hepatitis, allergies, hypotension, lipothymia, syncope, hypercholesterolemia, menorrhagia, viral hepatitis, fatty liver, cirrhosis of the liver, toxic liver, memory problems, psychasthenia, psoriasis

2) FIRE — Hypotension, right-sided cardiac insufficiency, memory problems, psychasthenia and melancholia.

Traditionally, the seeds of milk thistle were used to stimulate production of milk in nursing mothers, hence its familiar name. According to Christian legend, the Virgin Mary spilled milk while nursing the infant Jesus and left white streaks in its leaves. In Germany it was traditionally used to cure jaundice and to treat various biliary problems. It is also useful for treating phlegm congestion in the lungs. Culpepper recommended it to remove obstructions of the liver and the spleen, as well as to treat jaundice and expel stones.

The young plant is used as a spring tonic and blood cleanser. The seeds contain tyramine, an amino acid with antihistamine properties. The leaves have a bitter-warming flavor, supplementing the Liver and secondarily the Heart. It is prescribed for cirrhosis of the liver, for hepatitis and for all toxic liver symptoms; damage to the hepatic reticulo-endothelium, hepato-splenomegaly, hypotension, syncope and hypoestrogenic menorrhagia.

There is no known toxicity level. It regenerates damaged liver tissue by increasing the rate of protein synthesis for new cell regeneration as well as accelerating breakdown and removal of degenerated cells.

As an antioxidant, milk thistle can prevent damage to cell membranes from free radicals, thus protecting the system from environmental pollutants and ionizing radiation. It can be used as a preventive or antidote for amanita mushroom poisoning, even the deadly amanita phalloides. It inhibits prostaglandin synthesis during inflammation. It is useful for promoting liver regeneration for chemical damage of the liver found in former drug and alcohol abusers. Indicated symptoms include lethargy, postprandial drowsiness, depression, irritability, headaches, poor digestion and allergies. It is commonly used in Europe as a fundamental herb in the treatment of allergies.

MUGWORT *Artemisia vulgaris*

ACTIONS: Emmenagogue, tonic, stimulates secretion of pituitary gonadotropins (FSH and LH).

CONSTITUENTS: Essential oil rich in cineol, resin, tannin, mucilage, inulin. The leaves contain vitamins A, B1, B2 and C. The plant is extremely rich in iron.

FAMILY: Compositae.

FLAVORS: Pungent-cooling, bitter-cooling.

FIVE PHASE CATEGORIES: Wood yin, Earth yin, Metal yin.

PRINCIPAL INDICATIONS ACCORDING TO TERRAIN:

1) WOOD — Stimulates bile secretion, increases appetite, facilitates digestion; hypotension, syncope, epilepsy, hypoestrogenic amenorrhea, functional uterine bleeding, menstrual cramps, abortifacient (not without danger)

2) EARTH — Insufficient menses, amenorrhea, insufficiency of the corpus luteum due to anemia; antimicrobial, estrogenic and luteotropic.

The Latin name for mugwort, *artemisia,* comes from the goddess Artemis, protector of virgins and females suffering illness. Having slightly tonic properties, it has been used as an emmenagogue, diuretic and diaphoretic in the traditional medicine of Western Europe. Its oil is said to kill worms and to be beneficial for liver and jaundice and as a febrifuge. Culpepper used it as an antidote for opium poisoning. Native Americans used it as a vulnerary for wounds and used the fresh juice for poison oak irritation. In Russia, it has been used as a sedative for convulsions, epilepsy, neurasthenia, dysmenorrhea and labor pain.

The Japanese pounded it into glutinous rice to make *yomogi mochi,* a food favored for stamina and used traditionally by new mothers to stop postpartum blood loss, treat anemia and stimulate lactation. The leaves of mugwort were made into moxa, which is used in East Asian medicine to warm acupoints.

In East Asian medicine today it is used primarily as a hemostatic, but also as an antibacterial and digestive aid for promoting the secretion of gastric juices. It can be used for amenorrhea from general causes, including estrogen or luteal insufficiency, especially for women of the Wood yin and Metal yin constitutional type. It is uterolytic and helpful for painful spasms in dysmenorrhea. For the Wood yin constitutional type, it is used in neurological and psychiatric syndromes which originate with the liver, as well as hypotension, syncope, epilepsy and dyspepsia. It has been used the world over as a spring tonic.

TARRAGON *Artemisia dracunculus*

Actions: Eupeptic, vagolytic.

Constituents: Coumarin (herniarin); the essential oil contains phellandrene, ocimene and methylchavicol.

Family: Compositae.

Flavor: Sour-cooling, sour-warming.

Five phase categories: Wood yin, Earth yin.

Principal indications according to terrain:

1) Wood — Hyposecretion of bile and digestive juices; allergies.

2) Earth — Difficulties in digestion, dyspepsia, poor appetite, insufficiency of digestive secretions; calming of the parasympathetic nervous system.

Tarragon is a close relative of wormwood and of mugwort. It is called *estragon* in French, which derives from the Latin *dracunculus,* or "little dragon." It is often used in French cuisine, for example to make tarragon vinegar, a popular flavoring.

Therapeutically, it promotes the secretion of digestive juices and bile. In infusion, it is used for dispersing a repletion of Liver yang: flushing, irritability, bloodshot eyes and shoulder stiffness. Its extract, however, being simultaneously warming and cooling, can be useful for infections due to Liver vacuity, such as biliary and gastric hyposecretion. (See also Essential Oils Profiles)

HERBS FOR FIRE YANG PATHOLOGIES

FIRE YANG PROFILES - QUICK REFERENCE

BITTER ORANGE
nervousness
insomnia
digestive spasms

CHASTE TREE
menorrhagia
short cycle
anxiety
tachycardia

FEVERFEW
analgesic
anti-inflammatory

GINGKO
improves cranial circulation
improves memory

HAWTHORN
tachycardia
insomnia
anxiety

MEADOWSWEET
diarrhea
rheumatism
HBP
edema

MELILOT
hypertension
anxiety
insomnia
hot flushes

PASSIONFLOWER
insomnia
anxiety
hypertension

VALERIAN
insomnia
nervousness

WHITE WILLOW
calm fever
anxiety
insomnia
rheumatism

BITTER ORANGE *Citrus aurantium (var. amara)*

ACTIONS: Sedative (CNS), antispasmodic, expectorant, eupeptic, sympatholytic.

CONSTITUENTS: D-limonene, auraptene, auraptin, terpinol, linalool, hesperidin, myoinositol, bitter principles (naringine, aurantiamarine), vitamin C, vitamin B1, flavonoids. The flowers contain neroli essence, the trace elements manganese, cobalt, lithium, aluminum, phosphorus, magnesium, a bitter principle and flavonoid pigments.

FLAVOR: Bitter-cooling.

FAMILY: Aurantiaceae.

FIVE PHASE CATEGORIES: Fire yang, Wood yang.

PRINCIPAL INDICATIONS ACCORDING TO TERRAIN:

    1) FIRE — Tachycardia, anguish, nervousness, anxiety, insomnia, epilepsy.

    2) WOOD — Aerophagia, dyspepsia, digestive spasms, tachycardia of emotional origin, anxiety, insomnia.

In European phytotherapy, the flowers, leaves, rind and dried fruit of bitter orange are all extracted. Its nature is Fire yang and Wood yang, beneficial for cooling Liver Fire stemming from a repletion of Heart Fire (tachycardia, anguish, insomnia, epilepsy). The bitter-cooling effect is also beneficial as an antispasmodic for dyspepsia and aerophagia.

In East Asian medicine, the rind of the fruit is frequently used for abdominal pain and bloating with chest oppression, nausea and indigestion, and for sluggish digestive function in general. It is also indicated for borborygmus, intestinal cramps, coughs with abundant phlegm and other symptoms related to dampness. It has been shown to be effective in stopping the growth of staphylococcus *in vitro*. (See also Essential Oils Profiles)

CHASTE TREE *Vitex agnus castus*

ACTIONS: Sympatholytic, antispasmodic, estrogen antagonist, FSH inhibitor, luteotropic, galactagogue.

CONSTITUENTS: Aucubin, agnoside (iridoid glycosides), casticin, isovitexin, orientin (flavonoids), bitter principle containing viticin and castin, essential oil.

FAMILY: Verbenaceae.

FLAVOR: Sweet-cooling.

FIVE PHASE CATEGORIES: Fire yang, Wood yang.

PRINCIPAL INDICATIONS ACCORDING TO TERRAIN:

1) FIRE — Nervousness, genital excitation, dysmenorrhea; anti-FSH, sympatholytic, acne; stops excessive bleeding and corrects a shortened menstrual cycle.

2) WOOD — Neurotonia, globus hystericus, Liver depression, palpitations, tachycardia, dysmenorrhea, uterine fibroid hemorrhage, acne, genital excitation, mastosis and breast tenderness; anti-FSH properties, sympatholytic.

The berries of the chaste tree were once held in repute for securing chastity. For the sacred rites of Ceres, Athenian virgins would string their couches with the leaves. Its anaphrodisiac properties are legendary, and it was frequently used to treat nymphomania. In men, chaste tree can be used to treat impotence resulting from excessive sexual excitation.

The leaves and tops of the flowers have a sweet and cooling flavor. A stimulant of luteinizing hormone, it inhibits FSH production. It can be used to treat heart palpitations and tachycardia, epigastric tightness, globus hystericus, dysmenorrhea, liver depression, premenstrual syndrome, amenorrhea, polymenorrhea, bleeding fibromas and menorrhagia. It is a particularly useful herb for irregular menstrual cycles and for menstrual and premenstrual edema. Chaste tree has a regulating effect on milk production, stimulating lactation if there is insufficiency, but inhibiting lactation in the case of excessively high levels of prolactin. It is a very effective treatment for cystic breasts, as it normalizes the ratio of estrogen to progesterone.

FEVERFEW *Tanacetum parthenium*

ACTIONS: Anti-inflammatory, antifebrile, analgesic, estrogen antagonist.

CONSTITUENTS: Sesquiterpene lactones (parthenolide, camphor and several others), flavonoid glycosides (luteolin, apigenin).

FAMILY: Compositae.

FLAVOR: Bitter-cooling, sour-cooling.

FIVE PHASE CATEGORIES: Fire yang, Wood yang.

PRINCIPAL INDICATIONS ACCORDING TO TERRAIN:

    1) FIRE — Cluster headaches, anxiety, fever, arthritis, inflammation with pain.

    2) WOOD — Migraine headache, premenstrual headache, premenstrual or climacteric anxiety attacks.

Recently rediscovered because of well-publicized studies of its effectiveness for migraine, feverfew was known to the ancient Greeks and mentioned by Dioscorides as a potent anti-inflammatory. The name *parthenium* is a reference to its reputed use to save the life of someone injured in a fall from the Parthenon. John Hill's *Family Herbal* wrote that it was the best treatment for severe headaches. Culpepper recommended it for hysteria. More recently, an English double-blind study demonstrated its utility for rheumatoid arthritis pain as well as migraine headaches.

Feverfew has been used with success as a prophylactic for migraine, reducing frequency and severity of attacks and concomitant symptoms of nausea, vomiting and anxiety. In addition, it appears to have clinically desirable effects as an anti-inflammatory for arthritis, particularly rheumatoid arthritis, because of its prostaglandin-inhibiting properties. Its inhibition of platelet aggregation and secretion makes it potentially useful as an antithrombotic agent and invites comparison with aspirin.

A small percentage of patients report mouth ulcers and mild indigestion as side effects of use. It is recommended to begin with a low dose (40-50 mg/day) and to increase it gradually for ongoing use.

GINKGO *Ginkgo biloba*

ACTIONS: Circulatory stimulant, antitussive, parasympathomimetic.

CONSTITUENTS: Terpenes, flavones (rutoside, quercetol-3-rhamno-glucoside, kaempferol-3-rhamnoglucoside, quercetol, kaempferol, isorhamnetol), proanthocyanidins, ginkgolides, ginkgo heterosides (flavoglycosides), biflavones derived from apigenol, ginkgetol, isogingketol, ginkgolic acid, bilobol, heptacosanol, sitosterol.

FAMILY: Ginkgoaceae.

FLAVOR: Sweet-cooling, bitter-cooling.

FIVE PHASE CATEGORIES: Fire yang, Metal yin.

PRINCIPAL INDICATIONS ACCORDING TO TERRAIN:

1) FIRE — Vertigo, tinnitus, memory loss, altitude sickness, Raynaud's phenomenon, frostbite, hypertension, depression, lack of vigilance, cardiac hypoxia, diabetic retinopathy, cerebral vascular accident prophylaxis, arthritic and rheumatic conditions, coldness in the body, tinnitus.

2) METAL — Bronchitis, asthma.

An old species, having even survived the Ice Age, Charles Darwin called ginkgo a living fossil. The trees live as long as 1,000 years and seem to have a high resistance to 20th century pollution. Extracts from the leaves of the ginkgo tree are extremely rich in components that improve arterial and venous circulation, particularly in the brain, eyes, ears and limbs. Recently it has been widely publicized as a potential hope for Alzheimer's disease.

Though the use of ginkgo for circulation problems only dates back to research in France in the 1960's, the leaf extract has been used in China for respiratory complaints for thousands of years. It has been used successfully as a vasodilator and has been shown to scavenge free radicals, which may be responsible for its protective effect on vascular walls. It may also prove useful in treating brain allergies by restoring proper function of the blood-brain barrier in protecting the brain from pollutants and other toxins.

One of the ginkgolides, ginkgolide B, has been shown to prevent cardiac arrhythmias caused by myocardial ischemia as effectively as two widely used antiarrhythmic drugs. It also strengthens and restores nerve membranes and increases energy metabolism in nerve cells. It has a proven record as a useful antimicrobial and antitubercular agent.

Its chief clinical usage has been for treating peripheral circulation (Raynaud's disease), tinnitus, vertigo, altitude sickness and memory loss, for which it has a popular reputation. Recent experiments have been conducted using gingko in diabetic angiopathy. In France it is also used for varicose veins and varicose ulcers. It has been suggested for usage in protecting transplant organs from rejection. Ginkgo extracts in high doses have caused apparent side effects of headache and stomach upset. The standard dose is 50 mg three times daily.

HAWTHORN *Crataegus oxyacantha*

ACTIONS: Cardiac sedative, hypotensive, sympatholytic, febrifuge, diuretic and astringent, coronary dilator, chronotrope negative (strong), bathmotrope negative, antispasmodic.

CONSTITUENTS: Flavonoids (hyperoside, quercetin, vitexin, vitexin-rhamnoside), leukoanthocyanidins and its derivative crataeguslactone (containing crataegolic, ursolic and oleanolic acids), trimethylamine glycosides, saponins, procyanidins, choline, beta-sitosterol, ursolic acid, oleanic acid, chlorogenic acid, crataegolic acid, acantolic acid, caffeic acid, malic acid, citric acid, vitamins B2 and C, manganese, cobalt, iodine, lithium, selenium, vanadium and chromium.

FAMILY: Rosaceae.

FLAVORS: Sweet-cooling (tops of the flowers); bitter-cooling, sour-cooling (berries).

FIVE PHASE CATEGORIES: Fire yang, Wood yang.

PRINCIPAL INDICATIONS ACCORDING TO THE TERRAIN:

1) FIRE — Slows down and reinforces the heart's contractions, treats tachycardia, extrasystoles, arrhythmias; promotes vasodilation of the coronaries and sequela of infarctus; stimulates the venous walls (varices, varicose ulcers), diminishes arterial tension; diuretic; treats arterial hypertension, can reverse arteriosclerosis; diminishes diarrhea from a repletion of heat in the Small Intestine, inhibits the sympathetic tonus.

2) WOOD — Disperses the channels of the Liver and Gallbladder, calms the sympathetic nervous system, calms all sympathotonic spasms; acts as a central nervous system sedative, treats vertigo, tinnitus, anguish, insomnia, nocturnal terror, enuresis and hot flushes of menopause.

The flowers and berries of hawthorn are well known for their use as a cardiac sedative. Hawthorn is mainly used as a coronary dilator, increasing oxygen supply to the heart in most organic and functional heart troubles. Both the flowers and the berries are astringent and are also useful in decoctions to cure sore throats. Its berries have a bitter cold and sour cold flavor.

Hawthorn makes excellent fuel, producing the hottest wood fire known. It was considered more desirable than oak for oven heating. Charcoal made from it is said to melt pig iron without the aid of a blast.

Altogether, hawthorn comprises a medication that is excellent for repletion of Fire of the Heart (antispasmodic), treating such Fire yang symptoms as anguish, insomnia, hot flushes, vertigo and tinnitus. It is hypotensive and a vasodilator for coronary arteries, strengthening and slowing down the heart. While it is prescribed for tachycardia, extrasystoles, arrhythmias, arteriosclerosis and arterial hypertension, it is also useful for diarrhea and dysentery from heat of the intestines.   It is prescribed for precordial pain or oppression, dyspnea, rapid and weak heart contractions, cardiac hypertrophy and endocarditis.

In East Asian medicine, the haws of *Crataegus pinnatifida* are used for blood stasis, menstrual pain and postpartum lower abdominal pain as well as for precordial pain. Hawthorne is prescribed for intestinal bleeding and lower abdominal distention. It is used to increase stomach acidity to help digest meat and fats, and to treat bacterial dysentery and chronic enteritis. Often, in combination with other herbs, it is given to infants for poor appetite and indigestion. It is contraindicated for stomach ulcers with gastric hyperacidity. Chinese research has shown that flavones extracted from hawthorn can alleviate myocardial ischemia.

Crataegus oxyacantha is listed in European pharmacopoeias as a prophylactic agent for heart diseases. As a vasodilator, it reduces peripheral resistance and decreases heart rate and blood pressure from exertion. Not for acute cardiac insufficiency (where digitalis or lily-of-the-valley would be the therapy of choice), it can be taken over time to improve the functional tone of the myocardium and prevent arteriosclerosis. Externally, the berries are useful in treating angina and internally they are also useful for urinary tract and bladder lithiases.

The flavonoids of hawthorn can reinforce the crosslinking of collagen that forms connective tissue, and can prevent the release of proinflammatory substances such as prostaglandins, leukotrienes and histamine and thus help to prevent tissue destruction in inflammatory diseases of the soft tissues. Hawthorn potentiates the action of barbiturates.

MEADOWSWEET *Spiraea ulmaria*

ACTIONS: Antispasmodic, diuretic, antirheumatic, cardiotonic and sudorific.

CONSTITUENTS: Spireine, salicylic aldehyde, salicylic acid, methyl salicylate, gaultherine, spiraeoside, a flavonoid glycoside, flavonins, quercetin, citric acid, fatty acids, vitamin C, calcium, magnesium, iron, tannin and a sugar.

FAMILY: Rosaceae.

FLAVORS: Bitter-cooling, salty-cooling.

FIVE PHASE CATEGORIES: Fire yang, Wood yang, Earth yang, Water yang.

PRINCIPAL INDICATIONS ACCORDING TO TERRAIN:

1) FIRE — Arterial hypertension, arteriosclerosis, blotchiness, measles.

2) EARTH — Digestive malabsorption, chronic and acute diarrhea, digestive mycosis, obesity, cellulitis, arthrosis, rheumatism, arteriosclerosis, coronaropathy.

3) WATER — Oliguria, edema, urinary calculi, renal insufficiency, hypertension, general infections, fever, fibrositis, generalized rheumatism.

4) WOOD — Biliary calculi, arthritis.

Meadowsweet is an herb that was held sacred by the Druids. It was once known as mead wort because it was a flavoring used in the honey wine called mead.

In phytotherapy, the flowers, leaves and root are used. Having antispasmodic, diuretic, sudorific, antirheumatic (containing methyl salicylate) and cardiotonic properties, meadowsweet is useful for hypertension and arteriosclerosis, as well as other signs of heat from the heart such as blotchiness and reddishness. Its can be used as a diaphoretic for colds with a high fever, as a diuretic for edema of the limbs and abdomen and for urinary tract infections. The word "aspirin" is derived from the Latin name *spiraea*.

Meadowsweet reduces gastric hyperacidity and strengthens the Spleen yang (tonus of the digestive tract). Rich in salicylates, which have a reputation for causing irritation and even bleeding in the upper gastrointestinal tract, the plant's capacity to soothe digestive complaints is a good argument for using plant extracts in preference to isolating "active principles."

MELILOT *Melilotus officinalis*

ACTIONS: Sympatholytic, sedative, anticoagulant.

CONSTITUENTS: The extraction process yields coumarin, which comes from a glycoside (melilotoside); in the fresh plant, glucosides, resin, flavonoids and vitamin C.

FAMILY: Papilionaceae.

FLAVORS: Sour-cooling, sweet-cooling.

PRINCIPAL INDICATIONS ACCORDING TO TERRAIN:

1) FIRE — Arterial hypertension, arteriosclerosis, nervousness, anguish, insomnia, hot flushes.

2) WATER — Hypertension, sympatholytic action similar to reserpine; diuretic, anticoagulant; has astringent properties for treating cystitis.

3) WOOD — Varices, phlebitis, hot flushes, conjunctivitis, blepharitis.

Melilot, or sweet clover, received its name from mel, which is honey, and lot, which is lotus. It was called the honey lotus because of its popularity with bees. The flowering plant contains melilotoside, which yields the well-known anticoagulant substance coumarin. The development of the anticoagulant warfarin occurred as a result of the observation that cattle eating hay made from melilot suffered hemorrhages. It was used by Galen in a plaster for his imperial and aristocratic patients when they suffered from inflammatory tumors or swollen joints. Even today in some parts of Europe, the plant is used as a plaster and as an old-fashioned country remedy for relief of abdominal pains.

Culpepper used it externally for inflammation of the eye, for cataracts and for epilepsy. Internally, it relieves flatulence and in modern herbal practices it is prescribed to drain a repletion of Fire (arterial hypertension, arteriosclerosis) and to treat psychic troubles (nervousness, anguish, insomnia). Other indications include colic in infants, blepharitis and conjunctivitis.

PASSIONFLOWER *Passiflora incarnata*

ACTIONS: Sympatholytic, hypnotic, tranquilizer.

CONSTITUENTS: Alkaloids passiflorine, harmine, harmol, flavonic derivatives.

FAMILY: Passiflorae.

FLAVORS: Bitter-cooling, sweet-cooling.

FIVE PHASE CATEGORIES: Fire yang, Wood yang, Water yang.

PRINCIPAL INDICATIONS ACCORDING TO TERRAIN:

1) FIRE — Insomnia, excitability, anxiety, hypertension.

2) WOOD — Irritability, anger, anxiety, insomnia.

3) WATER — Excitation, insomnia, hypertension.

The name passionflower derived from the physical appearance of the flowers, which to the Spanish conquistadores resembled a crown of thorns. Thus it was named for the Passion of Christ rather than for any aphrodisiac qualities. The aerial portion of the plant, including the flowers, is used.

Passionflower contains an alkaloid called passiflorine, which appears to be somewhat similar to morphine in its activity. Known to be a depressant to the motor nerves of the spinal cord, it also increases the rate of respiration. The alkaloid harmine is a mild hallucinogen and is found in numerous psychotropic plants including *Banisteriopsis caapi*. Harmine is a MAO inhibitor and was used by the Nazis as a so-called truth serum. In large amounts, it depresses the central nervous system (CNS), and has been used to treat encephalitis.

Passionflower is indicated for cases of psychic agitation from repletion of Liver Fire (insomnia, irritability, anger, anguish). A diuretic and an antispasmodic, it has been used with some success in treating menstrual cramps. It is effective for treating mild cases of infant convulsions.

VALERIAN *Valeriana officinalis*

ACTIONS: Antispasmodic, sympatholytic, parasympatholytic, sedative, anticonvulsant.

CONSTITUENTS: Essential oil (sesquiterpenes, valerenic acid, valerenal, valeranone), monoterpenes, iridoid esters (including valepotriates, valtrate, isovaltrate, didrovaltrate, homobaldrinal), alkaloids, carboxylic acids.

FAMILY: Valerianaceae.

Flavor: Sour-cooling, bitter-cooling.

FIVE PHASE CATEGORIES: Fire yang, Wood yang, Water yang.

PRINCIPAL INDICATIONS ACCORDING TO TERRAIN:

    1) FIRE — anxiety, insomnia, tachycardia, arrhythmias, hot flushes, convulsions, epilepsy.

    2) WOOD — hot flushes, spasms, convulsions, insomnia, asthma.

    3) WATER — bladder and urethral spasms, asthma, insomnia, hypertension.

The ancient Greeks prescribed Valerian as a diuretic. In the Chinese and Ayurvedic traditions it was known peripherally. In Germany valerian (baldrian) is frequently prescribed by physicians as a sedative, and in most parts of Europe it has been well established as an herbal sedative for over two centuries.

Its main clinical indications are for the treatment of nervous stress, especially accompanied by muscle spasms, restlessness and insomnia. It is also useful to some degree for intestinal, bronchial and menstrual cramps. Its utility extends even to caffeine-induced insomnia, and for relaxing tachycardia of nervous origin. Because of its mild diuretic properties, care must be taken when recommending its use at bedtime for some patients.

Valerian root clears a repletion of Fire from the organism, especially from the Liver system. It is useful for menopausal hot flushes, insomnia, sore throats and asthma in Fire yang and Fire yin constitutional types. For Wood, Fire and Water yang types it has been used for treatment of epilepsy. However, its modern use has been only for spasms of the bladder and urethra in Water yang and Fire yang types.

WHITE WILLOW (EUROPEAN WILLOW) *Salix alba*

ACTIONS: Antirheumatic, antipyretic, anaphrodisiac.

CONSTITUENTS: Glycosides salicine and salicortine, tannins, mineral salts.

FAMILY: Salicaceae.

FLAVOR: Bitter-cooling.

FIVE PHASE CATEGORIES: Fire yang, Wood yang, Water yang.

PRINCIPAL INDICATIONS ACCORDING TO TERRAIN:

1) FIRE — rheumatic pain, insomnia, anguish, agitation, epilepsy, calms sexual excitation; calms elevated fever.

2) WOOD — arthritic pain, rheumatism, gallstones, gastralgia, excessive sexual excitation.

The bark of the willow tree has been used as a febrifuge at least since the time of the ancient Greeks. Its reputation as an anaphrodisiac also dates back to antiquity. It has been used to treat excessive genital excitation, nocturnal emission and nymphomania. A large tree with rough greyish bark, white willow has been administered traditionally as a tonic and astringent for dyspepsia and debility of the digestive organs, in convalescence from acute diseases, for worms, for chronic diarrhea and for dysentery. It treats arthritis (one of the components in the bark metabolizes to salicylic acid), gallstones and all types of neuralgias, as well as stomach pain from hyper-acidity.

HERBS FOR FIRE YIN PATHOLOGIES

FIRE YIN PROFILES - QUICK REFERENCE

BRIAR HIP (DOG ROSE)	anxiety chest pain fatigue anemia
CHICKWEED	fatigue anemia bronchitis weak kidneys
CINCHONA	cardiac weakness arrhythmias anorexia
ELECAMPANE	anxiety libido stimulant appetite
MOTHERWORT	chest pain oxytocic dysmenorrhea vertigo
SIBERIAN GINSENG	pituitary strengthener stamina

BRIARHIP (DOG ROSE) *Rosa canina*

ACTIONS: Cardiotonic, salidiuretic, astringent.

CONSTITUENTS: Vitamin C, flavonoid pigments, carotene, tannins.

FAMILY: Rosaceae.

FLAVORS: Sweet-warming (leaves and flowers), sour-warming (rose-hips).

FIVE PHASE CATEGORIES: Fire yin, Water yin.

PRINCIPAL INDICATIONS ACCORDING TO TERRAIN:

1) FIRE — angina pectoris, asthenia, anemia, profound anxiety, constipation, to stimulate the cerebrospinal tonus.

2) WATER — oliguria, renal calculi, constipation, asthenia, leukorrhea, chronic diarrhea, anemia, angina.

The leaves and flowers of the dog rose are sweet and warm and the fruits are sour and warm. The leaves have a tonic effect that is useful for fatigue and for viral maladies.

A toxic dose, the effect of a glucoside in the seeds, is comparable to a dose of digitalis and provokes the central nervous system to torpor, vertigo and headaches. The leaves and flowers in a sufficient dose have a therapeutic effect on anguish with sensations of emptiness in the chest, corresponding to a vacuity of Heart yang. Its mild diuretic effect is useful in treatment of lithiases (particularly phosphate and oxalic) plus its mild laxative action, which can be remarkable in treating constipation and oliguria in a Water yin constitution. Briarhip also has anti-inflammatory and astringent properties that can be used in treating angina.

This plant is the source of rose hips, which are well known for their wealth of vitamin C. Its astringent properties are useful for leukorrhea and diarrhea due to vacuity and cold, observed in Crohn's disease and phospho-oxalic lithiases.

CHICKWEED *Stellaria media*

ACTIONS: General tonic, cardiotonic.

CONSTITUENTS: Saponins, mineral salts; rich in iron, silica and potassium.

FAMILY: Caryophyllae.

FLAVOR: Sweet-cooling, salty-warming.

FIVE PHASE CATEGORIES: Fire yin, Water yin, Metal yin.

PRINCIPAL INDICATIONS ACCORDING TO TERRAIN:

1) **FIRE** — asthenia, hypotension, palpitations, anemia; excellent tonic for convalescents.

2) **WATER** — edema, glomerulonephritis, nephrotic syndromes, asystole, cardiac weakness, acute articular rheumatism, scarlatina, anemia.

3) **METAL** — bronchitis, pleurisy, coughs, colds, atonic bowel; to strengthen the lungs and bronchial tubes; used externally for skin conditions, especially burns, hemorrhoids and ulcers.

Chickweed is useful for treating palpitations, hypotension, asthenia and anemia. An excellent tonic for convalescent patients, it is a cholesterol cleanser that can be used long term to clear out cellulite, to treat obesity and for lipomas and other tumors. Some Native American tribes used it for colds and bronchial infections. In Japan, the juice of the chickweed plant is a folk remedy for gastric ulcer. Its main application in modern phytotherapy is as a cardiac tonic for arrhythmias and for depression.

CINCHONA (PERUVIAN BARK) *Cinchona succirubra*

ACTIONS: Febrifuge, antimalarial, bitter tonic, antispasmodic, astringent.

CONSTITUENTS: Quinine, hydroquinine, quinamine, cinchonine, cinchonidine, homocinchonidine, quinic acid, cincholannic acid, calcium oxalate, glucosides and starch.

FAMILY: Rubiaceae.

FLAVOR: Bitter-warming.

FIVE PHASE CATEGORIES: Fire yin, Earth yin, Water yin.

PRINCIPAL INDICATIONS ACCORDING TO TERRAIN:

1) FIRE — cardiac weakness, arrhythmia, delayed menses and delayed childbirth.

2) EARTH — anorexia, influenza, infections, malaria, diabetes.

3) WATER — delayed menstruation, diabetic emaciation.

Containing numerous alkaloids, the most famous of which is quinine (used as a treatment for malaria), cinchona has been used traditionally as a febrifuge, tonic and astringent, valuable for influenza, neuralgia and debility. The wood extract is used to cure drunkenness, and the powdered bark has been used in tooth powders because of its astringent properties. A toxic dose can be abortifacient. A small dose can be an effective appetite stimulant. It can be rapidly effective for relaxing leg spasms, especially nocturnal calf spasms. Cinchona is also used in the production of pastries, soft drinks, candy and ice cream.

In modern practice it is used mostly as a febrifuge for various infections and for influenza, anorexia, diabetic emaciation and cardiac arrhythmia.

ELECAMPANE *Inula helenium*

ACTIONS: Sympathomimetic, vagolytic, expectorant, alterative, choleretic, diuretic, pituitary stimulant.

CONSTITUENTS: Essential oil containing sesquiterpene lactones including alantolactone, very rich in inulin (up to 45%).

FAMILY: Compositae.

FLAVORS: Bitter-warming, pungent-warming.

FIVE PHASE CATEGORIES: Fire yin, Wood yin, Earth yin, Water yin, Metal yin.

PRINCIPAL INDICATIONS ACCORDING TO TERRAIN:

1) FIRE — hypotension, lipothymia, syncope from vagotonia; to stimulate the pituitary glands, testicular activity, FSH and LH-like activity.

2) WOOD — choleretic, immune stimulating; hepatomegaly, herpes; insufficient bile secretion.

3) EARTH — splenomegaly, gastroptosis, gastric atony, chronic diarrhea, hypothyroidism, insufficient hypophysial function, amenorrhea, impotence, frigidity.

4) WATER — oliguria, edema, glomerulonephritis, acute and chronic arterial hypertension.

5) METAL — bronchorrhea, pertussis, abundant expectoration, asthma, emphysema, tuberculosis, immunoallergic pneumopathies, sarcoidoses, anemia, leukorrhea, insufficient menses, amenorrhea, dermatoses, chronic diarrhea.

According to legend, elecampane first arose from the tears of Helen of Troy, as she was said to be carrying a sprig of elecampane when she was abducted by Paris; hence the name *Inula helenium*. Elecampane was considered one of the great medications by many of the great ancient doctors – Theophrastus, Dioscorides, Pliny, Albert the Great. Culpepper recommended elecampane for worms, gum problems and tooth decay.

Elecampane root has been used chiefly for coughs, consumption and pulmonary complaints, especially inflammatory conditions, because of its antibacterial properties. However, it is frequently used to clear phlegm from the digestive tract, to clear exudative skin disorders and as a constitutional treatment for strengthening and cleansing the mucosa of both the respiratory and gastrointestinal tracts.

In China, the species *Inula britannica* is used primarily for clearing phlegm and treating chronic coughs, nausea and vomiting. It is useful in hypotension and vagotonic syncope due to vagotonic reactions from sympathetic insufficiency. Elecampane stimulates the pituitary gland, which is associated with Fire. Its bitter-warm nature directly stimulates the Heart. In short, elecampane is an excellent plant for blood circulation, glandular insufficiency, and for deficient immunity. It is also useful for kidney symptoms including oliguria, edema and hypertension from renal insufficiency.

MOTHERWORT *Leonurus cardiaca*

ACTIONS: Cardiotonic, oxytocic, antispasmodic.

CONSTITUENTS: Alkaloids (leonurine A, leonurine B, stachydrine and betonicine), lauric acid, oleic acid, glucosides, flavonoids, resin and tannin.

FAMILY: Labiatae.

FLAVORS: Sour-warming, bitter-warming.

FIVE PHASE CATEGORY: Fire yin.

PRINCIPAL INDICATIONS ACCORDING TO TERRAIN:

1) FIRE — precordial pain, palpitations, cardiopathy, amenorrhea; oxytocin stimulating.

The flowers and leaves of motherwort are used traditionally in the West as a diaphoretic and antispasmodic, a tonic and an emmenagogue. It was considered especially valuable for weaknesses and disorders unique to women, having a calming effect on the nervous system. Ancients revered it for strengthening and gladdening the heart, so it was often used for hysterical complaints, for hysterical heart palpitations and fainting. Culpepper wrote of motherwort: "Venus owns this herb and it is under Leo. There is no better herb to drive melancholy vapors from the heart, to strengthen it and make the mind cheerful, blithe and merry."

In Russia it is known as a "heart herb," and is prescribed for heart conditions, amenorrhea, dysmenorrhea, insomnia, cardiac neurosis, goiter and epilepsy. Today in Europe, it is used as a cardiotonic and oxytocic, and for calming precordial pains with palpitations.

Motherwort is also a mild diuretic. It is used as an herb to excite the uterus, to promote uterine tonicity, and to stimulate the production of oxytocin. Its clinical uses include contracting and clearing the uterus after childbirth, relieving menstrual pain, improving circulation in the lower abdomen in the treatment of pelvic inflammatory disease, relieving edema due to nephritis, clearing blood and protein in the urine and treating blood in the urine from renal calculi. It is being used experimentally in China as a morning-after contraceptive. Other investigations in China have found that it decreases blood viscosity when injected and reduces the platelet aggregation rate.

Leonurus extract is used to relieve headaches, insomnia, vertigo and peripheral circulatory paresthesias. It can be used in place of valerian for calming the nervous system. In clinical trials it gave impressive results for treatment of numbness in the limbs, insomnia, headache and vertigo when used for blood stasis pathology.

SIBERIAN GINSENG *Eleutherococcus senticosus*

ACTIONS: Adaptogen, hypoglycemiant, endocrine regulator, CNS stimulant, gonadotropin stimulant, TSH stimulant.

CONSTITUENTS: Eleutherosides A, B, C, D, E, F, G, I, K, L and M (sterols, coumarins, saponins, triterpenes, among others); b-sitosterol, vitamin E, b-carotene, caffeic acid, oleanolic acid, essential oil, various sugars, copper.

FAMILY: Araliaceae.

FLAVORS: Bitter-warming, sweet-warming.

FIVE PHASE CATEGORIES: Fire yin, Wood yin, Earth yin, Metal yin, Water yin.

PRINCIPAL INDICATIONS ACCORDING TO TERRAIN:

1) FIRE — memory loss, hypovigilance, hypertension, decreased libido, altitude sickness, anemia, hypopituitarism.

2) WOOD — hypercholesterolemia, influenza, viral fatigue syndrome, thyroid hypertrophy.

3) EARTH — hyperglycemia, diabetes mellitus, leukocytosis, leukopenia, anemia.

4) METAL — chronic bronchitis, cough with sputum, altitude sickness, leukocytosis, leukopenia, thymus atrophy.

5) WATER — diseases caused by cold, fatigue, hypoadrenalism, tumors, low sperm count, decreased libido.

Siberian ginseng is most widely used in the former Soviet Union, where it is native to the steppes of Siberia. It has undergone clinical studies in Russia for over 25 years and was researched in large scale clinical trials of both healthy and sick subjects. It has been taken by Soviet deep sea divers, mine and mountain rescuers, climbers, explorers, soldiers and factory workers to resist stress while working hard under inhospitable conditions. Truck drivers and pilots take it to keep alert and to counteract the potentially dangerous side-effects of medications. Soviet cosmonauts have also taken it in space. Athletes take it to enhance their performance.

Eleutherococcus is listed in China's oldest pharmacopoeia, the Shen Nung herbal pharmacopoeia, and in the medicinal herb pharmacopoeia of the scholar Li Shih-Zhen of the Ming dynasty. It was prescribed to restore appetite, virility and vitality, strengthen the lungs, improve memory, concentration and muscle tone.

Siberian ginseng is classified as an adaptogen, meaning an herb that strengthens the body's adaptive capabilities (similar to alteratives). By its action on the hormone system and the central nervous system it can effectively counteract fatigue. Adaptogens are useful for people today who suffer the effects of stress and pollution.

The heterosides of eleutherococcus are antioxidant, inactivating free radicals and accelerating the mobilization of lipids and thus protective in radiation exposure. Eleutherococcus extracts have been shown to inhibit carcinogenesis in some cases, reduce hepatic cholesterol synthesis, normalize adrenal function, normalize production of both white and red blood cells, reduce serum cholesterol and prothrombin levels and reduce blood pressure and high blood sugar levels. It appears to have antiviral properties, particularly with the influenza virus. It stimulates the central nervous system, stimulates gonadotropic activity of the prostate and seminal vesicles, prevents diseases caused by cold and improves cerebral vascular activity. Due to the latter trait, it has been used to improve vision, color perception and hearing.

Clinically, it has been used as an expectorant and anti-inflammatory for chronic bronchitis, to speed up convalescence, to improve memory, concentration and stamina, to treat viral fatigue syndrome and influenza and to treat diabetes, hypertension, ischemic heart disease and male infertility.

HERBS FOR EARTH YANG PATHOLOGIES

EARTH YANG PROFILES - QUICK REFERENCE

AGRIMONY	obesity
	diabetes
	diarrhea
	stomatitis
BILBERRY	eye problems
	diabetes
	colitis
BURDOCK	diabetes
	lymphadenopathy
	skin problems
FUMITORY	obesity
	constipation
	HBP
	excitability
LIME TREE (TILIA)	anxiety
	fever
	stomach pain
WOODY NIGHTSHADE	skin disease
	rheumatism
	chronic bronchitis

AGRIMONY *Agrimonia eupatoria*

ACTIONS: Hypoglycemiant, astringent, diuretic, anti-inflammatory, cytophylactic.

CONSTITUENTS: Agrimonin A, agrimonin B, essential oil, vitamin K, tannin, nicotinamide, silicic acid, vitamin B complex, iron, bitter principle.

FAMILY: Rosaceae.

FLAVOR: Sour-cooling.

FIVE PHASE CATEGORIES: Earth yang, Metal yang.

PRINCIPAL INDICATIONS ACCORDING TO TERRAIN:

1) EARTH — obesity, diabetes, diarrhea, intestinal mycosis, asthma, gout, headaches, cataracts, tonsillitis, stomatitis, pharyngitis, aphthous ulcers, infected wounds, contusions, neuritis, cholecystitis with hyperacidity.

2) METAL — asthma, acute bronchopneumopathies with abundant expectoration, hemoptysis, diabetes, headaches, tonsillitis, dysentery, hoarseness, colds with fever, diarrhea, atonic bowel.

One of the most famous vulnerary herbs, agrimony enjoys a reputation as a cure for jaundice and other liver complaints. The Anglo-Saxons applied it to heal wounds, snake bites and warts. In the time of Chaucer, it was used with mugwort and vinegar in a mixture of pounded frogs and human blood as a remedy for internal hemorrhage. It is commonly used as a hemostatic, a cardiotonic, an antibacterial (gram-positive) and an anthelminthic (especially tapeworm).

Clinically, it is used as a hemostatic for nosebleeds, for hemoptysis, bloody stool, hematuria and uterine bleeding. The sour-cooling flavor calms heat of the Spleen and essentially treats diabetes, obesity and diarrhea from damp-heat excess of the Spleen. It is useful for treating asthma of the hot, moist type, mycotic infections and gout from the same origin (moisture and heat in the Spleen), in overweight Earth yang patients. It also has been used in the treatment of cataracts, tonsillitis, stomatitis and pharyngitis. Externally, it can be used for aphthous ulcers, infected wounds and contusions.

BILBERRY *Vaccinium myrtillus*

ACTIONS: Hypoglycemiant, antidiarrheic, hemostatic, antiseptic, circulatory stimulant.

CONSTITUENTS: Anthocyanosides, vitamin C and A, arbutin, myrtillin, tannin, citric and malic acids and the trace elements copper, magnesium, manganese, zinc, gold and silver (fruit); hypoglycemiant factor glucoquinine (leaves).

FAMILY: Ericaceae.

FLAVORS: Sour-cooling, sweet-cooling, salty-cooling.

FIVE PHASE CATEGORIES: Earth yang, Water yang.

PRINCIPAL INDICATIONS ACCORDING TO TERRAIN:

1) EARTH — colitis, *E. coli* bacillus, varices, hemorrhoids, dysmenorrhea, arteriopathy in the lower limbs, diabetic retinopathy, cataracts, diabetes; hypoglycemic action.

2) WATER — oliguria, uricemia, urinary colibacillus, arthritis, retinopathy, cataracts, glaucoma, macular degeneration.

Bilberry has been used in Russia for centuries as an astringent for gastritis and colitis. It is especially useful for soothing colitis, particularly after antibiotic therapy, and is considered to be one of the strongest agents against colibacillus. It can protect against gastric ulcers by reducing hyperacidity, by reducing transport time from the stomach to the duodenum, and by increasing gastric mucus secretion.

The fruits, traditionally used in the form of a syrup, have astringent properties, and are especially valuable in diarrhea and dysentery. The berries also are astringent; the leaves are a hypoglycemiant and have been used in the treatment of diabetes and as a diuretic. Bilberry treats the symptoms of Spleen repletion – arteriopathy, varices, hemorrhoids. It decreases capillary permeability and fragility, and is also used to treat thrombophlebitis and other forms of venous insufficiency, such as varicose veins. It has an activity similar to ginkgo in improving intracranial circulation.

In ophthalmology, bilberry is used for fragility of capillaries and ocular hemorrhages. The first reports of its effect on eyesight were during World War II when British RAF pilots reported dramatic improvements in night vision after ingesting bilberry jam. French researchers followed up on these reports, performing clinical trials. Their research concluded that bilberry acts by building up the retinal pigment, and is thus a useful agent for several types of eye disorders. It is often combined with vitamin E in the treatment of myopia, and improves both nighttime visual acuity as well as day blindness (hemeralopia). It has proven effective for retinitis pigmentosa, glaucoma, cataracts, diabetic retinopathy and macular degeneration.

Bilberry also shows promise as a treatment for joint inflammation because of its ability to decrease uric acid levels and its ability to prevent collagen destruction.

BURDOCK *Arctium lappa*

ACTIONS: Hypoglycemiant, antibiotic, diuretic, antifungal.

CONSTITUENTS: Essential oil (root), large quantities of inulin (up to 45 percent), iron, vitamin K, niacin, tannins; seeds contain a glycoside (arctiine).

FAMILY: Compositae.

FLAVORS: Sweet-cooling (root), bitter-cooling (leaves), sour-cooling (seeds).

FIVE PHASE CATEGORIES: Earth yang, Metal yang.

PRINCIPAL INDICATIONS ACCORDING TO TERRAIN:

1) EARTH — diabetes (stimulates insulin production), obesity, rheumatism, furuncles, staphylococcal infections of diabetes, buccal abscesses, dental abscesses, suppurative eczema, hyperuricemia, constipation, chronic swollen lymph nodes and glands.

2) METAL — important herb for drainage for all kinds of skin afflictions, infectious acne, complications of measles, swollen lymph nodes.

3) WOOD — choleretic and diuretic action comparable to artichoke, Wood terrain urinary tract infections.

One of the best blood purifiers, burdock has been used traditionally as an alterative, diuretic and diaphoretic. It is effective for skin diseases also and is often effective for eczema. Usually the root is employed, being traditionally harvested in the fall from two-year-old plants. The leaves and the seeds are also valuable. An infusion of the leaves imparts strength and tone to the stomach and is good for some forms of long-standing indigestion. Burdock seeds are considered by many to be a specific for all afflictions of the kidneys. In Chinese medicine, the seeds are used as a diuretic and antiphlogistic, as well as an antibacterial.

Clinically, the seeds are used in acute colds and influenza, for swelling in the throat, for infectious parotitis with constipation, for eczema, cough and suppurative types of inflammation. Experimentally, a water-soluble extract of burdock seed has proven to have a powerful effect in contracting the uterus.

Burdock is used to treat diabetes, obesity and rheumatism. The root is used in China for its antimicrobial properties. It is useful for treating acne, furunculoses, diabetic infections, buccal abscesses, dental abscesses, dermatoses and suppurative eczema, and for treating cutaneous staphylococcus infections and dermatoses in a hypopancreatic vagal insufficient terrain.

FUMITORY *Fumaria officinalis*

ACTIONS: Hypocholesterolemic, choleretic, cholagogue, stomachic.

CONSTITUENTS: Fumaric acid, fumaric acid salts, potassium, alkaloids (including fumarine, cryptocavine, cryptopine, corydaline, aurotensine, stylopine, sinactine, bulbocapnine), phlobaphene, yellow pigment, resinous substances, mucilage, bitter principle.

FAMILY: Fumariaceae.

FLAVORS: Salty-cooling, sour-cooling, salty-warming, bitter-warming.

FIVE PHASE CATEGORIES: Earth yang, Earth yin, Wood yang.

PRINCIPAL INDICATIONS ACCORDING TO TERRAIN:

1) EARTH — obesity, constipation, hypertension, gastritis, peptic ulcer, psychic excitability, insomnia, exanthematous skin lesions.

2) WOOD — biliary dyskinesia, icterus with retention, cholangitis, excess cholesterol and lipids, excess uric acid, hypertension.

3) FIRE — anti-inflammatory, antiserotonin, antiarrhythmia.

Fumitory is a depurative, laxative, bitter tonic, cholagogue and diuretic for Wood yang and Earth yang terrains. Of complex flavor, it is spicy-warm with ambiguous flavors of salty-cooling and sour-cooling fumaric acid, with a bitter warming property. When used in therapy, it efficiently drains the duodenal-pancreatic junction and is useful for icterus with retention; for cholangitis, biliary dyskinesia and hypertension, obesity; and for conditions of high blood fat such as hyperlipidemia, hypercholesterolemia, uricemia, exanthematous skin lesions and arthritis. As powerful as it is for drainage of the gallbladder, it also promotes secretion of bile when there is bile insufficiency. Fumitory is useful for states of psychic excitation and insomnia from repletion heat in the Spleen, characterized by obsessive thought, nausea, vomiting and diarrhea.

LIME TREE *Tilia europoea*

ACTIONS: CNS sedative, tranquilizer, antispasmodic, choleretic, emollient, sympatholytic, parasympathomimetic.

CONSTITUENTS: Essential oil with farnesol, mucilage, tannins, quercitroside, flavonic glycosides.

FAMILY: Tiliaceae.

FLAVOR: Sweet-cooling.

FIVE PHASE CATEGORIES: Earth yang, Fire yang, Wood yang.

PRINCIPAL INDICATIONS ACCORDING TO TERRAIN:

1) EARTH — dyspepsia, albuminuria, high cholesterol, arteriosclerosis; febrifuge; aids in the elimination of urea and uric acid; sympatholytic and parasympathomimetic.

2) FIRE — arteriosclerosis, insomnia, anxiety, depression, palpitations, anguish; febrifuge; aids in the elimination of urea, cholesterol and uric acid; sympatholytic and parasympathomimetic.

3) WOOD — biliary dyskinesia, hepatitis, gastralgia, nervousness, anguish, insomnia, vertigo, migraines; sympatholytic and parasympathomimetic.

Much used in Europe, stalks of dried lime flowers are kept in most French households for making *tilleul* tea. The honey from these flowers is highly prized in France for its flavor. The lime flowers are used only in infusion or in a water distillation as a household remedy for indigestion, nervous vomiting or heart palpitations. Prolonged baths prepared with the infused flowers are said to be good for hysteria.

Lime tree is used extensively in medicine and in liqueurs, enjoying a reputation for treating dyspepsia, for purifying the blood (urea, uric acid, cholesterol) and for treating arteriosclerosis. It is a central nervous system sedative, a tranquilizer and an emollient for the digestive tract. As a febrifuge it is especially good for cooling the entire system in cases of excessive heat as well as acute febrile conditions. The flowers and leaves are used to treat disorders of Earth yang, Wood yang and Fire yang. By draining the Fire of the Heart, it is useful for treating insomnia, anxiety, anguish, neurosis, hysteria, epilepsy, vertigo, migraines and apoplexy.

WOODY NIGHTSHADE *Solanum dulcamara*

ACTIONS: Depurative, diaphoretic, antirheumatismal, anti-infectious, vagolytic.

CONSTITUENTS: Alkaloid solanine, glucoside dulcamarine, resins, gum, starch, sugars.

FAMILY: Solanaceae.

FLAVORS: Bitter-cooling, sweet-cooling, pungent-warming.

FIVE PHASE CATEGORIES: Earth yang, Metal yang, Earth yin, Metal yin, Wood yin.

PRINCIPAL INDICATIONS ACCORDING TO TERRAIN:

    1) EARTH — rheumatism, weakened immunity, digestive mycoses, skin diseases from damp-heat.

    2) METAL — chronic bronchitis, pulmonary mycoses.

    3) WOOD — cervical lymphadenopathy, hepatosplenomegaly, herpes.

Woody nightshade is used to strengthen immunity and relieve congestion related to vacuity and coldness in cases such as tubercular cervical lymphadenopathy, hepatosplenomegaly and nightsweats. A febrifuge, it is used to induce a sweat in an acute febrile patient, but it can also stop nightsweats. It is also used for congestive skin problems due to damp-heat affecting the Spleen: psoriasis, eczema, furuncles and acne in the Earth yang constitution. It may be administered for treatment of herpes, including herpes progenitalia.

Woody nightshade is vagolytic and useful for drying secretions in acute and chronic bronchitis, and in pulmonary and digestive mycoses in the Earth yang and Metal yang constitutions. By opening up the venous circulation, it is effective for treating rheumatism in both yang and yin constitutional types.

Herbs for Earth Yin Pathologies

Earth Yin Profiles - Quick Reference

CHAMOMILE	anorexia dyspepsia
CENTAURY	dyspepsia flatulence parasites
FENNEL	stomachic flatulence colic
FOENUGREEK	fatigue lymphadenitis emaciation
GENTIAN	gastric ulcers chronic diarrhea anorexia
GERMANDER	damp disorders bronchitis gastritis
LICORICE	ulcers glandular weakness
MARIGOLD	oxytocic gastritis dysmenorrhea
OAK	diarrhea hemorrhage bronchitis
PROPOLIS	anti-inflammatory analgesic

CHAMOMILE *Anthemis nobilis*

ACTIONS: Eupeptic, carminative, bitter tonic, anti-inflammatory, sympatholytic, vagolytic.

CONSTITUENTS: Essential oil, esters of angelic acid, coumarin and flavonic heterosides, a glycoside (anthemisol), anthemic acid, glucosides, choline, inositol, fatty acids, sulphur, phosphorus, calcium and iron.

FAMILY: Compositae.

FLAVOR: Bitter-warming.

FIVE PHASE CATEGORY: Earth yin.

PRINCIPAL INDICATIONS ACCORDING TO TERRAIN:

1) EARTH — anorexia, dyspepsia, enteritis, digestive parasites (anthelminthic), anemia (insufficiency of erythrocytes), leukopenia, menstrual insufficiency and amenorrhea due to ovarian insufficiency, neuritis, facial neuritis, febrifuge; supplements the blood; calms the sympathetic and parasympathetic nervous systems.

2) WOOD — colic and biliousness in children, pediatric nervousness, insomnia, jaundice, headaches.

One of the most popular garden herbs, chamomile's reputation as a medicinal plant goes back to the Egyptians. Traditionally used as a tonic, stomachic, emmenagogue, anodyne and antispasmodic, it has also been used for nervous afflictions. It has a soothing sedative effect on the stomach and nervous system, and has been used for teething pain in children. In strong doses, however, it can be used as an emetic. It exerts an anesthetic effect on sensitive nerves comparable to colchicine, hence its use for neuritis and facial neuralgia. It is also traditionally said to be a preventive for nightmares. In Russia it is used for colds, stomach discomfort, colitis, eczema and as a sedative. In India it is used for pediatric stomach problems, as a sedative, for earaches, neuralgia, convulsions and tooth pain. The oil can also be used externally for rheumatic joint pain. (See Essential Oils Profiles.)

CENTAURY *Erythraea centaurium*

ACTIONS: Parasympathomimetic, carminative, anthelminthic (especially tapeworm), choleretic, febrifuge, aperitif, cicatrisant.

CONSTITUENTS: Bitter principles (including gentiopicrine) and a lactone (erythrocentaurin), minerals (6 percent), resin, alkaloids gentianine and erythricine.

FAMILY: Gentianaceae.

FLAVOR: Bitter-warming.

FIVE PHASE CATEGORIES: Earth yin, Metal yin, Wood yin.

PRINCIPAL INDICATIONS ACCORDING TO TERRAIN:

1) EARTH — anorexia, poor lymphatic circulation, dyspepsia, flatulence, swollen intestines, intestinal parasites, oozing eczema, gout; to stimulate the organism's defenses; to stimulate the exocrine secretions of the pancreas.

2) METAL — fatigue, lymphatic stagnation and congestion, eczema.

3) WOOD — stimulates bile secretion, hepatic congestion, fatty liver due to immune deficiency (hepatosplenomegaly), eczema.

The name centaury is derived from the legend of the Centaur Chiron, who used it for salving the wounds of Hercules. The stems and flowers of centaury are traditionally used as a stomachic and tonic. The "little gentian" has been popular since antiquity as a febrifuge. In Russia it has been used as an antipyretic, for high blood pressure, for liver and gallbladder problems and rheumatic joint pains. It is excellent for building up the immune system defenses, and along with St. John's wort and essential oil of pine, it could be useful for treating AIDS.

Acting on the liver and kidneys, it purifies the blood and kills worms, and is used for dyspepsia, for sluggish digestion, and for heartburn after eating. As a cicatrisant it is stimulating to the flesh (Spleen system); it supplements the yang of the Spleen to treat anorexia, asthenia and dyspepsia with flatulence. It is also used for treating the dampness of gout. A choleretic and stimulant of pancreatic secretions, it is used in cases of hepatosplenomegaly and eczema from dampness afflicting the Spleen, or from problems caused by parasites.

FENNEL *Foeniculum vulgare*

ACTIONS: Carminative, eupeptic, expectorant, antispasmodic, galactagogue, diuretic (azoturic), urinary antiseptic.

CONSTITUENTS: Vitamin A, B, C, mineral salts, a fatty oil, methylchavicol, foeniculine; the essential oil contains anethole, fenchone, estragole, a-pinene, limonene, anisaldehyde.

FAMILY: Compositae.

FLAVOR: Sweet-warming.

FIVE PHASE CATEGORIES: Earth yin, Water yin, Metal yin.

PRINCIPAL INDICATIONS ACCORDING TO TERRAIN

1) EARTH — digestive insufficiency, colic and pediatric abdominal pains.

2) METAL — intestinal colic, colitis, galactagogue.

3) WATER — oliguria, renal calculi, amenorrhea, frigidity, impotence, urinary infections.

Fennel leaf has primarily been used as a carminative. It has been called gripe water because of its traditional use to clear flatulence, particularly flatulence in infants. In India, it is used in after-dinner teas and condiments. The root is made into a tea for colds. In Arabic traditional medicine, it has been used for stomach and liver pains, for scrofula and to strengthen the eyesight. In classical Chinese medicine it is used primarily as a digestive aid and to harmonize the functions of the stomach and intestines. It reduces bloating and flatulence due to peristaltic insufficiency and acts as an antispasmodic, particularly for the smooth muscle of the stomach and intestines. It is also useful for supplementing the Kidney yang and dispersing coldness, relieving such symptoms as renal calculi and oliguria.

Fennel has a very smooth sweetness with a carminative and stomachic action. It is prescribed clinically for digestive insufficiency and for intestinal colic, and is also used for amenorrhea, frigidity and impotence. Its pediatric use has traditionally been as an expectorant in bronchitis and asthma as well as for colic. It should be used with laxatives for constipation in young or old patients with poor intestinal tonus. As a sedative and carminative, it is useful in treating excitable children who suffer from indigestion.

The essential oil has the same properties as the whole plant and is used to treat flatulence, intestinal spasms, anorexia nervosa and to stimulate lactation in nursing mothers.

FOENUGREEK *Trigonella foenum-graecum*

ACTIONS: Hypoglycemiant, adrenal cortex stimulant, digestive tonic.

CONSTITUENTS: Trigonelline (a derivative of nicotinic acid), choline; extremely rich in folic acid, vitamin B1; mucilage (30 percent), galactose, mannose, a steroidal saponin and a small amount of fatty oils, lecithin, magnesium, calcium, phosphorus and proteins; rich in fiber.

FAMILY: Leguminae.

FLAVOR: Bitter-warming.

FIVE PHASE CATEGORIES: Earth yin, Metal yin.

PRINCIPAL INDICATIONS ACCORDING TO TERRAIN:

1) EARTH — digestive aid, hypoglycemiant; to treat emaciation.

2) METAL — neuromuscular stimulation, emaciation, diabetic emaciation, poor nutrition, anemia, frigidity, impotence.

3) WATER — impotence, frigidity, lumbago, dysmenorrhea.

Foenugreek seeds, used medicinally for centuries, were held in high repute among the Egyptians, Greeks and Romans for medicinal and culinary purposes. In Egypt, the seeds were soaked in water until they swelled into a thick paste. For centuries, opera singers have used foenugreek for clearing excessive phlegm and mucus from the throat.

Foenugreek is said to be equal to quinine in preventing fevers. It is also effective for soothing the stomach and has been utilized for diabetes. It is indicated externally for cellulitis. A neuromuscular stimulant, it is especially recommended for emaciated types, for diabetic emaciation, for poor nutrition, anemia, frigidity and impotence. It assists weight gain by improving digestive absorption, clearing out mucus and intestinal plaque. It is a lymphatic detergent as well. Laboratory tests with rats have shown a decreased need for insulin when foenugreek seed extract is ingested, as it apparently inhibits transfer of glucose into the blood from the upper digestive tract.

In East Asian medicine it is classified as an herb to fortify the Kidney yang. It clears coldness and dampness, especially in the lower abdomen and reproductive system. It is used for leg heaviness and pains with muscle spasms, kidney pain, floating kidney and dysmenorrhea from coldness in the lower abdomen. In men, it treats impotence, chronic prostatitis and chronic lumbar pain.

GENTIAN *Gentiana lutea*

ACTIONS: Bitter tonic, aperitif, choleretic, astringent, febrifuge, sudorific, vagolytic, luteotropic.

CONSTITUENTS: Bitter glucosides gentiin, gentiamarin, gentiopicrin; gentianic acid, dextrose, levulose, sucrose, gentianose, gentiotriose.

FAMILY: Gentianaceae.

FLAVORS: Bitter-warming.

FIVE PHASE CATEGORIES: Earth yin, Metal yin.

PRINCIPAL INDICATIONS ACCORDING TO TERRAIN:

1) EARTH — gastric ulcers, anorexia, weight loss, fatigue, anemia, spleen congestion and swelling, malaria, amenorrhea, luteal insufficiency; dries dampness.

2) METAL — Chronic respiratory afflictions, chronic bronchitis, chronic diarrhea, Crohn's disease, malabsorption syndrome, colitis, vermifuge.

Gentian is vagolytic and luteotropic. Its leukocytogenic properties make it valuable in treating postinfectious asthenia, and for building strength and immunity in the chronically ill. Gentian is effective for anorexia, weakness, emaciation, anemia and depression.

It is useful as a febrifuge and gentle enough for pediatric use. Because of its antispasmodic (neurotropic) properties, it is helpful for pain relief, and is administered as a supplemental agent for the treatment of rheumatic pain with inflammation. It is the bitter agent in a variety of commercial aperitifs and digestive bitters.

GERMANDER *Teucrium chamaedrys*

ACTIONS: Antispasmodic, antidiabetic, antirheumatic, diaphoretic, diuretic.

CONSTITUENTS: Tannins, bitter principles and an essential oil.

FAMILY: Labiatae.

FLAVOR: Bitter-warming.

FIVE PHASE CATEGORIES: Earth yin, Metal yin, Wood yin.

PRINCIPAL INDICATIONS ACCORDING TO TERRAIN:

1) EARTH — asthenia, appetite disorders, influenza, infectious diseases, immune deficiency, hepatosplenomegaly.

2) METAL — asthenia, chronic bronchitis, bronchorrhea, chronic rheumatism.

3) WOOD — hepatosplenomegaly, sequelae of severe liver damage, insufficiency of hepatic cells.

Germander's reputation as a specific for gout goes back centuries; indeed, it was once cultivated for medicinal purposes. A slight aperiant as well as a tonic, germander is warm and bitter in flavor, and is indicated in cases of cold vacuity of the Spleen and for hepatosplenomegaly due to dampness. Excellent for drying out a damp terrain, it is especially good for drying out glairy mucus (the yin of the Spleen) that occurs in bronchorrhea and chronic bronchitis.

Germander is a fairly strong diaphoretic and is used for treating asthenia, anorexia, influenza and infectious diseases. In Arab countries it is prescribed to treat upper gastrointestinal problems such as ulcers. Germander extract has been shown to have a strong antiulcer activity in rats. In addition to strengthening a weak digestive tract, it is especially useful for aerophagia.

Recently in Europe it has been used as an aid in weight loss because of its ability to suppress appetite without hyperadrenal side effects or toxicity. The highest activity was exhibited in the water soluble extract.

LICORICE *Glycyrrhiza glabra*

ACTIONS: Anti-inflammatory, antiallergenic, immune strengthener, adrenal cortex stimulant, estrogenic, luteotropic, antispasmodic, antiulcerative, vagolytic, febrifuge, antitussive, aldosterone stimulant, MAO inhibitor.

CONSTITUENTS: Saponins, glycyrrhizin, glycyrrhetinic acid, isoliquritigenin, calcium and potassium salts of glycyrrhizic acid, asparagin, tannin, flavonoids, sugars, starch, resin, gum and a volatile oil.

FAMILY: Leguminosae.

FLAVOR: Sweet-warming.

FIVE PHASE CATEGORIES: Earth yin, Water yin, Metal yin.

PRINCIPAL INDICATIONS ACCORDING TO TERRAIN:

1) EARTH: — gastrointestinal ulcers and spasms, glossitis, stomatitis, herpes simplex infections, reduction of bacterial plaque on teeth.

2) WATER: — low immunity, depression, chronic infections, gonadal insufficiency, trichomonas infection.

3) METAL: — recurring and chronic respiratory tract infections, coughs.

Licorice root is a component in over 60 percent of Chinese and Japanese traditional herb formulas. By itself, it has been used to treat muscle spasms, especially those of the gastrointestinal tract (colic), stomach ulcers, glossitis and stomatitis. The drug carbenoxalone is derived from licorice and used to treat peptic ulcers. The action of licorice on the stomach and intestines is vagolytic and antihistamine. It fluidifies secretions of the bronchial tubes making it useful for treating bronchitis and tracheitis, especially in chronic cases including allergic types of bronchial asthma. It has been found to be as effective as codeine as an antitussive in experiments with cats. It is a safe expectorant for vagotonic, asthenic (Earth yin and Metal yin) children.

Licorice improves the metabolism of fats, and reverses the degeneration of liver cells by improving detoxification. This makes it useful for treating fatty livers, lowering cholesterol, and treating chronic hepatitis. It also improves immunity by increasing interferon production.

The glycoside glycyrrhizin has a molecular structure very similar to that of cortisone, which is responsible in part for the anti-inflammatory properties of licorice. It has been used topically for the treatment of eczema, and in eyedrops for treating conjunctivitis and blepharitis. In oral use, licorice is good for chronic gum infections and prevents bacterial plaque from adhering to the teeth.

Prolonged use of licorice can result in potassium loss, edema, and water retention. Thus prolonged use should be reserved for the Water yin type (vagotonic, hypogenital).

MARIGOLD *Calendula officinalis*

ACTIONS: Antispasmodic, diaphoretic, parasympathomimetic, emmenagogue, hypotensive, antiseptic, vulnerary and cicatrisant.

CONSTITUENTS: Flavonic pigments, terpenes (calendulozide B), saponins, resin, alcohols, bitter principle, essential oil containing carotenoids.

FAMILY: Compositae.

FLAVORS: Bitter-warming and cooling, sweet-warming and cooling.

FIVE PHASE CATEGORIES: Earth yin, Earth yang.

PRINCIPAL INDICATIONS ACCORDING TO TERRAIN:

1) EARTH — gastric ulcer, dysmenorrhea, chilblains, warts; benefits labor; can aid in inducing labor; stimulates parasympathetic tonus.

Both a stimulant and a diaphoretic, the flowering heads of marigold find use as a local remedy for conditions such as pain and swelling from a bee or wasp sting. A lotion made from the flowers is said to be useful for sprains and wounds, and a water distillation of the leaves treats inflamed and sore eyes. In external application as a cicatrisant and vulnerary, it is useful for removal of warts, and to treat tumors, warts, crevices (chapping), contusions and chilblains.

Used internally, it is said to prevent suppuration and is prescribed for chronic ulcers and varicose veins. Above all, marigold is emmenagogic and oxytocic. It is useful for dysmenorrhea and for gastric ulcers. It is sudorific, and can be used in both warm and cold types of infections. It has antibacterial, antifungal and antiparasitic (trichomonas) properties.

A therapist facing a clinical choice between arnica and marigold would choose arnica for cases of yang inflammations of the skin and tissues originating from heat, and marigold for the yin inflammations. For example, for a large, heavy-set patient exhibiting signs of diabetic infections from heat such as furuncles around the mouth and on the back, arnica would be the medicine of choice, whereas marigold would be used to treat juvenile acne, which is cold in nature. Marigold is also useful for eczema when taken internally.

OAK (COMMON OAK) *Quercus robur*

ACTIONS: Astringent, antidiarrheic, anthelminthic, hemostatic.

CONSTITUENTS: The bark contains tannins and bitter principles (quercitrin), the leaves contain glycosides (quercitrin and quercetol).

FAMILY: Cupuliferae (Fagaceae).

FLAVORS: Sour-warming, pungent-warming.

FIVE PHASE CATEGORIES: Earth yin, Metal yin.

PRINCIPAL INDICATIONS ACCORDING TO TERRAIN:

1) EARTH — acute diarrhea, chronic diarrhea, gastralgia, asthenia, gastroptosis, eczema, psoriasis, leukorrhea, malaria.

2) METAL — chronic bronchitis, hemoptysis, tonsillitis, diarrhea, rectocolitis, Crohn's disease, anal prolapse, anal fissures and fistulas, hemorrhoids, hypoasthenia, hair loss, chilblains, acrocyanosis, eczema, psoriasis.

As an astringent, the leaves, bark and acorns of oak have been used for hemorrhages, as well as in chronic diarrhea and dysentery, either alone or with aromatic herbs. Externally, oak has been used as a gargle for chronic sore throat; as a douche for leukorrhea; as a local application for bleeding hemorrhoids and for astringing loose gums; for loss of hair and for bathing the hands and feet in cases of chilblains and acrocyanosis (Raynaud's phenomenon).

Having flavors of spicy-warm and sour-warm, oak treats diarrhea, severe dysentery, hemorrhages (rectocolitis and Crohn's disease) severe gastralgia and gastroptosis, enuresis, asthenia, fevers and splenomegaly of malaria. Its nature is both cooling and warming. Externally, it is used for stomatitis, tonsillitis and dermatoses (eczema, psoriasis). Oak is used for hemoptysis, chronic bronchitis, hypoasthenia, leukorrhea, enuresis, anal prolapse, anal fissures, fistulas, hemorrhoids and other types of varicose veins. It is one of the best examples of a sour-warming flavor.

PROPOLIS *Propolis*

ACTIONS: Analgesic, disinfectant.

CONSTITUENTS: Waxes, resins and balsams, flavonoids (chrysine, galangine, pinocembrine, quercetin), cinnamyl alcohol, vanillin, kaempferid, acacetin, aromatic acids (benzoic, cinnamic, caffeic, ferulic, p-coumaric), coumarin, esculetol, essential oil (eugenol, guaiol, anethole, pineme), trace elements magnesium, zinc, aluminum, manganese, iron, copper, silicon, tin, nickel, etcetera), vitamin B complex.

FLAVOR: Sweet-warming, pungent-warming.

FIVE PHASE CATEGORIES: Earth yin, Metal yin.

PRINCIPAL INDICATIONS ACCORDING TO TERRAIN:

1) EARTH — Immune deficiency, infectious diseases, parasites.

2) METAL: — Respiratory infections, mucous and serous membrane infections, skin infections and wounds.

The use of propolis in healing goes back to time immemorial. Throughout their 6000 year civilization, the Egyptians used it medicinally as well as for the mummification of cadavers. A beehive product of greenish-brown to chestnut-brown color, it is composed of resins, gums and balsams made from the buds of trees, particularly poplar and birch. Propolis is Latin for "before the town (city)," a reference to its use as a barrier in defense of beehives. The *apis mellifica* (honey bee) uses it in the hive as a sanitary surface to prevent the growth of any bacteria, mold, fungi or parasites. It encases hive intruders that cannot be removed from the hive, sterilizing their decaying remains.

The Greeks used it to speed up the healing of wounds. Aristotle recommended it for all afflictions of the skin, wounds and suppuration. In Rome, every legionnaire carried a small amount of propolis with him to battle, not only for speeding up wound healing but for its analgesic action. Pliny recommended it for "expelling foreign objects, reducing swelling and softening hardened skin. It diminishes pain of the nerves, heals ulcers, abscesses, and often incurable furuncles." The Incas used it for febrile infections. It has been used in Soviet Georgia for buccal and dental infections. During the Boer War, the British used it directly on wounds as an antibiotic. Throughout history propolis has played an important role in veterinary medicine.

Propolis is a powerful analgesic. Based on his experiments with rabbits, Prokopovitch (USSR 1957) estimated that its analgesic strength is three times greater than cocaine and 52 times greater than novocaine. Frenkel, also in the USSR, used 10 to 30 percent concentrations of propolis, roughly equivalent to cocaine, for surgery of the nose, ear, stoma and dental roots, not only for its anesthetic properties, but to reduce the risk of postoperative infections.

It has inhibitory and lethal properties with a wide variety of fungi (nine species of candida alone), gram-positive, gram-negative and acid-resistant bacteria, and has proved its worth as a viricide, especially for herpes. In addition to its properties as a cicatrisant and analgesic used locally for wounds and infections, it is useful clinically for treating ear, nose and throat infections. It has been used successfully to treat chronic throat infections, several types of pneumonia, bronchial asthma and inflammations of the uterine cervix and vaginitis, including trichomonas vaginalis. Propolis also has properties of strengthening immunity by increasing antibody production. Its anti-inflammatory properties have been tested successfully in Poland where it is used for treating inflammation in rheumatic disease.

HERBS FOR METAL YANG PATHOLOGIES

METAL YANG PROFILES - QUICK REFERENCE

ASH	HBP
	constipation
	urinary calculi
BORAGE	dry bronchitis
	hemoptysis
	fever
	UTI
HOREHOUND	fever
	wet bronchitis
	arrhythmias
LUNGWORT	heat and dryness in the
	Large Intestine and Lung
	hemoptysis
MARSHMALLOW	heat and dryness in the
	Large Intestine and Lung
PERIWINKLE	HBP
	hyperglycemia
	tonsillitis
RHUBARB	purgative
	antibacterial

ASH *Fraxinus excelsior*

ACTIONS: Laxative, purgative, febrifuge, astringent.

CONSTITUENTS: Glycosides (fraxin, fraxetol, rutin), malic acid, resin, mineral salts, sugars, pigments, vitamins C and P.

FAMILY: Oleaceae.

FLAVORS: Bitter-cooling, sweet-cooling, sour-cooling.

FIVE PHASE CATEGORIES: Metal yang, Water yang, Fire yang, Earth yang.

PRINCIPAL INDICATIONS ACCORDING TO TERRAIN:

1) METAL — arterial hypertension, arteriosclerosis, hypercholesterolemia, uremia.

2) FIRE — urinary calculi, gout, rheumatism.

3) WATER — oliguria, urinary calculi, hypertension, arteriosclerosis; recommended as a medicine for longevity.

4) EARTH — arthritis, arteriosclerosis and rheumatism in a plethoric condition; stimulates sluggish lymph circulation.

Ash moves the bowels and relieves the pain of constipation. The bark is used for intermittent fevers and was once used in place of Peruvian bark (quinine) for malaria. The young leaves are used for arthritis, rheumatic pain and edema. It has also been used in the treatment of uremia (Cheynes-Stokes), arteriosclerosis and hypercholesterolemia. Ash stimulates a sluggish metabolism, stimulates secretions of the Islets of Langerhans and lowers blood cholesterol. In Russia it is used as a circulatory stimulant to warm the hands and feet, but it warms the entire body.

BORAGE *Borrago officinalis*

ACTIONS: Emollient (flowers), febrifuge, sudorific, demulcent, diuretic (stems and leaves).

CONSTITUENTS: High in potassium and calcium salts, mucilage, tannins.

FAMILY: Borraginae.

FLAVORS: Sweet-cooling, salty-cooling.

FIVE PHASE CATEGORIES: Metal yang, Water yang, Fire yang.

PRINCIPAL INDICATIONS ACCORDING TO TERRAIN:

1) METAL — acute bronchopneumopathies with heat and dryness, pulmonary abscesses, cutaneous eruptions, eruptive disorders such as measles, rubella.

2) WATER — repletion heat in the Kidney, oliguria, anuria, renal colic, nephritis, retention in the bladder, urinary tract infections; has an antagonistic action on the adrenals.

3) FIRE — coronaropathy, eruptive fevers, measles, scarlet fever, scarlatina.

According to legend, borage is the famous nepenthe of Homer, which brought about amnesia when drunk with wine. It has traditionally been used to discharge melancholy humors. Culpepper recommended it for a variety of conditions, including sore throat and consumption. It promotes the activity of the kidneys because its saline constituents include potassium, calcium and potassium nitrate, which having a "softening" effect on contracted kidneys. It has a relaxing effect on the heart, and its healing and regenerating effect on the lung is dramatic. Borage dissipates heat and heat from dryness (yin vacuity heat) in acute dry bronchial infections with hyperthermia and no perspiration (viral or bacterial); it also heals abscesses of the lungs. Midwives in England once used it as a galactagogue.

It is prescribed for measles, for rubella, eruptive fevers of Metal constitutions, and for scarlatina (eruptive fever of fire). It is good for pediatric fevers unaccompanied by perspiration.

HOREHOUND *Marrubium vulgare*

ACTIONS: Parasympathomimetic, febrifuge, expectorant, diuretic, loosens bronchial secretions, cardiac sedative.

CONSTITUENTS: Bitter principle (marrubine), tannin (marrubrin), essential oil, resin, saponiside, glucoside, choline, potassium, magnesium, calcium, iron, vitamin C.

FAMILY: Labiae.

FLAVORS: Pungent-cooling, bitter-cooling.

FIVE PHASE CATEGORIES: Metal yang, Water yang, Fire yang.

PRINCIPAL INDICATIONS ACCORDING TO TERRAIN:

1) METAL — respiratory infections, acute bronchial pneumonia, laryngitis, tracheitis, fevers, sore throat, bronchitis, asthma (diaphoretic), bacterial enteritis (typhoid).

2) FIRE — tachycardia, heart rhythm problems, menstrual insufficiency or amenorrhea due to venous congestion.

3) WATER — oliguria.

Horehound root has long been noted for its efficacy in lung troubles and coughs. According to Culpepper, when taken with orris root, it helps to expectorate thick phlegm from the chest. It is rich in potassium salts and in iron. Because of its purifying properties, it could be called a type of pungent-cooling and bitter-cooling herb, which is why it is prescribed for fevers and for respiratory affliction with heat and hot dryness, acute bronchopneumopathies, laryngitis and tracheitis. It has an antiarrhythmic action on the heart and is a diuretic in oliguria when the cause is dryness or heat and dryness.

Using it would be dangerous in cases of renal insufficiency due to Kidney vacuity. Traditionally it has been used for asthma, hysteria and sore throat and has been prescribed in large doses as a laxative to expel worms. Additionally, it has also been administered to counteract the effects of mercury poisoning. Dioscorides recommended its use as an emmenagogue.

LUNGWORT *Pulmonaria officinalis*

ACTIONS: Sudorific, emollient, diuretic.

CONSTITUENTS: Mucilage, tannins, mineral salts (especially silicon), silicic acid, allantoin, quercetin, kaempferol, vitamin C, saponins.

FAMILY: Borraginae.

FLAVOR: Sweet-cooling.

FIVE PHASE CATEGORIES: Metal yang, Fire yang.

PRINCIPAL INDICATIONS ACCORDING TO TERRAIN:

1) METAL — acute bronchial and pulmonary complaints, hemoptysis, hemorrhoids.

2) FIRE — palpitations, tachycardia.

Paracelsus valued lungwort for its effect on respiratory illness. Sweet and cooling, pulmonaria has a sudorific activity comparable to borage and specifically treats pulmonary afflictions stemming from heat and wind-heat, including acute bronchial and pulmonary problems, coughs, asthma, bronchitis, hemoptysis and pulmonary tuberculosis.

Its ability to resolve heat gives it heart-calming properties. Another name for the herb in French is "the cardiac herb." It is prescribed for agitation of the heart, palpitations and tachycardia. It is also indicated for hemorrhoids from heat of the Large Intestine, and externally for anal fissures and for chilblains. The leaves of the rosette are used.

MARSHMALLOW *Althaea officinalis*

ACTIONS: Emollient, sedative.

CONSTITUENTS: Mucilage, pectin, mineral salts, glucides, vitamin C, sugars, asparagine.

FAMILY: Malvaceae.

FLAVOR: Sweet-cooling.

FIVE PHASE CATEGORY: Metal yang.

PRINCIPAL INDICATIONS ACCORDING TO TERRAIN:

1) **METAL** — acute bronchial pneumonia, pharyngitis, laryngitis, acute dysentery, constipation, abscesses, furuncles, gingivitis and psychic excitability.

Marshmallow was mentioned in the writings of Dioscorides, Paracelsus, Galen and Pliny. The Greeks and Romans took marshmallow for acute and dry types of bronchopneumopathies, pharyngitis and laryngitis. The leaves, roots and flowers have traditionally been used for inflammation and irritation of the alimentary canal and of the urinary and respiratory organs. Externally, it was applied as a poultice to prevent mycosis and inflammation.

Sweet and cooling, it combats symptoms of heat and dryness in the lung, constipation due to heat and dryness of the large intestine, and acute dysentery. It is also prescribed for abscesses and furuncles in case of heat in the skin, for the teeth and for dental abscesses in gingivitis. The root calms teething pains in infants; it also has a sedative effect.

PERIWINKLE *Vinca minor*

ACTIONS: Sympatholytic, vagolytic, hypotensive, spasmolytic, vasodilator, astringent, hemostatic, vulnerary, stimulates FSH secretion, antigalactic.

CONSTITUENTS: Vincamine and vincristine (alkaloids), glucides, tannin, flavonoids, organic acids, pectin, mineral salts, vitamin C.

FAMILY: Apocynaceae.

FLAVORS: Bitter-cooling, sour-cooling.

FIVE PHASE CATEGORIES: Metal yang, Earth yang, Fire yang, Water yang.

PRINCIPAL INDICATIONS ACCORDING TO TERRAIN:

1) METAL — angina pectoris, coronary thrombosis, hypertension, epistaxis, hemoptysis, diabetes, glycosuria, hypoglycemiant action, tonsillitis.

2) EARTH — angina pectoris, coronary thrombosis, hypertension, diabetic vascular disease.

3) FIRE — angina pectoris, coronary thrombosis, hypertension, arteriosclerosis.

4) WATER — angina pectoris, coronary thrombosis, hypertension.

Periwinkle was once a favorite flower for making charms and love potions, and was believed to have the power to exorcise spirits. It is hypotensive, acting on the central nervous system and the peripheral circulation; a cerebral vasodilator and hypotensive, a coronary vasodilator, and a central nervous system sedative. It is adrenolytic and lowers the peripheral resistance. Its indications are for epistaxis and hemoptysis. In decoction it is used to treat glycosuria of diabetes and polydipsia. Other indications include vascular pathologies, hypertension, cerebral insufficiency, precordial pain and peripheral arteriopathy. Periwinkle has anticancer properties, especially the varieties that contain the anticancer alkaloid vincristine. Externally it is used for tonsillitis.

RHUBARB *Rheum rhaphonticum*

ACTIONS: Purgative, laxative.

CONSTITUENTS: Anthrones and dianthrones (emodin, rhein, aloe-emodin, rheum-emodin, chrysophanol, physcion), sennosides A-F, sennidin A, phenolic glucosides (lindleyin), gallic acid, cinnamic acid, tannins (rhatannin, glucogallin).

FAMILY: Polygonaceae.

FLAVORS: Bitter-cooling.

FIVE PHASE CATEGORIES: Metal yang, Wood yang.

PRINCIPAL INDICATIONS ACCORDING TO TERRAIN:

    1) METAL — constipation, dyspepsia, dysentery.

    2) WOOD — biliary dyskinesia, gallstones, high cholesterol, blood stasis.

Rhubarb is used as a purgative, a cathartic and as an anti-inflammatory. As a cathartic, it is known to accelerate peristalsis and to accelerate the elimination of feces, usually within about six hours of ingestion. Rhubarb extracts have been proven to be effective against such fungi as trichophyton, microsporum and epidermaphyton. It has marked antibacterial action *in vitro* against streptococcus, staphylococcus, diphtheria bacillus, typhus, paratyphus and pneumococcus, and has been found to prevent tumor formation in laboratory test animals.

Research in China indicates that certain components of rhubarb have an inhibitory effect on gram-positive bacteria. In Japan these components have been found to have bactericidal action against *bacterioides fragilis,* an intestinal bacteria that is sometimes pathogenic. *Bacterioides fragilis* has been found in large quantities in the gallbladders of patients with hepatic and gallbladder disease. Two components, lindleyin and isolindleyin, have been found to be as effective as aspirin and phenylbutazone for their anti-inflammatory and analgesic properties.

HERBS FOR METAL YIN PATHOLOGIES

METAL YIN PROFILES - QUICK REFERENCE

BLADDERWRACK
glandular stimulant
remineralizer
obesity
allergies
menopause

BLACK WALNUT
moistens secretions
colitis
parasites

COLTSFOOT
wet cough
bronchitis
laryngitis

GINGER
fever
nausea
bronchitis
anorexia
diarrhea

MALLOW
dry bronchitis
constipation

NETTLE
diarrhea
hay fever
kidney infections
gallstones

ST. JOHN'S WORT
immune system weakness
depression

YELLOW DOCK
diarrhea
dysentery
bleeding of lungs or bowels

BLADDERWRACK *Fucus vesiculosus*

ACTIONS: Remineralizer, glandular stimulant (especially thyroid).

CONSTITUENTS: Minerals: iodine (18-95 mg/100gm), bromine, manganese, copper, iron, magnesium and numerous trace elements; alginic acid, polysaccharide sulphates, phenolic components, free fatty acids, phospholipids, pigments, vitamins, mucilage.

FAMILY: Fucaceae.

FLAVORS: Salty-warming, sweet-warming.

FIVE PHASE CATEGORIES: Water yin, Earth yin, Metal yin.

PRINCIPAL INDICATIONS ACCORDING TO TERRAIN:

1) EARTH — obesity, constipation, anemia, hypothyroidism, excessive appetite and anorexia, lymphadenopathy, neuritis, paralysis.

2) METAL — anorexia, malnutrition, hypothyroidism, lymphadenopathy, chronic rhinopharyngitis, asthma, emphysema, demineralization, impotence, frigidity, chronic dermatoses.

3) WATER — asthenia, hypothyroidism, demineralization, rheumatic pain, arthrosis, polyarthritis, spondyloarthritis, collagenoses, frigidity, impotence, oligomenorrhea, amenorrhea.

Bladderwrack is a type of brown algae that can be used as a food, and is very similar in its properties to laminaria *(kombu)*, which is commonly eaten in Japan and some parts of China.   Bladderwrack is one of the best herbs for the treatment of obesity. It stimulates the activity of the thyroid and pituitary glands and the digestive tonus. It is useful for treatment of the pituitary-gonadal axis and for insufficiency of growth hormone. It is good for hypothyroid obesity and cellulite in Earth yin and Metal yin constitutional types. It strengthens the Lungs and can be used to strengthen an asthenic constitution of the Metal yin type.

Bladderwrack improves transit in the gastrointestinal tract because of the bulk provided by its mucilage content. The mucilage can absorb up to 100 times its weight in water, and can reduce the appetite just by filling the stomach. Even though it is frequently used in regimens for the treatment of obesity, it is effective in treating anorexia and asthenia, and even as a supplement in degenerative conditions, such as pulmonary tuberculosis, AIDS and cancer.

It is excellent in treating cases of blood vacuity: anemia, malnutrition, anergy, arthrosis, polyarthrosis, frigidity, impotence, amenorrhea, neuritis and paralytic conditions. Alginic acid, a component of bladderwrack, is said to remove heavy metals, such as lead and cadmium, from the body.

BLACK WALNUT *Juglans nigra, Juglans regia*

ACTIONS: Astringent, tonic, eupeptic, antibiotic (leaves), antifungal, anthelminthic (bark).

CONSTITUENTS: Tannins, bitter principle (juglone), fatty oil rich in linoleic acid, manganese, iron, iodine, copper, zinc, vitamins A, B1, B2, B6 and C, serotonin (nuts), naphthoquinone (leaves), ellagic acid, juglandin, juglandic acid.

FAMILY: Juglandeae.

FLAVORS: Sour-warming, bitter-warming.

FIVE PHASE CATEGORIES: Metal yin, Earth yin, Water yin.

PRINCIPAL INDICATIONS ACCORDING TO TERRAIN:

1) METAL — anemia, lymphatism, rachitism, tuberculosis, chronic diarrhea, Crohn's disease, rectocolitis, diabetes, leukorrhea, eczema, psoriasis.

2) EARTH — retarded growth, prepubescent obesity, leukorrhea, diarrhea, diabetes, dermatoses.

3) WATER — leukorrhea and dermatoses of the "wind-cold-damp" type (external usage); weeping eczema, cold abscesses, adenopathy of the neck, carbuncles, chilblains, acrocyanosis.

The fruit of the walnut tree, the "gland of Jupiter," is a specific for the brain. Dioscorides noted its excitatory effects and its engenderment of anger and discomfort of the head. One reason for this is that walnuts are high in serotonin, a chemical present in the brain and in the intestinal walls. A sudden discharge of serotonin in the organism results in acceleration of the heart, flushing, antidiuretic action (stimulation of bladder and the kidney yang) and an excitation of the peripheral nerve endings. An excitation and then depression of the motricity of the digestive tract can sometimes result in the occurrence of stomach pain. However, this excitation also stimulates mammary secretions – by stimulating the small intestine, oxytocin from the hypophysis and serotonin from the epiphysis.

The leaves contain vitamins A, B1, B2, B6. The shells are extremely rich in vitamin C. They are prescribed as an infusion for asthenic types, the aged and for infants. However, they are equally rich in zinc and copper and so are naturally useful in correction of retarded development.

Black walnut is useful for treating scrofula, lymphadenopathy, tuberculosis, anemia and rickets. It has antibiotic properties (naphthoquinone), destroys fungus, worms and parasites and has been used for syphilis, ringworm, eczema and even poison oak. Black walnut leaves are useful for all syndromes of wind, cold and dampness in the Earth yin and Metal yin constitutions when there is anemia, and also for chronic complaints of the digestive, skeletal and immune systems. Black walnut is useful for severe diarrhea of rectocolitis, and for Crohn's disease. Also, the leaves have hypotensive and hypoglycemic actions and thus can be used to treat diabetes.

In East Asian medicine, the dried nut is classified as a supplementing substance which strengthens the Lung and Kidney, warming the Lung, moistening the intestines and nourishing the blood. It is used for cough and asthma, in particular for chronic geriatric asthma or bronchitis due to adrenal insufficiency, administered two to three times daily for one to two months. As an expectorant and antitussive, it not only helps asthma but improves sleep and appetite. It is also used for lumbar pain and leg weakness resulting from Kidney yang vacuity (asthenia, hypoadrenalism). It is often added to kidney stone formulas to help with the pain. It helps with digestion and constipation in the elderly, but is best administered as other than a strong tea. It should not be used with a febrile cough.

In India, the bark is used as an astringent and anthelminthic, the leaves are used for eczema, worms, herpes and syphilis; the green hulls of the nut are used for worms and for syphilis and the kernels for dysentery, colic and as an aphrodisiac.

COLTSFOOT (TUSSILAGO) *Tussilago farfara*

ACTIONS: Emollient, expectorant, antitussive, vagolytic.

CONSTITUENTS: Mucilage, flavonoids, inulin, essential oil, phytosterol, arnidiol, faradiol, pigments, tannin, mineral salts, iron, calcium, potassium, sulphur, vitamin C.

FAMILY: Compositae.

FLAVORS: Bitter-warming, sweet-warming.

FIVE PHASE CATEGORY: Metal yin.

PRINCIPAL INDICATIONS ACCORDING TO TERRAIN:

1) METAL — cough, acute bronchitis, laryngitis, tracheitis, lymphadenitis, postinfectious fatigue, emphysema, silicosis.

Coltsfoot has been used since the days of Dioscorides in cigarette form or pipe form for asthmatics. Smoking the leaves to relieve a cough was also recommended by Galen, Pliny and Boyle. (The leaves are the basis for British herb tobacco which also includes betony, buckbean, chamomile, eyebright, lavender, rosemary and thyme.) Slightly bitter, sweet and mucilaginous, it is warming and has an odor like honey. It is thus an emollient agent that facilitates expectoration and dries up phlegm and is also slightly diaphoretic and tonic. In classical Chinese medicine it is used for vacuity and coldness of the lungs with dampness.

Coltsfoot treats coughs, acute bronchitis, laryngitis, tracheitis, lymphadenitis and tubercular adenopathy and is effective in the treatment of silicosis and emphysema. The controversy regarding the use of coltsfoot because of its pyrollizidine alkaloids has not been a major issue in Europe because many of the pharmaceutical manufacturers sell extracts from which the alkaloids have been removed. Pyrrolizidine alkaloids, found in coltsfoot, borage and comfrey, may cause liver damage from veno-occlusive disease. Individuals who imbibe frequent or numerous infusions of teas containing these herbs should be made aware of the possible danger.

GINGER *Zingiber officinale*

ACTIONS: Eupeptic, carminative, febrifuge, stimulant, antiphlogistic, antiprostaglandin.

CONSTITUENTS: Essential oil contains terpenes (cineol, borneol, citral, phellandrene), zingiberene, phenols (gingerol, zingerone, shogaol).

FAMILY: Orchidaceae.

FLAVOR: Pungent-warming.

FIVE PHASE CATEGORIES: Metal yin, Water yin, Earth yin.

PRINCIPAL INDICATIONS ACCORDING TO TERRAIN:

1) METAL — respiratory infections, bronchitis, influenza, bronchorrhea, pulmonary congestion, fever.

2) EARTH — anorexia, glairy diarrhea, deficient immunity, leukopenia.

3) WATER — impotence, urinary infections, glomerulonephritis.

Piquant, warm and aromatic, ginger root is used in classical Chinese medicine as a sudorific and eupeptic. When the root is desiccated, it is considered to have much stronger warming properties, and is used to warm the Stomach and the Lung, to discharge phlegm and to strengthen the yang functions of the body. It stimulates circulation and stimulates the sympathetic nervous system; it increases salivary and gastric secretions and strengthens peristalsis of the stomach and intestines. Clinically, it is used for nausea and vomiting caused by coldness of the Stomach; it also treats hiccups, abdominal pain and diarrhea. It removes gas, accelerates transport through the alimentary canal, soothes gas pains and in general has a calming effect. It stimulates appetite and has a slight detoxifying effect. In addition, it has antiulcerative properties, being especially beneficial for ulcers induced by an excess of hydrochloric acid (HCl).

Ginger can be prescribed for external symptoms of colds and for coughs with phlegm, where the phlegm is abundant and breathing is rapid. A cold constitution or a cold condition, such as amenorrhea due to insufficient circulation, functional bleeding or uterine bleeding stemming from adrenal insufficiency, will respond to ginger. Mixed with aconite, it makes a formula for treating shock. Although it has been used for morning sickness for centuries, caution should be exercised in using the dried form in pregnant women. The dried form of ginger is considered to have a stronger effect on the deeper circulation, whereas the raw ginger is said to act superficially at the exterior of the body and at the mucous membranes. It can also be used as a general immune tonic to prevent infections and for impotence. There is evidence that it is more effective than dramamine for motion sickness. In Ayurvedic medicine it is used as a carminative, for loss of appetite, rheumatism, allergies and as an aphrodisiac (see the Essential Oils Profiles).

MALLOW (BLUE MALLOW) *Malva sylvestris*

ACTIONS: Emollient, demulcent, laxative, antitussive, antigonadotropic.

CONSTITUENTS: Mucilage, anthocyanin, vitamins A, B1, B2 and C.

FAMILY: Malvaceae.

FLAVOR: Sweet-warming.

FIVE PHASE CATEGORIES: Metal yin, Earth yin.

PRINCIPAL INDICATIONS ACCORDING TO TERRAIN:

1) METAL — Bronchial pneumonia, chronic bronchitis, constipation, diarrhea, dermatoses; soothes the lungs.

2) EARTH — constipation, diarrhea, dermatoses, vaginitis; delays childbirth.

In 16th century Italy, mallow was known as omnimorbia, for it was considered useful for all afflictions. The Pythagoreans thought of it as a sacred plant for calming the spirit and cooling the body's passions.

Like marshmallow, mallow has a sweet and warm flavor. Therapeutically, the root, leaves and flowers can be used. As a laxative it is used for atonic constipation resulting from weakness of the large intestine and for diarrhea caused by coldness and vacuity. It is also used for coughs, dry respiratory irritations and chronic bronchitis. Externally, it is used for dermatoses, abscesses and as a douche for vaginitis with burning pain.

NETTLE *Urtica urens*

ACTIONS: Astringent, expectorant, antianemic.

CONSTITUENTS: Glucoquinines, protoporphyrin, coproporphyrin, histamine, tannins, carotene, gallic acid, acetylcholine, serotonin, silicon, potassium, calcium, iron, sulphur. There is an irritating level of formic acid until the plant is dried. Vitamins C, B2, E, K, pantothenic acid, folic acid, trace elements copper, zinc, manganese and nickel.

FAMILY: Urticaceae.

FLAVORS: Sour-cooling, salty-warming, sweet-warming, pungent-warming.

FIVE PHASE CATEGORIES: Metal yin, Wood yang, Water yin.

PRINCIPAL INDICATIONS ACCORDING TO TERRAIN:

1) METAL — fatigue, anemia, tuberculosis, dermatoses, enuresis, diarrhea, chronic enteritis, allergic rhinitis.

2) WOOD — biliary dyskinesia, biliary lithiases, hypercholesterolemia, arthritis, diabetes, urticaria, pruritus, hypoglycemiant action.

3) WATER — renal calculi, enuresis, chronic nephritis, chronic diarrhea.

Nettle combines both pungent and warm qualities with the astringent properties of sour-cold. In general, it is useful for improving respiration and cardiovascular tone, and as a blood tonic, hypoglycemiant and remineralizer; for treating weakness, anemia, diarrhea, stomach pain and chronic enteritis; for bronchial problems including asthma; for dermatoses, and for enuresis of kidney infections. It speeds the coagulation of blood, increases hemoglobin content and erythrocyte levels, and is a vasoconstrictor and tonic to the uterine muscles. The juice of the roots or leaves can be used, or the dry leaves can be inhaled in a cigarette or pipe. Externally, it is used as a styptic. In England, it is used for skin eruptions, eczema and nosebleeds as an external treatment. The American herbalist Jethro Kloss recommends its use on the scalp to restore hair color.

It is a very effective agent in the treatment of allergic rhinitis with symptoms of sinus congestion, nasal discharge, conjunctivitis, sneezing; itching and burning of the eyes, ears, nose and throat; facial edema, headache, wheezing and irritability. It should be combined with another agent when prescribed to strengthen liver function.

In Eastern Europe it is used for such complaints as anemia (nettle is very rich in iron), arteriosclerosis, muscular and joint rheumatism, edema, kidney and bladder infections, hemorrhoids, vomiting, skin diseases with itching, as a galactagogue and with vinegar for the pain of first degree burns.

ST. JOHN'S WORT *Hypericum perforatum*

ACTIONS: Sympathomimetic, immune stimulant, diuretic, antidepressant, astringent and antiseptic, antiviral, antiphlogistic, MAO inhibitor.

CONSTITUENTS: Polycyclic diones hypericin and pseudohypericin, flavonols (quercetin, hyperoside, rutin, methylhesperidin), xanthones, coumarins, phenolic carboxylic acids, phytosterols, n-alkanols (including octacosanol), essential oil.

FAMILY: Hypericaceae.

FLAVORS: Bitter-warming, sour-cooling.

FIVE PHASE CATEGORIES: Metal yin, Earth yin.

PRINCIPAL INDICATIONS ACCORDING TO TERRAIN:

1) METAL — diarrhea, urinary tract infections, nervousness, neurasthenia, depression.

2) EARTH — diarrhea, splenomegaly, dyspepsia, gastroptosis, lymphadenitis, depression, leukorrhea.

St. John's wort has attracted recent attention due to the alleged antiretroviral activity of its components hypericin and pseudohypericin. The use of these two chemicals has been shown to be effective in preventing the spread of retroviruses *in vitro* and *in vivo*. Experiments with these substances prevented the onset of leukemia induced by the FV (Friend leukemia) virus, and the oral administration of the substances reduced splenomegaly caused by FV. After treatment, no FV could be found in the spleen or blood of the animals. These two components also are able to cross the blood-brain barrier, which could make them useful for cerebral infections. For experimental treatment of AIDS, the French extracts are standardized at 0.18% hypericin at a daily dosage of 2-4 grams powdered herb or 50 drops alcohol extract three times daily.

In France, St. John's wort extracts are included in over-the-counter and prescription medications for mild depression. Traditionally, it has been used for nervous disorders, neurasthenia and depression. It contains xanthones that inhibit type A and B monoamine oxidase *in vivo*. St. John's wort has also been used for diarrhea, dyspepsia, splenomegaly, lymphadenitis, gastroptosis and as an anthelminthic. More recently it has been used for leukorrhea, especially with heat or cold dampness of the spleen and for peripheral neuropathy and problems in the peripheral circulation. It is a mild diuretic and urinary antiseptic.

Externally, the oil is used for burns, abrasions and muscle pain. It was used traditionally as a vulnerary and cicatrisant, although it can also have a photosensitizing effect. The essential oil has been used for bronchitis, asthma and pulmonary infections due to an insufficiency of the Lung yang. It can be used in an enema for colitis and is administered in an oil infusion as ear drops for congestion and inflammation in otitis media.

YELLOW DOCK *Rumex crispus*

ACTIONS: Bitter tonic, remineralizer, astringent, laxative, diuretic.

CONSTITUENTS: Anthracene derivatives, glucosides, tannins, tannoids, iron and phosphorus.

FAMILY: Polygonaceae.

FLAVORS: Pungent-warming, bitter-warming.

FIVE PHASE CATEGORIES: Metal yin, Earth yin.

PRINCIPAL INDICATIONS ACCORDING TO TERRAIN:

1) METAL — anemia, tracheitis, laryngitis, bronchitis, chronic rheumatism, constipation, diarrhea, dysentery, bleeding of the lungs or bowels.

2) EARTH — anemia, tracheitis, laryngitis, bronchitis, chronic rheumatism, constipation.

3) WATER — rheumatic conditions, demineralized terrain, cancer, glomerular tumors and swelling.

Yellow dock is rich in iron and thus can be prescribed for anemia, and for such lung problems as tracheitis, laryngitis and bronchitis. It is also prescribed for chronic rheumatism. It purifies the lymph system and thus is useful for scrofula and for chronic skin diseases, particularly for exudative sores. It can be an astringent for hemorrhoids and used as a laxative as well. As a laxative, it is somewhat weaker than rhubarb, but very seldom causes any pain or discomfort. It is also considered to have a positive effect as an alterative against malignancy and tissue necrosis. Yellow dock leaches arsenic from the body.

HERBS FOR WATER YANG PATHOLOGIES

WATER YANG PROFILES - QUICK REFERENCE

BLACK CURRANT	HBP urinary calculi gout
BLACK ELDER	UTI calculi hemorrhoids
BIRCH	nephrosis stones high urea cholesterol
DEVIL'S CLAW	arthritis anti-inflammatory rheumatic pain
REST HARROW	urinary tract infections calculi
SARSAPARILLA	strengthens sexual organs
SHEPHERD'S PURSE	kidney and bladder infections bleeding

BLACK CURRANT *Ribes nigrum*

ACTIONS: Salidiuretic, uricosuric, urinary antiseptic, antirheumatic, adrenal cortex stimulant.

CONSTITUENTS: Essential oil, glucides, rich source of gamma-linoleic acid, phycogenols, proline, hydroxyproline, cymene, pectin, sugars, rich source of vitamin C, anthocyanic pigments with vitamin P-like activity, numerous flavonic derivatives, trace elements manganese, copper, cobalt and sulphur.

FAMILY: Saxifragaceae.

FLAVORS: Salty-warming, sweet-warming (buds), sour-cooling, salty cooling (leaves and berries).

FIVE PHASE CATEGORIES: Water yang, Wood yin, Earth yin, Water yin, Fire yin, Earth yang, Fire yang.

PRINCIPAL INDICATIONS ACCORDING TO TERRAIN:

1) **WATER** — urinary calculi, hypertension, rheumatism, gout.

2) **EARTH** — dyspepsia, hypertension, obesity.

3) **FIRE** — arterial hypertension, gout, arthritis, rheumatism; circulatory problems, heavy leg.

Black currant is native to the Nordic regions. The word "ribes" comes from the Danish "ribs," a name for a currant grower. It did not appear in any pharmacopeia until the middle of the 17th century. By the second half of the 19th century, its use had spread to France. It is one of the best treatments for hypertension of a plethoric type with complications of obesity. The bark has also been helpful in urinary calculi, edema and hemorrhoids. The leaves are used in an infusion for urinary tract infections and for rheumatism. The leaves and the roots have a salty, sour flavor and are cooling. The fruit is eaten fresh and used in jams and liqueurs. It has a beneficial effect on the eyes and on the vascular system.

The leaves and buds of black currant yield a green essential oil, which contains significant quantities of cymene and vitamin C. Vitamin C, in combination with the flavonoids, is indispensable for the formation of collagen and in the formation of the vascular bed of the endothelium. It also assists in making steroids available from the adrenals and augments production of norepinephrine. Other derivatives of the plant help to maintain the integrity of the vascular system. Black currant inhibits liberation of proinflammatory hormones (e.g. histamine), stimulations secretion of catecholamines (e.g. norepinephrine) and enhances natural steroid production. As a mother tincture or glycerin macerate (gemmotherapeutic agent), the buds are frequently used to strengthen adrenal cortex function. It is one of the most powerful plant substances prescribed for this purpose. (See also Gemmotherapy Profiles.)

BLACK ELDER *Sambucus nigra*

ACTIONS: Purgative, emollient, anti-inflammatory, diuretic (volumetric, salidiuretic, uricosuric), prolactinogenic, sudorific, febrifuge.

CONSTITUENTS: Mucilage, potassium nitrate, tannins, alkaloids, vitamin C, essential oil with terpenes, glycosides (rutin and quercetin), the glucoside sambunigrin, flavonic and anthrocyanic pigments.

FAMILY: Caprifoliaceae.

FLAVORS: Salty-cooling, sweet-cooling.

FIVE PHASE CATEGORIES: Water yang, Water yin.

PRINCIPAL INDICATIONS ACCORDING TO TERRAIN:

1) WATER — urinary calculi, pyelonephritis, cystitis, urethritis, urinary retention, hemorrhoids, epilepsy, styes, dermatoses, furuncles, tuberculosis, asthma, respiratory infections, tonsillitis, chronic rheumatism, muscular pain and neuralgia.

Black elder was known to Hippocrates, Dioscorides, Pliny and Paracelsus and was treasured during the Middle Ages. There is a medieval belief that Judas was hanged on an elder tree. Another old tradition maintains that the cross of Calvary was made of elder.

The flowers, leaves and fruit of black elder all have medicinal value. The dried inner bark is salidiuretic, uricosuric, laxative and sudorific. The flavors of the bark are salty-cooling, sweet-cooling and mucilaginous. Black elder bark is the treatment of choice for grand mal or petit mal epilepsy. It is also used for pyelonephritis, urethritis, cystitis and urinary retention, and it cleanses the bladder of urinary calculi.

Both the bark and the root are strong purgatives, and if taken in larger doses, can be emetic. Culpepper recommended the root as a purgative. It has also been employed as a diuretic. Elder leaves are recommended for cooling and softening of all kinds of tumors, swellings and wounds. Externally, the leaves can be used for styes and for hemorrhoids.

BIRCH *Betula alba*

ACTIONS: Salidiuretic, azoturic, uricosuric.

CONSTITUENTS: Betulinol, glycoside (betuloside), tannins; trace elements fluorine, iodine, phosphorus, sulphur; an essential oil, saponiside, resin, bitter principle.

FAMILY: Betulaceae.

FLAVORS: Bitter-cooling (bark, leaves), pungent-warming (sap).

FIVE PHASE CATEGORIES: Water yang, Water yin, Fire yang, Earth yang.

PRINCIPAL INDICATIONS ACCORDING TO TERRAIN:

   1) WATER — oliguria caused by renal insufficiency, nephrotic colic and kidney stones, albuminuria, gout, arthritis, rheumatism, arterial hypertension.

   2) FIRE — arthritis, hyperuricemia, hypercholesterolemia, hyperazotemia, arteriosclerosis, obesity.

   3) EARTH — arthritis, hyperuricemia, hypercholesterolemia, hyperazotemia, arteriosclerosis, obesity.

Birch has a cooling influence, and is one of the best plant substances for treating uremia and oliguria. It is used in treatment of uremia from renal insufficiency and also hyperuricemia from repletion heat in the Bladder and Kidneys.

Birch is prescribed for edema and albuminuria, when the pathological manifestations are either renal and cardiac insufficiency, or renal and respiratory insufficiency. It treats gout and rheumatism, and is a reliable solvent for kidney and bladder stones, particularly oxalic and phosphatic stones. It can be used for diarrhea, dysentery, eruptive skin disorders and as a galactagogue.

It is a soothing gargle for sore throat and mouth sores. Externally, it is applied in the treatment of eczema.

See also the Essential Oils Profiles.

DEVIL'S CLAW *Harpagophytum procumbens*

ACTIONS: Antiarthritic, cholesterol-lowering.

CONSTITUENTS: Three monoterpenic bitter glucosides; flavonosides, saponosides, aucuboside-like glucoiridoids, harpagoside, procumbide, copper, magnesium, manganese, zinc, gold, silver.

FAMILY: Pedaliaceae.

FLAVOR: Bitter-cooling.

FIVE PHASE CATEGORIES: Water yang, Earth yang.

PRINCIPAL INDICATIONS ACCORDING TO TERRAIN:

1) WATER: — arthritis, rheumatism, rheumatoid arthritis, gout, acute tendinitis, bursitis, capsulitis, synovitis.

2) EARTH: — hypercholesterolemia.

Devil's claw originated in the savannahs of the Kalahari desert. Its red flowers are very beautiful, but it is the fruit, resembling a sharp claw, that evokes its name. It was known in the 19th century as *Uncaria procumbens,* because of its physical similarity to some types of uncaria. Its therapeutic usage began in South Africa with traditional healers, but its European discovery dates back to the turn of the century at the Hospital of Nababis, where German physicians began research into its use as an anti-inflammatory agent. Thus most of the available research on devil's claw has been done in the middle of this century in Germany. The only noted negative effect has been diarrhea from ingesting an excessive dose.

The root of devil's claw has significant anti-inflammatory and analgesic properties that are comparable to phenylbutazone, but without the negative effects. It lowers blood cholesterol and eliminates excess uric acid.

REST HARROW *Ononis spinosa*

ACTIONS: Urinary antiseptic, sudorific, depurative, salidiuretic.

CONSTITUENTS: Essential oil, flavonic glycoside (ononine), onocerine, ononide, ononcol, trifolirhizin, tannins, resin.

FAMILY: Papilionaceae.

FLAVORS: Salty-cooling, sour-cooling.

FIVE PHASE CATEGORY: Water yang.

PRINCIPAL INDICATIONS ACCORDING TO TERRAIN:

1) WATER — urinary lithiasis, uricemia, urinary infections, arterial hypertension, edema, cystitis.

The flowers, leaves and root of rest harrow have medicinal value. Used in all types of urinary lithiases and for cystitis, it also treats hypertension and renal edema in Kidney repletion cases. Traditionally, it was used as a medicine to subdue delirium. A tradition exists that this was the plant from which the crown of thorns was plaited for the crucifixion.

SARSAPARILLA *Smilax glabra, Smilax medicago*

ACTIONS: Depurative, diuretic (uricosuric and azoturic), stimulates LH secretion.

CONSTITUENTS: Steroid saponins (sarsaponin, smilasaponin, sarsaparilloside), sarsapogenin, smilagenin, sitosterol, stigmasterol, pollinastanol, paroaparic acid, sarsapic acid, oxalic acid, fatty acids, iodine, sulphur, magnesium, calcium, potassium, iron, resin and starch.

FAMILY: Liliaceae.

FLAVORS: Sweet-cooling, pungent-warming.

FIVE PHASE CATEGORIES: Water yang, Metal yin.

PRINCIPAL INDICATIONS ACCORDING TO TERRAIN:

1) **WATER** — nephritis, edema, gout, arthritis, rheumatism.

2) **METAL** — skin problems, flatulence, mild diaphoretic.

Sarsaparilla root has gone through several cycles of popularity in the last three centuries. A native of the West Indies, it was legendary among the conquistadores for conferring inner strength and virility. These actions are due to its ability to provide hormone precursors. Its traditional use is as a tonic and diuretic, but it was also used for the treatment of syphilis from the mid-16th century well into the 19th century. It was popular as a refreshment in 19th century America and used as a spring tonic in both the United States and Europe. Its most recent popularity is among bodybuilders, who use it in place of synthetic steroids because of its supposed testosterone content. Although its steroid saponin content may provide useful raw materials for the manufacture of sex hormones, there are conflicting opinions as to whether any type of smilax actually contains any testosterone or progesterone. In any case, there is no tradition that supports its use for building muscle mass.

It is useful for eliminating urea in uremia, for chronic nephritis with oliguria, for edema, arthritis, rheumatism and gout. Its Metal yin activities are related to its effects on the skin and Lungs. Its reputation for alleviating skin problems dates back to the 16th century when it was used for treating syphilis and leprosy. It has been used successfully in France for the treatment of genital herpes. Some smilax saponins have been shown to be useful for the treatment of psoriasis, but for most dermatoses it is not as effective as solidago, black walnut or violet. As a depurative and a treatment for psoriasis, there are indications that sarsaparilla acts as an endotoxin binder, which would make it useful as a general cleansing agent.

A type of smilax is used in China in combination with other herbs for leukorrhea with inguinal lymphatic swelling. Smilax preparations are treatment of choice for primary stages of syphilis in many parts of China.

SHEPHERD'S PURSE *Capsella bursa-pastoris*

ACTIONS: Parasympathomimetic, sympatholytic, arterial vasodilator, venous vasoconstrictor, astringent, hemostatic, uterotonic, oxytocic, salidiuretic, thyroid inhibitor.

CONSTITUENTS: Saponiside, tannins, malic, acetic, citric and fumaric acids, choline, tyramine, aminophenol, choline, acetylcholine, histamine, flavonoids (diosmin), resins, potassium, calcium, vitamins C and K.

FAMILY: Cruciferae.

FLAVORS: Salty-cooling.

FIVE PHASE CATEGORY: Water yang.

PRINCIPAL INDICATIONS ACCORDING TO TERRAIN:

1) WATER — arterial hypertension, metrorrhagia, menorrhagia, hemorrhoids, hematuria, epistaxis, hemoptysis, venereal infections, orchitis, psychic excitation, epilepsy.

2) WOOD — hyperthyroidism; distinct thyroid inhibiting activity.

The salty and cold flavor of shepherd's purse calms repletion heat, so it has cardiovascular indications for hypertension and gynecological indications as a vasoconstrictor and hemostatic with activity similar to ergot. It is indicated for metrorrhagia of menopause, endometritis originating from the heat of blood stasis and for uterine fibromas. Shepherd's purse is also useful for treating venereal infections and problems of the genitals. It is one of the best specifics for stopping hemorrhages of all kinds, from the stomach, the lungs, the uterus or from the kidneys. It has been used as a decoction for hematuria, hemorrhoids, chronic diarrhea and dysentery, and is used locally for nosebleeds. During the first World War it was used to stop bleeding from wounds. It is also a good postpartum hemostatic.

In Water yang and Fire yang types, it calms hyperexcitability of repletion heat in the Lungs causing epistaxis, hemoptysis or epileptic seizures.

Shepherd's purse is also extremely important for treating inflammations and ulcerated conditions of the bladder. It increases the flow of urine and helps to discharge any mucus (i.e. clears turbidity of the urine). It is useful for urinary lithiases, as well as for inflammations.

In England, the juice has been used as a local treatment for otitis externa. In Russia, it is used for genitourinary problems, venereal disease and for gastritis, diarrhea and dysentery.

HERBS FOR WATER YIN PATHOLOGIES

WATER YIN PROFILES - QUICK REFERENCE

BEARBERRY
: urinary tract infections
diarrhea
prostatitis

GOLDENROD
: urinary tract infections
rectocolitis
Crohn's disease
acne
herpes

HEATHER
: urinary tract infections
bacterial

HORSETAIL
: urinary tract infections
demineralization
spasmophilia
diabetes

MADDER
: warms Kidney and Heart
nephrosis
calculi
HBP

MOUSE EAR
: renal insufficiency
poor eyesight
rheumatism

SEA HOLLY
: weak kidneys
weak libido
edema

YARROW
: nephrosis
diabetes
stimulates sexual organs

BEARBERRY *Arctostaphylos uva ursi (uva-ursi)*

ACTIONS: Salidiuretic, urinary antiseptic.

CONSTITUENTS: Arbutin (7-9 percent), glycosides (arbutoside, methyl arbutoside), quercetin, allantoin, tannins, hydroquinolone, mineral salts;ellagic, malic, gallic and citric acids, a resin (urvone).

FAMILY: Ericaceae.

FLAVORS: Sour-cooling, bitter-warming.

FIVE PHASE CATEGORIES: Water yin, Water yang.

PRINCIPAL INDICATIONS ACCORDING TO TERRAIN:

1) WATER — regulates and calms inflammation of the kidneys and the bladder; acute cystitis, prostatitis, urethritis, pyuria, acute pyelonephritis, urinary retention of the bladder, hematuria due to lithiases, urinary incontinence, enuresis, glomerulonephritis, leukorrhea, metrorrhagia, menorrhagia, acute infectious diarrhea, gonorrhea, cervical ulceration.

The dried leaves of the bearberry are the only part of the plant that is used medicinally. They should be gathered only in the morning after dew has dried in good weather.

Bearberry is powerfully astringent and has been traditionally used in diseases of the bladder and kidney, strengthening and imparting tone to the urinary passages. Bearberry is prescribed for leukorrhea, urinary incontinence, enuresis and glomerulonephritis resulting from cold dampness, and is frequently used to treat inflammatory diseases of the urinary tract. It disperses turbidity in the urine. It also has an antiseptic effect on the mucous membranes of the urinary tract, the genitalia and the uterine lining. Bearberry is administered to contract the uterus following childbirth. In addition, the leaves have a hypoglycemic effect, and have been used along with bilberry to treat diabetes. Large doses have been found to cause nausea and tinnitus.

GOLDENROD *Solidago virga aurea*

ACTIONS: Salidiuretic, azoturic, uricosuric, astringent.

CONSTITUENTS: Essential oil, saponins, tannins, flavonic pigment, citric, oxalic and tartaric acids.

FAMILY: Compositae.

FLAVORS: Bitter; sour-cooling and warming, salty-warming and cooling.

FIVE PHASE CATEGORIES: Water yin, Wood yang, Water yang.

PRINCIPAL INDICATIONS ACCORDING TO TERRAIN:

1) WATER — oliguria, urinary infections, glomerulonephritis, chronic diarrhea, rectocolitis, Crohn's disease, chronic acne, furuncles, chronic eczema.

2) WOOD — acne, herpes and eczema.

Goldenrod is effective in a wide variety of kidney problems. It can be used to treat warm syndromes such as oliguria, glomerulonephritis, urinary tract infections and gram-positive bacterial and viral infections of the kidney. The salty-warming nature makes it possible to treat diarrhea, rectocolitis, Crohn's disease and chronic enteritis, which originate with vacuity of Kidney yang.

In Russia it has been traditionally used for cystitis, diarrhea and amenorrhea. It is good for treating all infections of the skin which are due to liver malfunction, such as acne, herpes, eczema, chronic acne, furuncles and psoriasis. Goldenrod is astringent and diuretic, useful for stones in the bladder. As a spray and given internally, it has been of great value in diphtheria.

HEATHER *Calluna vulgaris*

ACTIONS: Urinary antiseptic, astringent, salidiuretic.

CONSTITUENTS: Flavonoid glycosides (quercitrin, myricitrin), resin (ericoline), essential oil (ericinol), tannins, fumaric and citric acids, arbutin.

FAMILY: Ericaceae.

FLAVORS: Sour-cooling, sweet-warming.

FIVE PHASE CATEGORIES: Water yin, Water yang.

PRINCIPAL INDICATIONS ACCORDING TO TERRAIN:

1) WATER — proteinuria, chronic nephritis, colibacillosis, urinary tract infections, pyelonephritis, cystitis, prostatitis, phosphaturia, oxalic and phosphatic calculi, enuresis, acne.

The flowering tops of heather have a variety of medicinal effects on the kidney, being useful for infections due to either heat or xold. Heather relieves uremia due to hyperfunction and inflammation or to xold, such as proteinuria, and is recommended for chronic nephritis, pyelonephritis, colibacillosis, *klebsiella* and for phosphatic and oxalic urinary calculi. It is effective for enuresis in cold and vacuous terrains.

Heather is also used for oliguria of acute pyelonephritis, for acute cystitis with pyuria (damp-heat), and for prostatitis with congestion (damp-heat). It has a sedative effect; it calms heart palpitations and can be used to relieve menstrual pain. It can be used for acne in Wood and Water constitutions.

HORSETAIL *Equisetum hiemal, E. arvense*

ACTIONS: Salidiuretic, hemostatic, remineralizing agent, astringent.

CONSTITUENTS: Extremely rich in silica (60 percent), 15 percent selenium and calcium with the trace elements magnesium, manganese, lithium, potassium, copper and cobalt, saponoside (equisetonin), glycosides (isoquercitrin), tannins, nicotine, bitter principle and organic acids.

FAMILY: Equisetaceae.

FLAVORS: Sour-cooling, sweet-cooling, salty-cooling.

FIVE PHASE CATEGORIES: Water yin, Wood yang, Water yang, Metal yin, Earth yin.

PRINCIPAL INDICATIONS ACCORDING TO TERRAIN:

1) WATER — edema, oliguria, ascites, glomerulonephritis, cystitis, nephrotic syndromes, osteoporosis, demineralization, pathological calcification, Paget's disease, amenorrhea, diabetes.

2) WOOD — hemorrhages, metrorrhagia, epistaxis, hematuria, spasmophilia, tetany.

3) METAL — immune deficiency, scrofulosis.

4) EARTH — diabetes, immune insufficiency, chronic rheumatism.

Horsetail is used for urinary tract infections from cold dryness or cold dampness (glomerulonephritis, cystitis) with oliguria, edema and ascites. It is prescribed for amenorrhea and for problems with bone mineralization, such as osteoporosis and Paget's disease. A diuretic, it is good for treating nephrotic syndromes and nightsweats due to vacuity of Kidney yang (hypoadrenalism). It has also been found beneficial for kidney stones and is used generally for kidney afflictions, edema and ulceration of the bladder and the urinary passages.

Applied externally, it will stop the bleeding of wounds and quickly heal them. It is good for nervousness in a Water yin terrain and is useful for tissue regeneration. Partly due to its high silica content, it is considered especially beneficial to the nails and skin and for promoting lymphatic drainage Traditionally, it was used in the treatment of tuberculosis.

Internally, it can be used to treat hematemesis and bleeding during pregnancy. As a gargle, it is useful for treating aphthous ulcers. As a foot bath, it is good for excessively damp feet.

Chinese medicine considers horsetail to be sweet, slightly bitter and neutral in temperature, and to influence the Lung, Liver and Gallbladder systems. Its functions include clearing wind heat, calming eye spasms, muscle spasms and inflammation and promoting diuresis. In combination with chrysanthemum flower and other herbs, its primary use in China is to treat eye afflictions, acute conjunctivitis with corneal opacity, acute dacry-ocystitis and swelling of the eyelids.

Horsetail is also used for "smoothing" the liver (spasmophilia). The Russians use horsetail as a diuretic and for cardiac edema. It is used there for liver conditions, and has been used experimentally to chelate lead from the system.

Only the barren stems are used medicinally.

MADDER *Rubia tinctorum*

ACTIONS: Salidiuretic, azoturic, laxative.

CONSTITUENTS: Anthraquinone heterosides, ruberythric acid, galiosine, munjistine, purpuroxanthine; citric, tartaric and malic acids.

FAMILY: Rubiaceae.

FLAVORS: Sweet-warming, pungent-warming.

FIVE PHASE CATEGORY: Water yin.

PRINCIPAL INDICATIONS ACCORDING TO TERRAIN:

1) WATER — osteoporosis, demineralization, oliguria, nephrotic syndromes, chronic glomerulonephritis, chronic renal insufficiency, renal calculi, arterial hypertension.

The root of madder reddens the bones of animals who eat it, hence the name "rubia." Hippocrates prescribed it as a diuretic. It is azoturic in proteinuria and hypotensive. Prescribed in nephrotic syndromes and in chronic glomerulonephritis, as well as chronic renal insufficiency, it is very useful for phosphocalcic kidney stones. Because of its choleretic effect, it has laxative properties. It is also antibacterial and antifungal for urinary infections. An emmenagogue, it has been employed by the Arabs for centuries to facilitate childbirth. Madder is reputed to be effective in amenorrhea, jaundice and edema. It is also a useful treatment for osteoporosis in the Water yin terrain.

MOUSE EAR *Hieracium pilosella*

ACTIONS: Salidiuretic, azoturic, anti-infectious (Enterococcus, brucella).

CONSTITUENTS: Mucilage, tannins, umbelliferone, flavones, resin, manganese.

FAMILY: Compositae.

FLAVORS: Bitter-warming, sour-cooling.

FIVE PHASE CATEGORIES: Water yin, Earth yin, Wood yang.

PRINCIPAL INDICATIONS ACCORDING TO TERRAIN:

  1) WATER — asthenia, oliguria, edema, renal insufficiency.

  2) EARTH — chronic rheumatism, epistaxis, brucellosis.

  3) WOOD — uremia, biliary insufficiency, myopia; to strengthen the eyesight.

The name *Hieracium* derives from the Greek word *Hierax,* or "sparrowhawk," because it was believed that this bird sucked the juice of the plant to sharpen its vision. Indeed, traditionally it was said that drinking the fresh juice would improve vision. Collected in May and June when in flower, it was dried and powdered and applied externally for epistaxis.

Mouse ear is administered in the treatment of water retention and obesity. It can be prescribed as a diuretic for oliguria, edema, renal and cardiorenal insufficiency with hypertension, and uremia. It has anti-inflammatory properties, and is also useful in asthenia and cellulitis. Its warming energy dries out excessive dampness of the Spleen and Kidney. It exerts a tonic action on the heart and on the kidney yang. A choleretic and cholagogue, it lowers the blood cholesterol level.

SEA HOLLY *Eryngium campestre*

ACTIONS: Salidiuretic, azoturic.

CONSTITUENTS: Saponins, essential oil, mineral salts (potassium, sodium, calcium).

FAMILY: Umbelliferae.

FLAVORS: Salty-warming.

FIVE PHASE CATEGORY: Water yin.

PRINCIPAL INDICATIONS ACCORDING TO TERRAIN:

1) WATER — edema, oliguria, ascites, nephrotic colic, urinary calculi, chronic glomerulonephritis, nephrotic syndromes, jaundice, amenorrhea, frigidity, impotence, aphrodisiac activity.

The root of the sea holly is harvested in autumn, dug from plants that are at least two years old. Traditional lore maintained that it helped with "melancholy of the heart." Boerhaave, a Danish physician, recommended sea holly for bladder diseases and for maintaining good health of the kidney.

One of the best plants for oliguria, edema and renal insufficiency with uremia and ascites, it is used for nephrotic colic, chronic glomerulonephritis and other nephrotic syndromes. It clears up uric acid deposits. Additionally, it is an emmenagogue with a reputation as an aphrodisiac, and useful for frigidity and impotence. It can be prescribed in the treatment of jaundice. It promotes expectoration, and is also administered in cases of paralysis and chronic nervous disorders.

YARROW *Achillea millefolium*

ACTIONS: Spasmolytic (sympatholytic and vagolytic), anti-inflammatory, luteotropic, astringent, diaphoretic, immune stimulant.

CONSTITUENTS: Essential oil (cineol, eugenol, proazulene), resin, tannins, glycosides, quercetin, caffeic acid, salicylic acid, camphor, bitter principle (achilleine), organic acids, potassium, phosphorus, azotic substances. Among the 120 or so chemical compounds that have been isolated from yarrow, the sesquiterpene lactones, flavonoids, chamazulene and the alkaloid achilleine are considered to be responsible for most of its medicinal properties.

FAMILY: Compositae.

FLAVORS: Sour-cooling, bitter-warming.

FIVE PHASE CATEGORIES: Water yin, Wood yang, Fire yang.

PRINCIPAL INDICATIONS ACCORDING TO TERRAIN:

1) WATER — enuresis, lithiasis, glomerulonephritis, nephrotic syndromes, intermittent fevers, auto-immune disorders, bronchial asthma, amyloidosis, diabetes, dysmenorrhea, amenorrhea, sequela of terror; stimulates the testicles, luteotropic action.

2) WOOD — diarrhea, biliary lithiases, renal lithiases, arthritis, gout, hemorrhoids, allergic asthma, allergic rhinitis, varicose veins, heavy leg, amenorrhea or insufficient menstrual flow, dysmenorrhea.

3) FIRE — menopausal disorders, arteriosclerosis.

4) EARTH — intestinal spasms, gastritis, enteritis, gastric ulcers, diarrhea.

According to legend, the association of *Achillea* with Achilles is because of the account by Gerard which tells us that Achilles used yarrow to stanch the bleeding wounds of his soldiers. In ancient times it was referred to as *herba militaris,* and during World War I it was used as an emergency hemostatic.

It stops intestinal or pulmonary hemorrhage, is a vasodilator of cutaneous blood vessels, helps to restore the elasticity of blood vessel walls and lowers peripheral resistance. It is excellent for uterine bleeding, since it is antihemorrhagic and stimulates progesterone production. A stimulant to the veins, it is used for thrombotic conditions of the veins. A mild aromatic decoction of the whole yarrow plant is useful for bleeding piles.

Yarrow inhibits the formation of arterial plaque. It is a pelvic decongestant for the treatment of cervicitis and endometritis. An immune stimulant, it catalyzes the activity of the bone marrow. In general, it is also good for kidney disorders. With its warm and cold properties and activity on the kidney, it is prescribed for urinary calculi and for gout as well as for inter-mittent fevers. It is indicated for nephrotic syndromes, amylosis, autoim-mune disorders, chronic glomerulonephritis, oliguria, enuresis and for amenorrhea from cold or from great fright or terror.

Yarrow has been used traditionally for dispelling melancholia. English herbalists have used it for stomach cramps and loss of appetite. In France it is used for gallstones because of its choleretic action. Russian herbalists have also used it for gastric ulcers, inflammation, dysentery, colds and coughs. It is especially good for colds at their onset. It expels gas from the stomach and is good for diarrhea in infants. It is reputed to prevent bald-ness if the head is washed with it.

SHORT PROFILES OF OTHER COMMONLY USED PLANTS

(alphabetically listed)

Arnica	Belladonna	Bistorte	Blackberry
Black Horehound	Blessed Thistle	Boldo	Bryonia
Buckthorn	Butcher's Broom	Calendula	Canadian Fleabane
Celery	Cherry	Colchicum	Combretum
Cramp Bark	Datura	Digitalis	Drosera
Ephedra	False Hellebore	Gelsemium	Goat Rue
Groundsel	Hellebore	Henbane	Hepatica
Honeysuckle	Hops	Horseradish	Ivy
Kelp	Khella	Lespedeza	Lily, White
Lily-of-the-Valley	Lotus	Lycopus	Maize
Menyanthe	Mulberry	Mullein	Oat, Wild
Olive	Opium	Orthosiphon	Pellitory-of-the-Wall
Poppy, Red	Raspberry	Rauwolfia	Sand Spurry
Scarlet Pimpernel	Senna	Snakeroot	Star anise
Violet	Woundwort		

ARNICA *(Arnica montana):* Earth yang. Vulnerary, anti-inflammatory, spas-molytic, nerve sedative, cholagogue, cerebral stimulant, anticoagulant. Useful for treating peripheral neuropathy and its pain in diabetes. Arnica is a histamine antagonist at the level of the muscles. It is indicated for states of nervous hyperexcitability (central and medullar), and for neurological afflictions such as toxic polyneuritis, neurotoxic side effects of pharmaceuticals, poliomyelitis, syringomyelitis, amyotrophic lateral sclerosis, multiple sclerosis and various types of coma (hyper-glycemic, hyperthermic, hypothermic, azotemic). Arnica tincture clears damp phlegm and can be used with maize for gout crises. It is also use-ful for vomiting and aqueous diarrhea. It disperses blood heat, and has been used popularly as an abortifacient and as an emmenagogue. As an emmenagogue, it is useful for a Spleen yang constitution with obesity and an excess of dampness, and for hyperluteal amenorrhea. The mother tincture is toxic in a dose greater than 30 drops a day. Arnica is used in a higher dilution and homeopathically in treating nervous system disorders. A good bactericide and fungicide, it will treat dermatological infections. Arnica is contraindicated for pregnancy.

BELLADONNA *(Atropa belladonna):* Earth yin, Metal yin. Vagolytic. It opposes the muscarinic effects of acetylcholine. As it is highly toxic, it must be used allopathically in a low dose and with respect to its contraindications. Containing the alkaloid atropine, it dilates the pupils, increases heart rate, elevates blood pressure and inhibits secretions of salivary, gastric, intestinal and sweat glands. It relaxes the smooth muscles of the stomach, intestines, bladder and gallbladder, and dilates the bronchial tubes. It can be a useful adjunct to botanical treatment of visceral spasms, asthma, pertussis, spastic constipation, hypersudation and urinary incontinence. Effects of overdose are sympathotonic: tachycardia, dryness of the mouth, retention of urine, flaccid constipation, hyperthermia, hallucinations, delirium, then coma with tremor and convulsions. Contraindications are glaucoma, prostate hypertrophy, cardiac or coronary insufficiency, hypertension and paralytic ileus.

BISTORT *(Polygonum bistorte):* Earth yin, Water yin, Metal yin. A powerful tonic, astringent, antihemorrhagic, antimycotic. As an astringent, bistort is used for diarrhea, hemorrhoids, leukorrhea and metrorrhagia. It is a pelvic decongestant, especially with mycoses of the pelvic organs. As an Earth yin herb it is used for stomatitis, aphthous ulcers, splenomegaly and diabetic polydipsia. As a Metal yin and Water yin herb, it is used to treat tuberculosis, bronchitis with abundant secretions, pharyngitis, intermittent fevers, prostate congestion, urethritis and enuresis.

BLACKBERRY *(Rubus fructicosus):* Earth yang. Hypoglycemiant, astringent, antithrombotic, hemostatic, anti-inflammatory (buds). Blackberry leaves and stems are used as an extract or mother tincture for throat infections including streptococcus. They have a strong effect on draining the tonsils and are used for pancreatic drainage. As a gemmotherapy extract, it is used for senile osteoporosis and as an anti-inflammatory for arthritis. As a mother tincture or decoction it is used for the treatment of diabetes. Its hypoglycemiant effect is because it drains the pancreas. It is effective for leukorrhea due to dampness of the Spleen. As a mouthwash it is good for glossitis, stomatitis and aphthous ulcers.

BLACK HOREHOUND *(Ballota fetida, Ballota nigra):* Wood yang, Fire yang. Sympatholytic, parasympathomimetic, antispasmodic, sedative. Treats symptoms of Liver Fire and its subsequent transformation to Heart Fire. Used for tachycardia, neurotonic conditions, irritability, anxiety, phobias, instability, insomnia, hysterical hearing loss, psychological problems of menopause, spasmophilia and paroxysms of pertussis.

BLESSED THISTLE *(Cnicus benedictus):* Earth yin, Metal yin. Vagolytic, febrifuge, anti-inflammatory, antirheumatic, eupeptic, galactagogue, diuretic (volumetric and uricosuric), sudorific. Blessed thistle has antibiotic activity against brucellosis, colibacilloses and klebsiella.

Excellent for migraine headaches and as a mild cardiac stimulant, it is used as well to treat anorexia, arthritis, neuritis, depression, memory loss, nervous obsessions, melancholia and insomnia in an Earth yin or Metal yin type of constitution where there is indication of poor nourishment, splenomegaly or lymphadenitis.

BOLDO *(Peumus boldus):*   Wood yang.   Choleretic, cholagogue, hypnotic. Used for liver drainage.   Boldo is used as a digestive aid by Chilean Indians.   It possesses a remarkable effect of draining engorged bile ducts. It stimulates digestion and bile secretion, and is used to treat biliary and urinary tract stones.   Very effective for insomnia of a Wood yang nature.

BRYONIA *(Bryonia dioica):*   Metal yin, Earth yin.   Powerful purgative, cholagogue, expectorant, antirheumatismal.   Bryonia is highly toxic, and a violent purgative.   It has a warming effect on such conditions as bronchorrhea, pulmonary congestion, polyarthritis, ankylosing spondylitis, cold vacuity chronic diarrhea due to malabsorption, chronic infections, rectocolitis, Crohn's disease and the like.   Its purgative properties are useful in treating pleurisy, pneumonia, peritonitis, pericarditis or pertussis in the Metal yin and Earth yin constitutions.   Overdose of bryonia can result in intestinal hemorrhage, or choleriform diarrhea if ingested by a patient with a damp heat condition.

BUCKTHORN *(Rhamnus frangula):*   Metal yin, Earth yin.   Cholagogue, laxative, purgative.   Buckthorn is a gentle laxative that is used for stomach pain, nausea, vomiting and constipation.   It is suitable for children or people with weak intestines.

BUTCHER'S BROOM *(Ruscus aculeatus):*   Wood Yang, Water yang.   Pelvic decongestant, diuretic (volumetric and natriuric), venotonic, vasoconstrictor (arterial and venous), anti-inflammatory, antiedematous.   Butcher's broom is used to treat prostate hypertrophy, prostatitis, gynecological infections (especially salpingitis), hemorrhoids, urinary tract infections and arteritis.

CALENDULA *(Calendula officinalis):*   Earth yang, Earth yin.   Antispasmodic (parasympathomimetic), sudorific, emmenagogue, hypotensive, vulnerary, uterolytic, oxytocic, adrenal cortex stimulant (internal), antiseptic, anti-inflammatory (especially digestive mucosa), epitheliogenic (external or internal), estrogenic (external).   Calendula is useful externally in all of the dermatoses: staphylococcus infections, furuncles, anthrax, acne, diabetic skin infections and warts. It is one of the best vulnerary antiseptics. For internal use, its Earth yang functions are hypotensive and vasodilating, for gastric ulcers due to Stomach heat, dysmenorrhea from blood heat or blood vacuity; it is choleretic, relieving high estrogen levels in Liver depression.   Its Earth yin functions include treatment of gastric ulcers, dysmenorrhea and tumors.   Calendula has anticancer properties. It is emmenagogic, oxytocic and uterolytic.

CANADIAN FLEABANE *(Erigeron canadensis):*   Water yin, Water yang, Earth yin. Antidiarrheic, diuretic (salidiuretic, volumetric, uricosuric), pelvic decongestant, antirheumatic, anti-inflammatory, astringent.   Canadian fleabane is useful for treating chronic nephrotic syndromes, glomerulonephritis with proteinuria, chronic diarrhea, leukorrhea and metrorrhagia. It has been used in Canada as a vermifuge and an antihemorrhagic. It is helpful for rheumatic pain. The essential oil contains human growth hormone.

CELERY *(Apium graveolens):* Water yin, Wood yin. Diuretic (salidiuretic), eupeptic, choleretic. Celery is used to treat oliguria, kidney stones, albuminuria, uremia, edema and ascites in the feeble Water yin constitution. Since the Middle Ages it has been administered to treat melancholia. It is also used for chronic respiratory insufficiency as in asthma and emphysema. It gently drains the liver, so that the patient is not overwhelmed with detoxification, but it improves liver function in a patient with chronic weakness in the liver and kidney systems.

CHERRY (CHERRY LAUREL) *(Prunus cerasus):* Water yin, Water yang. Diuretic, laxative. An extract from the stems is used to treat obesity, hypertension and rheumatism in the heavier yang type, but also hypertension with edema, renal insufficiency and cardiac insufficiency in the yin constitution.

COLCHICUM *(Colchicum autumna):* Earth yin. Peripheral analgesic. Also called meadow saffron, colchicum is used for gout crises and peripheral neuralgia. It has antiviral properties, but is highly toxic.

COMBRETUM *(Combretum raimbaultii, Combretum micranthum):* Wood yang. Cholagogue, choleretic, diuretic. Combretum (kinkeliba) is used for constipation, to clear gallstones and in the treatment of cirrhosis of the liver. It is a powerful cholagogue of last resort, used in gastrointestinal and respiratory infections and in the complications of mumps, such as orchitis or pancreatitis. A species of combretum is used to treat opium addiction in China.

CRAMP BARK *(Viburnum opulus):* Wood yang, Fire yin. Parasympathomimetic, sympatholytic, hemostatic, antispasmodic (musculotrope). Cramp bark is used for the pain of dysmenorrhea, threatened abortion (or other endometrial hemorrhage), arteriosclerosis and tachycardia.

DATURA *(Datura alba, Datura stramonium):* Water yin, Metal yin. Strongly vagolytic, sedative, hypnotic, antalgic. Toxic, it should be administered knowledgeably. Used like henbane. It has been used for Parkinson's disease and asthma. It contains the same alkaloids hyoscyamine, scopolamine and atropine that give the herb its anticholinergic properties. Traditionally, the powdered leaf was smoked in asthma powders, which were administered to relieve bronchial spasms. Scopolamine is hallucinogenic.

DIGITALIS *(Digitalis purpurea):* Fire yin. Cardiotonic, diuretic. Digitalis is used to treat arterial hypotension, cardiac insufficiency, arrhythmia and tachycardia. The contraindications for digitalis are Basedow's disease, cerebral hemorrhage, neurotonia and any condition of repletion of Heart yang or blood heat. As it is highly toxic, it should be administered with care.

DROSERA *(Drosera rotundifolia):* Metal yin. Antispasmodic, vagolytic, antibiotic, antitussive. Drosera alleviates vagotonic bronchial spasms. It is one of the best remedies for cough and is used for pertussis, laryngitis, chronic bronchitis, and asthma.

EPHEDRA *(Ephedra vulgaris, et al):* Wood yin, Fire yin, Metal yin, Water yang, Water yin. Sympathomimetic, diaphoretic, vasoconstrictor, bronchodilator, adrenal medulla stimulant, volumetric diuretic. Ephedra has been used in classical Chinese medicine as a diaphoretic for acute stages of bronchopulmonary diseases, for acute episodes of dyspnea and as a diuretic for edematous and arthritic conditions. In Europe it is used for respiratory problems and for cardiac disorders such as hypotension and bradycardia. Misuse or careless prescription of ephedra exposes the patient to the unpleasant side effects of its potential toxicity.

FALSE HELLEBORE *(Adonis vernalis):* Fire yin. Cardiotonic, diuretic (salidiuretic, azoturic). Also called adonis, false hellebore is used to treat chronic cardiopathy, valvulopathy, myocarditis, pericarditis, arrhythmias and cardiorenal insufficiency. Like digitalis and strophanthus, it slows the heart rate, reinforces the cardiac tonus and accelerates the speed of conduction. It is toxic and the daily adult dose should be limited to 60 drops a day of the mother tincture.

GELSEMIUM *(Gelsemium sempervirens):* Wood yang. Parasympathomimetic, emmenagogue, antimigraine, sedative. Gelsemium is effective for treating tics, neuralgia, menstrual pain, asthma and allergic rhinitis. It is specifically effective for facial neuralgia. Toxic to the respiratory system in a strong dose, the daily dose of the mother tincture of gelsemium root should not exceed one gram.

GOAT RUE *(Galega officinalis):* Earth yang. Diuretic (volumetric), sudorific, hypoglycemiant. Stimulates the secretion of pituitary gonadotropins and prolactin. Goat rue is used as a hypoglycemiant to treat diabetes. It stimulates prolactin production in the pituitary and activates pancreatic function, and is also used to treat circulatory problems like arteritis and arteriosclerosis.

GROUNDSEL *(Senecio vulgaris):* Earth yin, Metal yin. Parasympathomimetic, astringent, expectorant, emollient, emmenagogue. Through its cholinergic activity, groundsel is a uterine sedative. It is useful for amenorrhea in women who have blood vacuity, anemia or low estrogen levels. If taken over a prolonged period of time, it is toxic to the liver.

HELLEBORE *(Veratrum album):* Wood yang, Fire yang, Earth yang, Water yang, Wood yin. Hypotensive, analgesic, sedative. Hellebore is used in serious cases of hypertension such as eclampsia. It exerts its influence on the carotid sinus rather than on the blood vessels. It is considered to be a specific for hyperthyroidism (Basedow's) and the resulting trembling, spasmophilia or chorea. Hellebore has a strong relaxing effect on striated muscles. Leclerc reported its effectiveness for paranoid schizophrenia and the incoherent soliloquies of melancholia. It has also been used for manic episodes. It was once given to thieves to extinguish aggressiveness and combativeness. The hypotensive action of hellebore is not due to any influence on the blood vessels or ganglions, but on the vasoregulating centers of the carotid sinus. Hellebore is also hypothermic. Once called "vegetal arsenic," hellebore is quite toxic. Nausea is a sign of toxicity. Maximum adult dose is 50 drops per day of the mother tincture.

HENBANE (Hyoscyamus niger): Water yin, Metal yin. Vagolytic, sedative, hypnotic, antineuralgic. Henbane is used almost identically to datura (*Datura alba, Datura stramonium*). Containing the alkaloids atropine, hyoscyamine and scopolamine, it is a central nervous system sedative useful for anxiety, depression, agitation and alcoholic delirium. Because of its influence on the extrapyramidal nervous system, it is useful for the treatment of chorea and tremor of Parkinsonism. It is used for asthma and for bronchial, gastric, intestinal and vascular spasms because of its vagolytic activity. Externally it is used for rheumatic pain, especially neuritis. Oil of henbane combines with belladonna, black nightshade (*Solanum nigrum*), *Datura stramonium*, essential oils of lavender, peppermint, rosemary and thyme, and a base oil such as olive to make "tranquil balm." For internal use, all the precautions in using belladonna should be observed, as it has toxic effects if prescribed incorrectly.

HEPATICA (Hepatica nobilis): Wood yang, Wood yin. Diuretic, astringent, emollient. Hepatica is indicated for biliary and urinary stones. It is said to nourish the nerves in the treatment of degenerative nerve disorders such as multiple sclerosis, medullar degeneration, neuralgic amyotrophy, peripheral neuropathy and collagenoses. Toxic in high doses, the maximum adult dose is 30-50 drops per day of mother tincture.

HONEYSUCKLE (Lonicera caprifolium, Lonicera periclymenum): Water yin, Fire yin. Diuretic (salidiuretic), antiseptic, sudorific, febrifuge, oxytocic. The flowers and leaves are antibiotic *in vitro* against colibacillus, staphylococcus, hemolytic streptococcus, typhus, meningococcus, pneumococcus and tubercule bacillus. It is antiviral (influenza) and antimycotic (ringworm). In classical Chinese medicine it is used to clear pathogenic heat. Clinically, it is used for tonsillitis and streptococcal infections, especially with oliguria, or complications such as pyelonephritis. Through its diuretic action, it is also effective for acute articular rheumatism. The leaves have been used to accelerate childbirth.

HOPS (Humulus lupulus): Wood yin, Earth yin. Bitter tonic, eupeptic, sympatholytic, estrogenic, antiandrogenic, febrifuge. Hops is used for anemia, gastric hyposecretion, lymphadenopathy, cervical tubercles, hepatosplenomegaly and as a sedative for insomnia. It is also used to treat eczema and herpes. Its estrogenic activity has been used to treat prostate adenoma as well as various female disorders, and its antiandrogenic properties have been used in the treatment of Stein-Leventhal syndrome in which there is an excess of androgens that results in luteal insufficiency, ovarian cysts, infertility, hirsutism, acne and adrenal hyperplasia.

HORSERADISH (Cochlearia officinalis, Cochlearia armorica): Metal yin, Earth yin. Astringent, digestive stimulant. Used for advanced cases of bronchitis and asthma with hypersecretion and dilatation of the bronchial tubes.

The vitamin C and iodine content are important factors in its beneficial effects on lymphatism and hypothyroidism. It is used for treating neuritis (especially from dampness), leukorrhea and rheumatism, and is indicated for patients suffering alternating constipation and diarrhea.

IVY *(Hedera helix):* Earth yin, Metal yin, Wood yang. Respiratory antispasmodic, cholagogue, emmenagogue (estrogenic and gonadotropin stimulating), vasoconstrictor, pelvic decongestant, anticellulite, analgesic. Ivy is used for acute bronchitis in adults, chronic bronchitis, laryngitis, tracheitis and pertussis. As a vasoconstrictor it is used for phlebitis and digestive hemorrhage. It is useful for the pain of dysmenorrhea, neuropathies and rheumatism, and is effective for removing cellulite from the pelvic area.

KELP *(Laminaria saccharina):* Earth yin, Metal yin, Water yin. Glandular stimulant, remineralizer. Also known as *kombu,* laminaria is used to treat obesity and cellulite by nourishing the thyroid function. It is also used for retarded development. Rich in minerals, it is a nutrient for various deficiencies and useful in treating anorexia, emaciation, asthenia, lymphatism, anemia, frigidity and impotence. It strengthens a weak constitution in treating chronic complaints like asthma, emphysema, sinusitis, arthritis, collagenoses, chronic dermatoses, amenorrhea, oligomenorrhea, hypothyroidism, polyneuritis and paralysis. It is a useful adjunct for treating autoimmune disorders and degenerative diseases, including cancer.

KHELLA *(Amni visnaga):* Wood yang, Fire yang, Water yang. Sympatholytic, vagolytic, antispasmodic (smooth muscles), diuretic (volumetric and urinary antispasmodic), coronary dilator. An antispasmodic agent used for renal colic and cardiac arrhythmia.

LESPEDEZA *(Lespedeza capitata):* Water yang, Water yin. Diuretic (uricosuric), hypoglycemiant. Lespedeza lowers levels of uric acid and blood sugar. It is also used for uremia with oliguria of chronic nephritis.

LILY, WHITE *(Nymphea alba):* Wood yang, Fire yang, Water yang. Sympatholytic and vagolytic, anticonvulsive, antispasmodic, astringent, hypnotic and anaphrodisiac. White lily is used for insomnia, excessive sexual excitation, convulsions from cortical hyperexcitation, cystalgia and pyelonephritis. It calms Liver Fire, Heart Fire and the hyperadrenalism of anxiety states.

LILY-OF-THE-VALLEY *(Convallaria majalis):* Wood yang, Fire yang, Fire yin, Water yin. Antispasmodic, sympatholytic, cardiotonic, diuretic (salidiuretic). Lily-of-the-valley is mainly used to treat extrasystoles, neurotonic tachycardia, arrhythmias, arterial hypotension, valvulopathies, anxiety and cardiac disorders related to hyperthyroidism. It slows down and reinforces the strength of heart contractions. It should be prescribed knowledgeably to avoid potential toxicity.

LOTUS *(Lotus corniculatus):* Fire yang. Antispasmodic, central nervous system sedative. Lotus is used to treat tachycardia, anxiety, depression, insomnia. It is sympatholytic and musculotropic and a neurotropic antispasmodic.

LYCOPUS *(Lycopus europaeus):* Fire yang. Thyroid inhibitor, pituitary inhibitor (TSH, gonadotropins, prolactin), sympatholytic. Lycopus is also known as wolfstrap or gypsy weed. It is used to treat tachycardia and arrhythmias, especially when associated with hyperthyroidism. It has a hormonal influence in treating various prostate and ovarian disorders.

MAIZE *(Zea mays):* Earth yang, Earth yin, Water yang, Water yin. Diuretic (volumetric, azoturic, uricosuric, natriuric), choleretic, cholagogue, TSH inhibitor, hypocholesterolemiant, hypoglycemiant. Extracts of cornsilk are diuretic and are used to relieve the pain of rheumatism and gout. As a diuretic, it is also useful for nephritis, cardiac insufficiency and edema. Maize is used to treat obesity, high cholesterol and arterial hypertension. The germ oil of maize inhibits the development of arterial plaque. It has a strong influence on the pancreatic-duodenal junction and is used to treat hepatitis and cholecystitis.

MENYANTHE *(Menyanthes trifoliata):* Earth yin, Metal yin. Bitter tonic, sympathomimetic, vagolytic, emmenagogue, diaphoretic. Like gentian, menyanthe is both vagolytic and sympathomimetic. It is used to treat dyspepsia, aerophagia, intestinal swelling, gastritis, anorexia and postprandial headaches. As a diaphoretic, it is used to treat intermittent fevers and acute viral infections. It is indicated for amenorrhea in women with vacuity of the blood or the Spleen.

MULBERRY, BLACK *(Morus nigra):* Earth yang. Hypoglycemiant, astringent. Black mulberry is used almost exclusively as a hypoglycemiant for the treatment of diabetes. It influences the endocrine functions of the pancreas (insulin secretion of the Islets of Langerhans).

MULLEIN *(Verbascum thapsus):* Fire yin, Earth yin, Fire yang, Water yin. Sympatholytic, vagolytic, papaverine-like smooth muscle relaxant, digitalis-like cardiotonic, anti-inflammatory of the respiratory and gastrointestinal mucosa, antispasmodic (musculotrope and neurotrope), emollient, sudorific, diuretic. Mullein is used for gastrointestinal inflammations such as gastritis and pancreatitis, for gastrointestinal spasms, to fluidify bronchial secretions and as a cardiotonic for tachycardia and arrhythmias. It can be used externally as a compress for earaches in acute otitis media.

OAT, WILD *(Avena sativa):* Metal yin. Thyroid stimulant, estrogen stimulant, hypolipemiant, hypoglycemiant. It treats osteoporosis, not only as a remineralizer, but also as a hormone regulator. It is used for asthenia and weight loss in diabetes, for hypothyroidism of the Metal yin constitution, anemia and anorexia. Wild oat stimulates sexual organ function in cases of impotence, luteal insufficiency and infertility. It is also useful for calming tachycardia and insomnia in the asthenic Metal yin type.

OLIVE *(Olea europaea):* Earth yang. Sympatholytic, hypotensor, hypoglycemiant, hypolipemiant, diuretic (volumetric and azoturic), coronary vasodilator; used for drainage of the biliary ducts and the pancreas. Extracts from the leaves and the bark are used to treat diabetes and associated vascular pathology. It is often used to protect the heart from coronary occlusion and to reverse arteriosclerosis. It is also used to treat uremia and arterial hypertension.

OPIUM POPPY *(Papavera somniferum):* Metal yang. Sympatholytic, antiarrhythmic, narcotic, analgesic, central nervous system depressant. Opium contains numerous alkaloids and is subject to restrictions in Europe, although not as severely as in the U.S. Its sedative and depressant actions have most often been utilized for severe coughs and for diarrhea. As a narcotic it has traditionally been used for all types of pain. One of its alkaloids, papaverine, relaxes smooth muscles, especially of the biliary and digestive systems. As an aerosol, it alleviates the bronchial spasms of asthma. Papaverine is also a vasodilator of the cerebral arteries and the genitals. Its potential toxicity recommends its prescription by a competent practitioner.

ORTHOSIPHON *(Orthosiphon stamineus):* Wood yang, Water yang, Fire yang. Cholagogue, diuretic (salidiuretic, uricosuric, azoturic), lowers cholesterol. Orthosiphon is used for urinary tract infections, uremia, obesity, gallstones, arthritis and gout. It is also used for obesity and edema associated with obesity.

PELLITORY-OF-THE-WALL *(Parietaria officinalis):* Wood yang, Water yang. Diuretic (salidiuretic, azoturic), emollient. Pellitory-of-the-wall is used for stones, both biliary and urinary. It reduces swelling of the bladder and is used to treat glomerulonephritis, pyelonephritis, cystitis, hemorrhoids, eclampsia, acute rheumatism and skin infections.

POPPY, RED *(Papavera rhoeas):* Metal yang, Fire yang. Vagolytic, antispasmodic, sedative, antitussive. Red poppy calms smooth muscle spasms, drains lymph congestion, and is useful for treatment of coughs, fevers, insomnia and excitability. It is particularly indicated for insomnia of children and the elderly, but it is useful for all ages. Also a pelvic decongestant.

RASPBERRY *(Rubus idaeus):* Water yin. Salidiuretic, laxative, antithrombotic, antihemorrhagic. Raspberry leaves are also astringent. They are good for flaccid constipation and are safe for pregnancy. In fact, they are often used before and during pregnancy to enrich the blood with iron and to improve pelvic circulation. Raspberry is one of the few laxative herbs safe for constipation during pregnancy. Useful for dysmenorrhea, aphthous ulcers, tonsillitis, oliguria and anemia.

RAUWOLFIA *(Rauwolfia serpentina):* Fire yang, Water yang. Sympatholytic, adrenolytic, central nervous system sedative. Commonly known as Indian snakeroot, it is the source of the alkaloid reserpine, which was the first pharmaceutical tranquilizer. It is used for hypertension in sympathotonic subjects. Rauwolfia slows the heart rate and is effective for calming atrial fibrillation without affecting renal drainage, and is also useful for acute states of anxiety and excitation. In Ayurvedic medicine it is prescribed as a treatment for snakebite as well as a sedative. Other uses include as a febrifuge, antiepileptic and for diarrhea. To avoid the potential of toxic side effects, it should be administered by a knowledgeable practitioner.

SAND SPURRY *(Arenaria rubra):* Water yang. Diuretic (volumetric, uricosuric). Used for acute nephritic colic. It is an excellent herb for the elimination of uric acid.

SCARLET PIMPERNEL *(Anagallis arvensis):* Wood yang, Wood yin, Fire yin, Water yin, Earth yin. Antispasmodic, estrogenic, salidiuretic, mycostatic, diaphoretic. Scarlet pimpernel is used for nephrotic syndromes, for ascites, bronchorrhea and for digestive, respiratory or cutaneous mycoses. It is also a mild cardiac stimulant and has been used for right-sided cardiac insufficiency and depression. Other indications include rhinitis, allergic asthma and hepatic insufficiency. It is toxic and should not be given to an adult at a dose exceeding 45 drops per day of the mother tincture.

SENNA *(Cassia angustifolia):* Metal yang, Water yang. Purgative. Senna purges the bowel by means of inhibiting the reabsorption of water from the colon, and by stimulating peristalsis. It is contraindicated for intestinal inflammation, pelvic congestion or pregnancy.

SNAKEROOT *(Aristolochia clematitis):* Earth yin, Metal yin. Emmenagogue (stimulates FSH), oxytocic, anti-inflammatory. Aristolochia comes from the Greek words meaning "better labor." It is useful in obstetrics for delayed or protracted labor, and can also be used for amenorrhea or dysmenorrhea with muscular pains. Snakeroot increases the phagocytic power of leukocytes and is useful for infections of the reproductive system. It is prescribed for asthma in a Metal yin constitution.

STAR ANISE *(Illicium verum):* Earth yin. Carminative, eupeptic. Star anise has very similar functions to green anise and is sometimes used in its place.

VIOLET *(Viola tricolor):* Wood yang, Metal yin. Diuretic (volumetric), laxative, depurative, diaphoretic, anticoagulant, antipruritic. Violet is frequently used for treating skin problems, for example, juvenile acne, herpes, urticaria, eczematous varicose ulcers, chronic psoriasis and eczema. It is a tonic to the venous system, and is effective for treating hemorrhoids, phlebitis and constipation. It has antiallergic and anti-inflammatory properties and also treats arthritis and rheumatism with oliguria.

WHITE HELLEBORE *(Veratrum album):* See HELLEBORE.

WILD OAT: See OAT, WILD.

WOUNDWORT *(Stachys palustris and Stachys sylvatica):* Wood yang. Strong emmenagogue; oxytocic, sympatholytic, parasympathomimetic, antispasmodic, hypotensive, sedative. Woundwort treats dysmenorrhea, amenorrhea, ovaritis, metritis and Liver depression associated with menopause. Woundwort is oxytocic, and therefore contraindicated in pregnancy. It is useful for visceral spasms from sympathotonia and for the treatment of essential hypertension.

COMMONLY USED ESSENTIAL OILS

The essential oils profiled in this section can also be classified according to five phase categories and neuroendocrine categories. In general, they have wide-ranging properties. Because about one third of them can be classified as three or more of the five phases, they are listed here alphabetically. Certain oils do have more specific five phase tropisms, but most of them have multiple properties, both yang and yin. Many of them are also paradoxically warming and cooling. Anyone who has felt camphor or wintergreen on the skin can understand this simultaneous warming and cooling effect. Some of the oils, such as the phenolics, which are high in phenols, are quite hot. These include cinnamon, clove, savory, oregano, thyme and nutmeg. The phenolic oils should not be used topically except in small amounts as a rubefacient.

Some oils are from different parts of the same plant. For example, bitter orange, also known as bigaradier, is from the peel of *Citrus aurantium var. amara.* The essence of the young leaves and immature fruits is called *petit grain,* and the essence of the flowers is called neroli. The essence terebenthine, which means turpentine, is distilled from the resin of different species of conifers including *Pinus sylvestris*, but essence of pine is distilled exclusively from the needles of *Pinus sylvestris*.

Below is a list of the main essential oils profiled in this section with key indications to assist in familiarizing the practitioner with their use.

Profiles of Commonly Used Essential Oils

Anise (Green) — gas (aerophagia, meteorism), headaches, chest tightness.

Basil — gastrointestinal spasms, nervous fatigue.

Bitter Orange — tachycardia, insomnia, gastric spasms.

Cajeput — pulmonary, intestinal and urinary antiseptic.

Chamomile (German) — pain, digestive difficulties.

Caraway — gastric spasms, nervous stomach.

Chenopodium (Wormseed) — intestinal parasites.

Cinnamon — fatigue, weak digestion, weak libido.

Clove — fatigue, loss of memory, depression, colitis, weak libido.

Coriander — carminative, antispasmodic; anorexia.

Cypress — menstrual pain, hemorrhoids, irritability, cough.

Eucalyptus — bronchitis, sinus headache, fever.

Everlasting — expectorant, antispasmodic (coughs); contusions (external).

Fennel — sluggish digestion, gas, nervous vomiting, anorexia.

Garlic — asthma, arteriosclerosis, hypertension, parasites.

Geranium — uterine hemorrhage, gastric ulcer, fatigue.

Ginger — anorexia, poor immunity, diarrhea, fever.

Hyssop — chronic bronchitis, sinusitis, depression, leukorrhea.

Juniper — fatigue, diabetes, urinary lithiasis, gout.

Lavender — anxiety, depression, respiratory problems, headaches.

Lemon — infections, blood hyperviscosity, hemorrhage, acid stomach.

Marjoram — nervous fatigue, headaches, tachycardia, gastric pain.

Melissa (Sweet Balm) — anxiety, asthma, indigestion, vertigo.

Myrrh — astringent, disinfectant, clears phlegm.

Myrtle — chronic bronchitis or sinusitis, urinary antiseptic.

Niaouli — chronic bronchitis or sinusitis, urinary antiseptic.

Oregano — bactericidal; to fluidify bronchial secretions, diarrhea.

Peppermint — fatigue, headaches, menstrual pain, gastric spasms.

Pine — infections, impotence, asthma, bronchitis, cystitis.

Ravensare — all types of viral infections, nervousness; expectorant.

Rosemary — headaches, asthma, gallstones, vertigo, memory loss.

Sage — proestrogenic; autoimmune disorders, hepatosplenomegaly

Sandalwood — urinary tract infections, diarrhea, impotence.

Sassafras — mental fatigue, syphilis, urinary tract infections.

Savory — mental fatigue, impotence, diarrhea, gastritis, colic.

Tarragon — gastrointestinal spasms and pain, hiccups, parasites.

Terebenthine — chronic bronchitis, hemorrhage, gallstones, gout.

Thuya — pelvic decongestant, cystitis, weak immunity.

Thyme — fatigue, respiratory and intestinal infections, cough.

Ylang Ylang — hypertension, tachycardia, impotence.

ANISE (GREEN) *Pimpinella anisum*

ACTIONS: Carminative, stomachic, antispasmodic, galactagogue.

CONSTITUENTS: Anethole, choline, malic acid.

NEUROENDOCRINE PROPERTIES: Parasympatholytic, stimulates prolactin secretion.

PRINCIPAL INDICATIONS ACCORDING TO TERRAIN:

1) EARTH — stomach and intestinal pain and spasms, menstrual pain, precordial pain ("false angina"), hiccough, aerophagia, bronchial spasms, insufficient lactation, frigidity and impotence.

Earth yin in quality, green anise has a warming, sweet flavor, warming the yang of the Spleen and the Lung. It has long been used as an aperitif in alcohol extracts, including the well-known French aperitif *Pastis*. Extremely useful for intestinal and gastric pain and spasms, especially infant colic, it is also effective for menstrual pain, cardiac pain and bronchial spasms in an Earth Yin constitutional type or condition (Spleen dampness or Spleen vacuity). It is used to strengthen the libido and for insufficient lactation, and has mild diuretic properties.

Powerfully vagolytic, green anise in a strong dose is a potent analgesic, but an excessive dose is stupefying and can cause epileptiform seizures. Nine to twelve drops a day is a dose in the normal range for most indications. For chest pain and spasms, it is more effective to take a lower dose more frequently, e.g., one or two drops six times a day.

BASIL (SWEET) *Ocymum basilicum*

ACTIONS: Antispasmodic, sedative, galactagogue.

CONSTITUENTS: Essential oil contains eugenol, thymol, estragol, lineol, linalool, camphor; the leaves contain tannins.

NEUROENDOCRINE PROPERTIES: Sympatholytic, parasympatholytic, stimulates adrenal cortex.

PRINCIPAL INDICATIONS ACCORDING TO TERRAIN:

1) WATER — asthenia, anxiety, insomnia, amenorrhea, gout, paralysis.

2) EARTH — dyspepsia, gastric spasms, indigestion, intestinal infections, headaches, vertigo, epilepsy, neuritis, amenorrhea; to delay onset of childbirth.

3) METAL — whooping cough, intestinal infections, anosmia, amenorrhea.

Originally from India, basil is used throughout the world as a culinary herb. It has been prescribed as a sedative for calming hysteria, to help nursing mothers produce milk and as an antispasmodic, particularly for gastrointestinal spasms. Pungent and sweet in flavor, it is good for afflictions related to nervousness, for example, insomnia, mental fatigue, headache and nervous disorders of the gastrointestinal tract.

BITTER ORANGE (BIGARADIER) *Citrus amara*

ACTIONS: Antispasmodic, central nervous system sedative, antisclerotic (removes arterial plaque), antihemorrhagic.

CONSTITUENTS: Geraniol, linalool, nerol, indole, jasmone, anthranylic and phenylacetic benzoic esters.

NEUROENDOCRINE PROPERTIES: Sympatholytic, thyroid inhibiting, CNS sedative.

PRINCIPAL INDICATIONS ACCORDING TO TERRAIN

1) WOOD — insomnia, anxiety, digestive spasms, chronic diarrhea.

1) FIRE —insomnia, tachycardia, palpitations, angina pectoris, epilepsy, depression, anorexia.

Wood yang and Fire yang in nature, bitter orange has a bitter-cooling flavor affecting both Liver Fire and Heart Fire. It is indicated for tachycardia (it diminishes the force of the heart's contractions), insomnia and arrhythmias. It is also useful as an antispasmodic for cases of aerophagia and gastric indigestion.

CAJEPUT *Melaleuca leucadendron*

ACTIONS: General antiseptic, antispasmodic, sedative, antiparasitic (vermifuge).

CONSTITUENTS: Cineol, pinene (levorotatory), terpineol, aldehydes, eucalyptol (50 to 60 percent).

NEUROENDOCRINE PROPERTIES: Sympatholytic, parasympatholytic, oxytocic, uterolytic.

PRINCIPAL INDICATIONS ACCORDING TO TERRAIN:

1) **METAL** — bronchitis, enteritis, dysentery, asthma, nervous vomiting, chronic laryngitis and pharyngitis

1) **WATER** — cystitis, urethritis, menstrual pain, gout, rheumatism.

Cajeput oil is Metal yin and Water yin in nature. Its flavor is pungent and warm, rendering it useful for all afflictions of the Lung or Kidney stemming from either cold vacuity or heat repletion, such as bronchitis, laryngitis, pharyngitis or asthma when there is a moderate fever, perspiration and chills. It is therapeutic for cold and vacuous conditions of the large intestine, and according to Valnet can be used to treat cystitis and urethritis.

Externally, it treats dermatoses (acne, psoriasis), dental and auricular neuralgia and rheumatism. Its antispasmodic activity when taken internally is due to its sympatholytic and vagolytic activity. It is also oxytocic.

CHAMOMILE (GERMAN) *Matricaria chamomilla*

ACTIONS: Anti-inflammatory, analgesic, antispasmodic, carminative, eupeptic, aperitif, immune stimulating, sudorific, anticoagulant.

CONSTITUENTS: Azulene (1 percent), ethers of capryllic and monilic acids.

NEUROENDOCRINE PROPERTIES: Sympatholytic, mildly proestrogenic.

PRINCIPAL INDICATIONS ACCORDING TO TERRAIN:

1) EARTH — Anemia, neuritis; strengthens immunity, improves appetite and digestion; sedative particularly for infants and small children. Externally: inflammatory conditions of skin and mucosa.

German chamomile has an Earth yin nature and is bitter and warm. It is often used externally for its anti-inflammatory properties. An important constituent, azulene, which is responsible for the blue color of the oil, has shown powerful *in vitro* bacteriostatic activity against staphylococcus, hemolytic streptococcus and proteus vulgaris. It has often been used for skin inflammations, eczema, varicose ulcers, vulvar pruritus and urticaria.

Internally, it is more frequently used in the form of an extract or an infusion, but it can also be used as an oil. It will treat repletion heat or cold in the Spleen and supplement the blood. Clinically, it is indicated for anemia, amenorrhea, leukocytosis, anorexia and neuritis pain (especially for facial neuralgia). It is not used for yang types of neuropathies such as diabetic neuropathy or gout.

Sympatholytic, German chamomile has a general calming effect on the nervous system, soothing anxiety in excitable patients. It is similar enough in action to Roman chamomile *(anthemis nobilis)* that they are often prescribed interchangeably for internal use. German chamomile has stronger anti-inflammatory properties, but is much more expensive than Roman chamomile.

CARAWAY *Carum carvi*

ACTIONS: Digestive stimulant, antispasmodic, carminative, galactagogue, emmenagogue, anthelminthic.

CONSTITUENTS: Carvone, carvene, carvacrol.

NEUROENDOCRINE PROPERTIES: Parasympatholytic, mildly proestrogenic, prolactin stimulant.

PRINCIPAL INDICATIONS ACCORDING TO TERRAIN:

1) EARTH: — digestive spasms, gastroptosis, intestinal parasites (vermifuge), amenorrhea, oligomenorrhea, insufficient lactation, indigestion.

Caraway is sweet, pungent (spicy) and warm with an Earth yin nature. It is useful for dyspepsia and intestinal parasites and supplements the yang of the Spleen (digestive tonus). An emmenagogue, it treats amenorrhea or oligomenorrhea. It relieves gastric and intestinal spasms in cases of vagotonia and is also good for aerophagia or general indigestion.

CINNAMON *Cinnamomum zeylanicun*

Actions: Sympathomimetic, adrenal cortex stimulant, carminative, astringent, antibacterial.

Constituents: Essential oil is 80 percent cinnamic aldehyde; furfural, cinnamic acid, terpenes, eugenol, methyl-amyl ketone, cinnzeylanol, cinnzeylanin, calcium oxalate, tannins. Chinese cinnamon (*cinnamomum cassia*) does not contain eugenol or methyl-amyl ketone, but is rich in cinnamic aldehyde, o-methoxycinnamic aldehyde, cinnamyl acetate, phenyl-propyl acetate, cinncassiol A, cinncassiol A 19-glucoside, cinnzeylanol, cinnzeylanin, sugars and tannins.

Neuroendocrine properties: Stimulates adrenal cortex; oxytocic, anti-spasmodic, sympathomimetic.

Principal indications according to terrain:

1) Earth — influenza, parasitosis, digestive mycosis, fatigue following an infectious illness, spastic colitis, obsessions; contracts the uterus for labor (oxytocic), stimulates sexual appetite, stimulates central nervous system.

2) Metal — influenza, hemoptysis, melancholy; stimulates psychic functions.

Antiseptic with a sweet-warming flavor, cinnamon is a stimulant of the nervous system and the intestines having an oxytocic function. It contains the phenolic eugenol, which is both antiseptic and anthelminthic. It has strong antiseptic qualities and is capable of killing typhoid bacillus. In addition, it rectifies both cold and heat of the Spleen and is prescribed for parasites, postinfectious exhaustion, colds and influenza, amenorrhea, insufficiency of the libido, colitis on the right side from cold vacuity of the Spleen and digestive mycoses and hemoptysis from cold vacuity of the Lungs. As a general stimulant, cinnamon treats psychic troubles such as obsession and melancholia. It stops vomiting, relieves flatulence and as an astringent is useful for diarrhea and for uterine hemorrhage. In Ayurveda, it is used for coughs, sinusitis, anorexia and rheumatism. *Cinnamonum cassia* is a frequent substitute.

Cinnamomum cassia is also referred to as Chinese cinnamon. It possesses many of the same qualities and constituents, but is somewhat inferior. The cassia bark yields from 1 to 2 percent of volatile oil somewhat resembling that of *Cinnamomum zeylanicum*. It is cheaper and more abundant than the Ceylon variety and is the only official oil of cinnamon in the United States and German pharmacopeias. Its market value depends on the percentage of cinnamic aldehyde that it contains. In classical Chinese medicine, *Cinnamomum cassia* is considered to enter the Heart, Lung and Bladder channels. The branch is used as an antiphlogistic, for acute onset of colds and fevers with perspiration, as an analgesic because of its warming and antispasmodic qualities, an eupeptic because of its stimulation of saliva and gastric juice secretion. It is antibacterial and antiviral, having been shown to restrain the growth of the influenza virus, and to kill ringworm *in vitro*. The bark is used to warm a frigid terrain, stimulate the immune system and endocrine functions and to stimulate digestion.

CLOVE *Eugenia caryophyllata*

ACTIONS: Oxytocic, aphrodisiac, parasympathomimetic.

CONSTITUENTS: 80 percent eugenol, acetyl-eugenol, caryophyllin (sesquiterpene), vanillin, naphthalene.

NEUROENDOCRINE PROPERTIES: Sympatholytic, parasympathomimetic, oxytocic.

PRINCIPAL INDICATIONS ACCORDING TO TERRAIN:

1) WATER — severe fatigue, anergy, depression, melancholia, loss of memory, impotence, frigidity, diarrhea from chronic maladies of the intestines, Crohn's disease, hemorrhagic rectocolitis, headaches, urinary tract infections, edema, renal insufficiency, dental caries, deafness.

2) METAL — pulmonary infections, tuberculosis, anorexia, parasites, aerocolitis, chronic diarrhea.

Clove oil is sweet-warming and pungent-warming, supplementing the Kidney yang as well as the Lung yang. It is used in the treatment of physical and psychic anergy, asthenia, depressive states, melancholia and deficiencies of the memory. It strengthens the body's immunity, and can be used as a treatment for pulmonary tuberculosis, Crohn's disease and hemorrhagic rectocolitis. It is specifically indicated for headaches, congenital deafness, and deafness due to senescence. It is prescribed for cases of edema due to renal insufficiency and is also used in preparation for childbirth. During childbirth labor it has an effect similar to oxytocin. It is also useful for impotence and frigidity.

In classical Chinese medicine it is used as an eupeptic and to warm the Kidney yang. It warms the limbs, regulates peristalsis, controls flatulence and stimulates gastric secretions. In combination with several other herbs (including fennel, atractylodes alba, codonopsis, citrus peel and raw ginger), it regulates digestive insufficiency and chronic gastroenteritis when there is abdominal pain, coldness of the hands and feet, vomiting and diarrhea It relieves chest oppression in a patient with a slow, feeble pulse. It is also used in China in some anticancer formulas.

It is antibacterial for dysentery bacillus, cholera bacillus, staphylococcus and pneumococcus. As an antibacterial it is stronger than bichloride of mercury *in vitro*. It is also antiviral against the influenza PR8 virus, and it is useful both for hiccoughs due to coldness of the stomach, and for diarrhea in weak asthenic patients.

In large doses clove is an emetic. A solution of clove used topically is effective for ringworm. It is three to four times stronger than phenol as a topical antiseptic.

CORIANDER *Coriandrum sativum*

ACTIONS: Antispasmodic, carminative, stimulant.

CONSTITUENTS: Coriandrol, geraniol, pinene, cineol, terpinene.

NEUROENDOCRINE PROPERTIES: Parasympatholytic, bulbar stimulant (medulla oblongata).

PRINCIPAL INDICATIONS ACCORDING TO TERRAIN:

1) **EARTH** — aerophagia, painful digestion, flatulence, intestinal spasms, depression.

Coriander has a flavor that is both sweet and pungent with a warming influence. Its stimulating properties have made it a choice of remedies for conditions of shock and prostration in severe diseases. There is a risk of nervous system damage and anuria if administered in too high a dose (normal dose is 1 to 3 drops two or three times daily).

A normal dose is indicated for dyspepsia, flatulence and intestinal spasms. It stimulates libido and memory and can relieve nervous system complaints such as vertigo and epileptic seizures (supplements the yin). It is also indicated for anorexia nervosa and depression.

CYPRESS *Cupressus sempervirens*

ACTIONS: Astringent, pulmonary antiseptic, bronchial antispasmodic, antisudorific and lymphatic tonic, antibacterial (gram-positive), antihemorrhagic, capillary protector, pelvic decongestant, vagolytic.

CONSTITUENTS: d-pinene, d-campene, d-sylvestrene, cymene, a ketone, sabinol (a terpenic alcohol), valerianic acid, camphor.

NEUROENDOCRINE PROPERTIES: Parasympatholytic, proestrogenic, antispasmodic.

PRINCIPAL INDICATIONS ACCORDING TO TERRAIN:

1) WOOD — hepatic infections, hepatomegaly (fatty liver), menstrual difficulties from insufficient estrogen, varices, hemorrhoids, hemorrhages, enuresis.

2) EARTH — pertussis, enuresis, hypoestrogenic insufficiency, menstrual insufficiency; calms the parasympathetic nervous system.

3) METAL — lung infections, coughs, loss of voice, hemoptysis, pertussis, enuresis; calms the parasympathetic nervous system.

Although the essential oil of cypress is primarily used, the cones or nuts of cypress are useful for treating symptoms of hepatic insufficiency, infections and hepatomegaly, in accordance with its parasympatholytic properties. It also can be used to treat dysmenorrhea and metrorrhagia from insufficient estrogen. It is administered to stop hemorrhage in cases of dysentery, hemoptysis, hematemesis, hemorrhoids and gingivitis. It acts as an antispasmodic for bronchial spasms, ovarian spasms and metrorrhagia. As a vagolytic agent and antisudorific it is used in respiratory complaints such as hemoptysis of pneumonia, spasmodic cough, loss of voice and pertussis, especially when there is lymph stagnation accompanying these conditions. It has proven utility in childhood nocturnal enuresis. Externally it has been prescribed for hemorrhoids.

EUCALYPTUS *Eucalyptus globulus*

ACTIONS: Antiseptic of the respiratory tract, astringent, hemostatic, antispasmodic, antibiotic and hypoglycemiant.

CONSTITUENTS: Eucalyptol, cineol, phellandrene, aromadendrene, eudesmol, pinene, camphene, valeric, butyric aldehydes, ethyl and amyl alcohols.

NEUROENDOCRINE PROPERTIES: Hypoglycemiant.

PRINCIPAL INDICATIONS ACCORDING TO TERRAIN:

1) **METAL** — pulmonary infections, bronchial infections, colds, influenza, complications of measles, diabetes, arteriosclerosis, hypertension.

2) **FIRE** — scarlatina, diabetic arterial hypertension and arteriosclerosis, neuralgia, headaches.

3) **EARTH** — gastric atony, diabetes, malaria, rheumatism, influenza.

4) **WATER** — urinary and kidney infections, diphtheria.

The flavor of eucalyptus and warm and slightly bitter, followed by a fresh, cool sensation. Prescribed for bronchial and pulmonary bacterial and viral infections, for colds, infections related to asthma and complications of measles, it is also used externally for sinusitis. It has a hypoglycemiant action and is used in France to treat diabetes. It is a urinary antiseptic for gram-positive (streptococcus, staphylococcus) and gram-negative bacteria (colibacillus). For therapeutic inhalations, eucalyptus is frequently combined with other oils such as pine, thyme, lavender or mint.

EVERLASTING *Helichrysum italicum*

ACTIONS: Anticoagulant, epitheliogenic, antiviral, expectorant.

CONSTITUENTS: Terpenes and sesquiterpenes (almost 50 percent sesquiterpenes).

NEUROENDOCRINE PROPERTIES: Vagolytic, sympatholytic, antispasmodic (musculotrope).

PRINCIPAL INDICATIONS ACCORDING TO TERRAIN:

1) **METAL** — expectorant for respiratory phlegm congestion, pertussis, bronchitis, acute respiratory viral infections.

2) **FIRE** — topical epitheliogenic, dissolves hematomas, scar tissue, antisclerotic, stimulates growth of new tissue, bruises, contusions, pelvic decongestant, dysmenorrhea, bartholinitis.

3) **WOOD** — muscle spasms, respiratory antispasmodic, pertussis, high cholesterol, cirrhosis.

One of the best agents for wounds and trauma, everlasting is excellent for dissolving hematomas, even old ones, clearing out scar tissue and stimulating growth of new tissue. It is used for all spasms, and is a strong respiratory antispasmodic and expectorant. It stimulates growth of hepatic cells and lowers blood cholesterol. As a pelvic decongestant it is used for bartholinitis, dysmenorrhea and locally for cervical dysplasia.

GARLIC *Allium sativum*

ACTIONS: Pulmonary and intestinal antiseptic, general tonic, hypotensive, diuretic, vermifuge.

CONSTITUENTS: Sulphurous glucosides, allicin, garlicin, allistatin I and II, allyl oxide, iodine, silicon.

NEUROENDOCRINE PROPERTIES: Sympatholytic, hypotensive, thyroid stimulant.

PRINCIPAL INDICATIONS ACCORDING TO TERRAIN:

1) FIRE — arterial hypertension, tachycardia, edema of the legs, arteriosclerosis.

2) METAL — pulmonary pathology, intestinal pathology

2) WATER — rheumatism, gout, oliguria.

Garlic grows wild throughout the Mediterranean countries and is cultivated in France. Since antiquity it has been used as a condiment. The Egyptians held it in high esteem as did Galen. Garlic was considered a panacea by the Hebrews, the Greeks and the Romans.

Garlic treats all types of respiratory infections including pertussis. It has cardiotonic properties and thyroid-stimulating properties that make it useful as a general stimulant. It acts as a vasodilator for the peripheral circulation, lowering the blood pressure and slowing the pulse rate. It is effective for arterial hypertension, cardiac fatigue and arteriosclerosis, and can reduce cardiac edema in the legs. It has utility for all disorders due to hypercoagulability of the blood: varices, phlebitis, etcetera.

Garlic is effective for a variety of infectious diseases such as influenza, diphtheria, typhus and all kinds of bronchopulmonary infections including asthma, emphysema, pertussis and tuberculosis. It can effectively lower a fever in an acute infection. It aids digestion by helping to digest heavy foods, and is a potent antiparasitic agent, useful for dysentery and other types of diarrhea related to intestinal parasites. It can be useful for intestinal cramps and other types of digestive pain. In addition, it dissolves uric acid and urinary lithiases; it stimulates diuresis, providing relief of rheumatism and gout.

GERANIUM *Pelargonium roseum, P. odorantissimum*

ACTIONS: Astringent, hypoglycemiant, diuretic, antiviral, sympathomimetic, epitheliogenic.

CONSTITUENTS: Phlobaphene, isokaempferid, various polyphenol and flavonoid compounds.

NEUROENDOCRINE PROPERTIES: Adrenal cortex stimulant, hypoglycemiant.

PRINCIPAL INDICATIONS ACCORDING TO TERRAIN:

1) EARTH — stomatitis, glossitis, aphthous ulcers, gastroenteritis, diarrhea, anemia, metrorrhagia, eczema, diabetes; head lice (externally).

2) WATER — asthma, listlessness and fatigue, adrenal insufficiency, glomerulonephritis, nephrotic syndromes, tonsillitis and slow healing of bone fractures.

Earth yin and Water yin, with bitter-warming and sweet-warming flavors, geranium is therapeutic for diarrhea, gastroenteritis and metrorrhagia due to vacuity of the Spleen. It also has mild tranquilizing properties. Used clinically for severe gastritis from gastrectomy and severe diarrhea from rectocolitis and Crohn's disease, it can improve digestive absorption in wasting and malnutrition from diabetes and can be used externally for stomatitis, glossitis or aphthous ulcers.

Geranium is a powerful but gentle treatment for urinary infections in a vacuous Water terrain where there is adrenal cortical insufficiency. It can be used to treat all nephrotic syndromes, especially acute or chronic glomerulonephritis. Its astringent properties extend to treatment of hemoptysis and uterine hemorrhage in a Water yin terrain, and for uterine hemorrhage when there is a strong psychological factor. It is also said to have some anticancer properties. It is useful as a douche for cervical dysplasia and for condyloma. Since ancient times it has been considered to be one of the best vulneraries and cicatrisants.

GINGER *Zingiber officinale*

Actions: Eupeptic, carminative, febrifuge, stimulant, antiphlogistic, antiprostaglandin.

Constituents: Essential oil contains terpenes (cineol, borneol, citral, phellandrene), zingiberen, phenols (gingerol, zingerone, shogaol).

Neuroendocrine properties: Stimulates glucocorticoid production.

Principal indications according to terrain:

1) Metal — respiratory infections, bronchitis, influenza, bronchorrhea, pulmonary congestion, fever.

2) Earth — anorexia, glairy diarrhea, deficient immunity, leukopenia.

3) Water — impotence, urinary infections, glomerulonephritis.

Ginger can be used as an essential oil for most of the applications listed in the previous section (Herbs for Metal Yin Pathologies). However, the essential oil is particularly useful as a digestive aid and febrifuge, and also externally for rheumatic pain.

HYSSOP *Hysopus officinalis*

ACTIONS: Vagolytic, expectorant, eupeptic, stimulant, antiseptic, diaphoretic.

CONSTITUENTS: Thuyone, pinocamphone, phellandrene, borneol, limonene, geraniol.

NEUROENDOCRINE PROPERTIES: Sympathomimetic, parasympatholytic, bulbar stimulant (medulla oblongata), spasmolytic.

PRINCIPAL INDICATIONS ACCORDING TO TERRAIN:

1) METAL — chronic bronchitis, asthma, allergic rhinitis, tuberculosis, colic pain, leukorrhea, dermatoses.

2) WATER — urinary lithiases, depression, anergy, arthritis, cancer.

Hyssop was a sacred herb to the ancient Hebrews. Hippocrates recommended its use for pleurisy, Dioscorides recommended it for asthma. Its flavor is bitter and salty with a warming effect. Prescribed for treatment of asthma, chronic bronchitis, allergic rhinitis and even tuberculosis, it is also used for gastric pain and colic, eruptive fevers, dermatoses (acne, eczema and psoriasis), intestinal parasites, arthritis and urinary lithiases (phosphatic and oxalic) and leukorrhea. It is helpful for treating depression in a Water yin terrain and is supposed to have a normalizing influence on a cancerous terrain.

JUNIPER *Juniperus communis*

ACTIONS: Eupeptic, hypoglycemiant, diuretic, diaphoretic, antibacterial (wide spectrum), anti-inflammatory, anthelminthic, antiviral.

CONSTITUENTS: Essential oil contains camphene, terpineol, alpha-pinene, cadinene, organic acids, invert sugar; berries contain a bitter principle. The berries are rich in the catalytic trace elements potassium, magnesium, iodine, lithium and phosphorous.

NEUROENDOCRINE PROPERTIES: Hypoglycemiant.

PRINCIPAL INDICATIONS ACCORDING TO TERRAIN:

1) **EARTH** — dyspepsia, postprandial somnolence, diabetes, arteriosclerosis, eczema, psoriasis, hypoglycemiant action.

2) **WATER** — urinary infections, cystitis, renal calculi, glomerulonephritis, hypoglycemiant action, strengthens adrenals.

Oil of juniper has traditionally been used as a diuretic, stomachic and carminative for indigestion, flatulence and for diseases of the kidney and bladder. It has Earth yang, Water yang and Water yin properties. Essentially, it is an antiseptic and digestive, stimulating gastric acid secretion. Its flavors are sweet-cooling and spicy-warming. It is useful for treating dyspepsia and postprandial somnolence, hence diabetes, arteriosclerosis, eczema and psoriasis. The oil can be rubbed into rheumatic joints for pain relief and can be vaporized to use for bronchitis. It is a urinary antiseptic as well as a diuretic and improves circulation in the pelvic area; thus it is useful in relieving low back pain. Juniper should not be taken in cases of acute kidney disorders.

LAVENDER *Lavandula officinalis, L. angustifolia*

ACTIONS: Cardiotonic, antispasmodic, analgesic, antibacterial (gram-positive), diaphoretic, vulnerary.

CONSTITUENTS: Essential oils linalool, cineol, pinene, limonene, geraniol, borneol and herniarin, a hydroxy-coumarin.

NEUROENDOCRINE PROPERTIES: Central nervous system sedative, sympatholytic, parasympatholytic.

PRINCIPAL INDICATIONS ACCORDING TO TERRAIN:

1) **FIRE** — hypertension, arrhythmias, tachycardia, excitability, anxiety, intestinal spasms.

2) **WOOD** — headaches, leukorrhea, acne.

3) **EARTH** — acidic hyposecretion, dyspepsia, digestive parasitosis, typhoid fever, leukorrhea, all types of infestations.

4) **METAL** — asthma, bronchitis, spasmodic coryza, pulmonary infections, whooping cough, depression.

5) **WATER** — cystitis, oliguria, renal infections, depression.

The name of lavender comes from the Latin *lavare,* to wash, implying its use from antiquity as a bath scent, and perhaps even as a disinfectant. It is Fire yang, Fire yin, Wood yin, Earth yin, Metal yin, Water yin and cardiotonic. Bitter and warming, lavender supplements the yang of the Heart. It is an antispasmodic, both musculotropic and neurotropic; it relieves neuralgia pain, and is a central nervous system sedative. It can be used to treat hypertension and correct problems with the cardiac rhythm. Because of its sympatholytic properties and because it is an arterial vasodilator, it lowers blood pressure. It is also a pulmonary antiseptic, and has a strong anti-infectious influence for streptococcus infections. Additionally, it calms digestive spasms due to vagotonia and is used for renal and hepatobiliary drainage. Externally it is often used as stimulant, tonic and antispasmodic.

LEMON *Citrus limonum*

ACTIONS: Antiseptic, antirheumatismal, cholagogue, hemostatic, astringent.

CONSTITUENTS: Pinene, limonene, phellandrene, camphene, linalool, linalyl acetate, geranyl acetate, citral, citronellal.

NEUROENDOCRINE PROPERTIES: Sympathomimetic.

PRINCIPAL INDICATIONS ACCORDING TO TERRAIN:

1) WOOD — biliary dyskinesia, gastric hyperacidity, gallstones, venous pathology, high cholesterol, rheumatism, arthritis, jaundice, vomiting, asthma, bronchitis, gout, rheumatism, fevers.

2) FIRE — myocardial congestion, arterial hypertension, arteriosclerosis, plethora, hyperviscosity of the blood, hemorrhage, fevers.

3) EARTH — leukopenia, acute infectious diarrhea, pancreatic insufficiency, obesity, malaria, anorexia, gastric hyperacidity, gastric ulcer, asthma, bronchitis.

4) METAL — pulmonary tuberculosis, typhus, asthenia, anorexia, bronchitis, asthma.

5) WATER — urinary lithiases, osseous tuberculosis, gout, rheumatism.

Lemon has properties of Wood, Fire, Earth, Metal and Water. Its flavors are both sour-cooling and sweet-warming. It has strong powers as a solvent not only for phlegm and dampness, but also for hyperviscosity of the blood, including hypercholesterolemia and phlebitis, and can even be used to dissolve stones of the biliary or urinary tract. It promotes the flow of bile and lowers stomach acidity, and in fact is helpful for all types of congestive disorders and for many types of infections, having been commonly used for diphtheria, typhus and malaria. When prescribed for infections, it also activates the white blood cells.

MARJORAM *Origanum marjorana*

ACTIONS: Hypotensive, vasodilator.

CONSTITUENTS: Essential oil contains thymol, carvacrol, origanene and tannin.

NEUROENDOCRINE PROPERTIES: Sympatholytic, parasympathomimetic, spasmolytic.

PRINCIPAL INDICATIONS ACCORDING TO TERRAIN:

1) FIRE — agitation, insomnia, anxiety, anguish, visceral spasms of sympathetic origin, cluster headaches, spasmophilia, epilepsy; stimulates the parasympathetic and disperses the sympathetic nervous system.

2) WOOD — headaches, migraines, globus hystericus, sympathetic nervous system hyperactivity, stomach spasms, epigastric spasms, violent spasmodic intestinal pain, palpitations, tachycardia, spasmophilia, seasonal allergic asthma; stimulates the parasympathetic and calms the sympathetic nervous system.

The flavor of marjoram is bitter-cooling. Essentially, its sympatholytic action is due to its parasympathomimetic effects of reducing or calming spasms of sympathetic origin, such as headaches, migraines, cluster headaches, globus hystericus, yang-type asthma, tachycardia, palpitations, epigastric tension, stomach pain, nausea and intestinal spasms. It calms Heart Fire in the treatment of epilepsy. The Greeks used it for rheumatic pain. It is also considered to be an anaphrodisiac, and has been used as an external application for sprains and bruises and as an emmenagogue.

MELISSA (LEMON BALM, SWEET BALM) *Melissa officinalis*

ACTIONS: Sedative, eupeptic, choleretic, carminative, antispasmodic, emmenagogue, anaphrodisiac, diaphoretic, febrifuge.

CONSTITUENTS: Essential oil containing linalool, citronella, citral, geraniol, aldehydes, resin, tannins, succinic acid.

NEUROENDOCRINE PROPERTIES: Parasympatholytic, antispasmodic (musculotrope).

PRINCIPAL INDICATIONS ACCORDING TO TERRAIN:

1) EARTH — dyspepsia, obsession, digestive spasms, anorexia nervosa.

2) FIRE — nervous crises, emotionality, memory problems, excessive worry, fainting, insomnia, cardiac arrhythmia.

3) WOOD — headaches, emotional instability, neurosis, tinnitus, vertigo, asthma, hysteria, nymphomania, insomnia, painful menses.

Traditionally, the flowering stems and leaves of melissa are used which have flavors both bitter and sweet with a citrus-like odor. Melissa is classified Earth yang, Wood yang and Fire yang, having a cooling and calming effect on the Fire of the Liver. It is used for treating asthma, neuroses, hysteria, nervous anguish, nymphomania, tinnitus and vertigo and is an excellent plant for treating the vertigo of Menière's syndrome. The Arabs used it for depression. It has also been used to expel retained placenta and stimulate the onset of delayed menses.

MYRRH *Commiphora myrrha*

ACTIONS: Astringent, anti-inflammatory, immune stimulant, epitheliogenic.

CONSTITUENTS: Resin (myrrhin), volatile oil, organic salts, potassium sulphate, benzoate, malate and acetate.

PRINCIPAL INDICATIONS ACCORDING TO TERRAIN:

1) **METAL** — phlegm drainage of mucous membranes, bronchitis, urinary tract infections, pharyngitis, gingivitis, skin ulcers.

Myrrh increases the number of leukocytes. It clears phlegm from the mucous membranes of the bronchial tube and from the genitourinary tract. As a disinfectant and astringent, it is used for problems of the mouth and throat. Because of its disinfecting, immune system stimulating and epitheliogenic properties, it greatly accelerates the healing of wounds. It is used for coughs (orally or as incense), pharyngitis and gingivitis (as mouthwash), gangrenous ulcers and hemorrhoids (externally), dyspepsia (orally) and diphtheria (aerosol).

MYRTLE *Myrtus communis*

ACTIONS: Anti-inflammatory, antiseptic, astringent, antitussive.

CONSTITUENTS: Pinene, myrtenol.

NEUROENDOCRINE PROPERTIES: Mild stimulant of adrenal cortex.

PRINCIPAL INDICATIONS ACCORDING TO TERRAIN:

1) METAL — bronchitis, sinusitis, rhinitis, dermatoses, hemorrhoids.

2) WATER — urinary tract infections, nephrosis.

Myrtle has sour-warming and pungent-warming flavors. It is useful in treating respiratory problems including bronchorrhea, acute or chronic bronchitis in an asthenic or elderly patient and chronic rhinitis with a clear watery discharge. Its antiseptic qualities are also useful for kidney hypofunction, urinary tract infections and mycoses.

Being very gentle and non-irritating to sensitive mucous membranes, myrtle can be used externally and internally for hemorrhoids in an asthenic patient, and as a douche for numerous gynecological complaints including vaginitis, cervicitis, cervical dysplasia, condyloma and leukorrhea. It is also used externally and internally to treat eczema and psoriasis.

NIAOULI *Melaleuca viridiflora*

ACTIONS: Pulmonary and urinary antiseptic, expectorant, antibacterial (wide spectrum), mucous membrane analgesic.

CONSTITUENTS: Eucalyptol, terpinol, pinene, limonene, citrene, terebenthine, esters of valerianic, acetic and butyric acids.

PRINCIPAL INDICATIONS ACCORDING TO TERRAIN:

1) METAL — sinusitis, rhinitis, pharyngitis, bronchitis, pertussis, tuberculosis, dysentery, intestinal parasites.

2) WATER — cystitis, urethritis.

Having simultaneously pungent-warming and cooling properties, niaouli is one of the best respiratory antiseptics with pronounced effects on the rhinopharyngeal region. In combination with myrtle, it effects a strong synergy for drying the bronchial tubes and nasal passages.

Niaouli is also helpful for treating dysentery, particularly when there is aqueous diarrhea. Like myrtle, it is also a urinary tract disinfectant in urethritis and cystitis. It has some analgesic and antirheumatic properties. Externally it is an excellent antiseptic and cicatrisant.

OREGANO *Origanum vulgare*

ACTIONS: Pulmonary antiseptic, antispasmodic, antifungal.

CONSTITUENTS: Rich in phenols carvacrol and thymol; geranyl acetate, cymene, terpinene, origanene.

NEUROENDOCRINE PROPERTIES: Antispasmodic, sympatholytic, parasympathomimetic.

PRINCIPAL INDICATIONS ACCORDING TO TERRAIN:

1) METAL — acute or chronic bronchitis, asthma, tuberculosis, diarrhea, amenorrhea.

2) EARTH — sluggish digestion, indigestion, aerophagia, gastric or intestinal spasms, anorexia nervosa, rheumatic pain, amenorrhea.

Oregano is a strong antimicrobial agent particularly useful in respiratory infections marked by thick heavy secretions, irritable spasmodic cough, tuberculosis and asthma. It stimulates the stomach in patients with sluggish digestion or aerophagia, and strongly stimulates the pancreatic secretions. It is recommended for anorexia nervosa and is very effective for intestinal gas and for killing intestinal parasites. It is used for treating amenorrhea in the Metal yin or Earth yin constitution and is also used both internally and externally for relieving rheumatic pain. Externally, it can be used with a variety of other substances for pain relief, but should be used in a maximum strenght of five percent.

PEPPERMINT *Mentha piperata*

ACTIONS: Carminative, choleretic, peripheral vasodilator, central nervous system stimulant, emmenagogue, fungicide, antibacterial (wide spectrum), antipruritic, analgesic.

CONSTITUENTS: Essential oil (50 to 85 percent) menthol, menthone, jasmone, sesquiterpene alcohols, aldehydes, a-pinene, cineol, l-limonene, camphene, acetylmenthol, piperitone, piperitenone.

NEUROENDOCRINE PROPERTIES: Sympatholytic, parasympatholytic, antispasmodic, antigalactic.

PRINCIPAL INDICATIONS ACCORDING TO TERRAIN:

1) **METAL** — respiratory infections, bronchorrhea, fatigue, menstrual insufficiency; stimulates sexual appetite.

2) **EARTH** — anorexia, gastralgia, digestive spasms, fatigue, menstrual insufficiency, poor sexual appetite, impotence, frigidity, trembling, neuritis.

3) **WOOD** — biliary insufficiency, chronic hepatitis, headache, hypertension, menstrual insufficiency, trembling, neuritis.

Hippocrates proclaimed that peppermint was an aphrodisiac. Like coriander, its pungent warm flavor imparts a sense of freshness into the mouth. Peppermint is strengthening; it stimulates the appetite and relieves gastric pain and digestive spasms through its vagolytic action. Its strengthening effect on the lungs makes it useful in respiratory infections caused by weakness and cold with excessive bronchial secretions. It can also soften hardened bronchial secretions. The use of peppermint is contraindicated for subjects who present signs of heat repletion in the Spleen (gastric pain and ulcers).

Peppermint stimulates the central nervous system and has a choleretic activity, which makes it useful for biliary insufficiencies, chronic hepatitis, frontal orbital headaches, amenorrhea, impotence and trembling due to neuropathy. In Western Europe, it is classically used as an antispasmodic for dyspepsia, flatulence, colic, diarrhea, nausea and heartburn. It is also used for other types of sudden pains and for cramps in the abdomen, being especially useful for cramps and hiccups in children. Wide use has been made of peppermint in treating cholera and diarrhea.

In China, it is considered anti-inflammatory, analgesic, eupeptic, anticolic and antibacterial, having been shown to be useful in treating human tubercle bacillus and typhus. In classical Chinese medicine it is used for external invasion of wind and heat resulting in onset of fever, perspiration, headache, bloodshot eyes, soreness and swelling in the throat. In the form of an external compress, it can be used to relieve a headache. It is also useful for treating sunstroke, fever, thirst and elimination of dark cloudy urine. The anesthetic properties of peppermint oil on peripheral sensory nerves render it useful externally as an analgesic and antispasmodic. Since it has been found to diminish the secretions of lactating mothers, it should be avoided by nursing mothers.

PINE *Pinus sylvestris*

ACTIONS: Respiratory and urinary antiseptic.

CONSTITUENTS: Essential oil (pinene, phellandrene), resin, glucosides, glycosides (pinicrine, coniferoside, piceine), terebenthine, bornyl acetate.

NEUROENDOCRINE PROPERTIES: Adrenal stimulant (particularly cortex) sympathomimetic.

PRINCIPAL INDICATIONS ACCORDING TO TERRAIN:

    1) WATER — cystitis, prostatitis, pyelonephritis, impotence; stimulates the sympathetic tonus, stimulates the adrenals.

    2) METAL — respiratory infections (expectorant and anti-inflammatory), rhinitis, laryngitis, pharyngitis, tracheitis, bronchitis, asthma.

Pine is Water and Metal in nature. The sap, wood, needles and cones are a respiratory and urinary antiseptic. It is bitter-warming and pungent-warming, thus indicated in urinary infections due to heat and for pyelonephritis, cystitis and prostatitis due to cold.

Administered for the treatment of impotence, pine has been used traditionally as a remedy for kidney and bladder dysfunction and for rheumatic disorders and mucous membrane and respiratory diseases. The Native American Navajo tribe used pine needles for colds and upper respiratory tract infections. Externally, it has been used in the form of liniment plasters and inhalants. As an external application it is also been found useful in treating chronic eczema and psoriasis.

RAVENSARE *Ravensara aromatica*

ACTIONS: Cardiotonic, expectorant, choleretic, stomachic, antispasmodic (neuromuscular), antiviral, immune stimulant.

CONSTITUENTS: Monoterpenes: a-pinene, b-pinene; sesquiterpene: b-caryophyllene; a-terpinol; terpenyl acetate; 1,8-cineol.

NEUROENDOCRINE PROPERTIES: Stimulates pituitary function (ACTH, gonadotropins, prolactin, oxytocin).

PRINCIPAL INDICATIONS ACCORDING TO TERRAIN:

1) METAL — viral respiratory infections, sinusitis, rhinitis, rhinopharyngitis, influenza, viral enteritis, colitis.

2) WOOD — shingles, muscle pain, influenza, pertussis, ophthalmic herpes, amenorrhea, dysmenorrhea, irregular menses.

3) FIRE — chest pain, cardiac arrhythmia, anxiety.

Used mostly for viral infections such as viral chronic fatigue syndrome, influenza, viral enteritis, varicella, herpes, sinusitis, rhinitis, pharyngitis and neuromuscular fatigue, ravensare reduces glandular swelling and relieves neuromuscular pain. For respiratory infections such as rhinopharyngitis and influenza or even pertussis, it is a strong expectorant.

It is effective both internally and externally for shingles and is effective for ophthalmic herpes. It can also be used to treat amenorrhea, dysmenorrhea, irregular menses, stomach pain, colitis, chest pain, cardiac arrhythmia, dyspnea, bronchitis, lumbar pain and general body aches and pains. Ravensare is also an effective agent for nervous insomnia.

ROSEMARY *Rosmarinus officinalis*

ACTIONS: Cholagogue, lymphatic tonic, vascular analeptic, antibacterial (colibacillus), diaphoretic, epitheliogenic (including mucous membranes), diuretic (uricosuric), choleretic.

CONSTITUENTS: Essential oil rich in terpenes (borneol, cineol, pinene and esters), tannic acid, camphorous resin, saponiside, choline.

NEUROENDOCRINE PROPERTIES: Stimulates the adrenal cortex; anti-inflammatory, antispasmodic, parasympathomimetic, antalgic, antineuralgic, sympatholytic.

PRINCIPAL INDICATIONS ACCORDING TO TERRAIN:

1) WOOD — tension headaches, fatigue, icterus with retention, viral hepatitis, hypercholesterolemia, hypotension, syncope, neurological problems, migraines, Menière's syndrome, tinnitus, epilepsy.

2) FIRE — anguish, palpitations, bradycardia, cardiac insufficiency, apathy, hypotension, depression.

3) METAL — bronchitis, asthma, respiratory infections.

4) WATER — fatigue, loss of memory, hypotension, overexertion, impotence, frigidity.

The flowers and leaves of rosemary are traditionally used for alleviating headache, colic, colds and nervous diseases. Rosemary was used in the Middle Ages for catarrh of the lungs and large intestine. It has an age-old reputation for strengthening the memory and enhancing mental alertness. When rubbed and smoked together, rosemary and coltsfoot leaves have been considered good for asthma and other infections of the throat and lungs.

Both sour-cooling and sweet-warming, rosemary is indicated for all pathology related to the Liver and Gallbladder and any manifestations of a repletion of Liver yang including jaundice, palpitations, vertigo, tinnitus, Menière's syndrome and epilepsy. It is used in infectious Liver problems that originate from vacuity of the Liver as well, such as hypotension, bradycardia, chills, depression, asthenia and neurological problems related to hypertonicity. Its ability to elevate blood pressure and heart rate stems from its stimulating effect on the adrenals and the heart.

The sweet and spicy flavors stimulate the Kidney yang, which also affects hypotension along with adrenal cortex insufficiency, impotence and frigidity by strongly stimulating the testicles and ovaries. They also stimulate the yang of the Lung making it useful for asthma, bronchitis and other respiratory infections. It is a Wood yang plant, but its action is also of the sweet-warming type, which stimulates the adrenals and corresponds to the parasympathomimetic activity. It can have abortifacient properties in large doses.

The oil is also used externally as a rubefacient and is added to liniments as a fragrant stimulant. An oil or infusion can be used in the bath to calm sympathotonia and has been used for relief of rheumatic pain. Rosemary has antioxidant properties and extracts are being developed for use as a natural food preservative.

SAGE *Salvia officinalis*

ACTIONS: Astringent, emmenagogue (estrogen stimulant), antigonadotropic, sympathomimetic, parasympathomimetic, hypertensive, antispasmodic, antibacterial (gram-positive), hypoglycemiant, psychoanaleptic, vascular analeptic, antigalactic, central nervous system stimulant, adrenal cortex stimulant.

CONSTITUENTS: Essential oil contains thujone, cineol, borneol, camphor, pinene, salvene. The extract contains the trace elements copper, magnesium, manganese, zinc, gold, silver, rosemarinic acid, labiatenic acid, oleanolic acid, ursolic acid, flavonoids, saponins and bitter principles.

PRINCIPAL INDICATIONS ACCORDING TO TERRAIN:

1) EARTH — low immunity, autoimmune disorders, gastritis, intermittent fevers, splenomegaly, sterility, absence of menses, estrogenic action.

2) METAL — asthma, acute or chronic bronchitis, intestinal spasms and inflammations.

3) WATER — urinary tract infections, oliguria, enuresis, arterial hypotension, adrenal cortex insufficiency.

4) FIRE — hypotension, cardiac weakness.

5) WOOD — fatty liver of immune origin, hepatomegaly, neurological maladies.

Sage, known as the sacred herb, has been prized as a longevity elixir. The name "salvia" means "savior."   A stimulant, astringent, tonic and carminative, it has also been used for dyspepsia. It is very useful as a stimulant tonic in debility of the stomach and nervous system, and in general for weak digestion. Its action is remarkable in stopping perspiration and drying up salivation and breast milk. The Chinese valued it, giving it preference to their own tea. It has been considered a useful medicine for liver complaints, kidney troubles, hemorrhages from the lung or from the stomach, and for colds in the head. A cup of strong infusion is said to be good for relieving nervous headaches. The dried leaves have been smoked in pipes as a remedy for asthma.

Sage is one of the strongest proestrogenic herbs and is therefore useful for symptoms of menopause, especially nightsweats. It has been prescribed for nightsweats in tuberculosis patients because of its strong astringent properties. It is also useful for inflammations and spasms of the intestinal tract. Having an aromatic, sweet and slightly bitter-warming flavor, sage is indicated for gastritis, colic, chronic diarrhea, impotence and frigidity, as well as for intermittent fevers, splenomegaly and paralyses. Earth yin, Metal yin, Water yin, Fire yin and Wood yin, it supplements vacuity of the blood, as well as vacuity of the yang of the Spleen, Lung, Kidney, Heart and Liver. It is considered effective for autoimmune disorders, since it affects the coolness and warmth of the five organs.

SANDALWOOD *Santalum album*

ACTIONS: Urinary antiseptic, aphrodisiac.

CONSTITUENTS: Santanol, fusanol, santalic acid, teresantalic acid.

PRINCIPAL INDICATIONS ACCORDING TO TERRAIN:

    1) WATER — urinary tract infections, impotence, frigidity.

    2) METAL — chronic bronchitis, chronic or severe diarrhea.

Sandalwood has a salty-warming flavor with a bitter tang. It is indicated for all types of urinary tract infections in vacuous or replete patients, especially colibacillus and gonococcus. It is used for treating impotence or frigidity, chronic bronchitis, tuberculosis or chronic diarrhea.

SASSAFRAS *Sassafras officinale*

ACTIONS: Antirheumatic, diuretic (salidiuretic, uricosuric), diaphoretic, pulmonary and urinary antiseptic.

CONSTITUENTS: Safrol, pinene, phellandrene, eugenol, camphor.

PRINCIPAL INDICATIONS ACCORDING TO TERRAIN:

1) WATER — urinary tract infections, syphilis, physical and mental fatigue, rheumatism, gout.

2) METAL — respiratory infections; cleanses skin in dermatoses.

Sassafras is renowned for its diaphoretic properties. Its flavor is pungent and warming, but it is also effective for infections of the respiratory or urinary systems that have an abundance of heat. Its main application in addition to diaphoresis is for rheumatic conditions and skin pathology. It is recommended to strengthen the genitourinary system and is used to treat syphilis; it is considered to be a powerful stimulant for treating physical and mental fatigue. It has both internal and external application as an anti-inflammatory for rheumatism and gout.

SAVORY (WINTER) *Satureia montana*

ACTIONS: Antispasmodic, sympathomimetic, adrenal stimulant, expectorant, antibacterial (wide spectrum, including staphylococcus), antifungal, antiviral, antiprotozoal, cerebral stimulant, antidiarrheic.

CONSTITUENTS: Carvacrol, cymene, terpenes, cineol, thymol.

NEUROENDOCRINE PROPERTIES: Stimulates gonadotropin release; adrenal cortex stimulant, sympathomimetic, parasympatholytic.

PRINCIPAL INDICATIONS ACCORDING TO TERRAIN:

1) METAL — respiratory infections, asthma, bronchitis, chronic colitis, intestinal colic, chronic diarrhea.

2) EARTH — chronic gastritis, retarded development, sterility, impotence, frigidity; stimulates the activity of the testicles and ovaries.

3) WATER — asthenia, anergy, impotence; stimulates the activity of the testicles and ovaries.

Savory is Earth yin, Water yin and Metal yin in nature, with bitter-warming and pungent-warming flavors. Vagolytic for spasms of the stomach and intestine that originate from cold vacuity, it is used in cases of gastritis, colic and chronic diarrhea. It is very useful in cases of impotence and frigidity due to gonadotropin insufficiency, and for sterility. As well, it is excellent for most types of mycosis. A powerful adrenal cortex stimulant for improving overall immunity, and a powerful cerebral cortex stimulant for dementia, it is one of the strongest essences for building up a weak immune system.

TARRAGON *Artemisia dracunculus*

ACTIONS: Stomachic, vagolytic, antispasmodic, vermifuge.

CONSTITUENTS: Estragol (60 to 70 percent); terpenes: ocimene, phellandrene, etcetera (15 to 20 percent).

NEUROENDOCRINE PROPERTIES: Vagolytic, estrogenic.

PRINCIPAL INDICATIONS ACCORDING TO TERRAIN:

   1) EARTH — epigastric distress, amenorrhea, dysmenorrhea, intestinal parasites.

Tarragon is especially good for epigastric distress such as stomach pain from gastritis, hiccoughs or aerophagia. It stimulates sluggish peristalsis, and is used to treat flatulence, intestinal fermentation, intestinal parasites, and anorexia. It has also been used for rheumatic pain and dysmenorrhea.

TEREBENTHINE
(ESSENCE OF PINUS PINASTER & OTHER CONIFERS)

ACTIONS: Expectorant, balsamic, respiratory and urinary antiseptic.

CONSTITUENTS: Terpenes, acids and alcohols of high molecular weight.

NEUROENDOCRINE PROPERTIES: Adrenal cortex stimulant, sympathomimetic.

PRINCIPAL INDICATIONS ACCORDING TO TERRAIN:

1) METAL — acute and chronic bronchitis, asthma, leukorrhea, intestinal parasites, constipation.

2) WATER — urinary tract infections: pyelonephritis, cystitis, urethritis; urinary stones, chronic rheumatism aggravated by cold and dampness, arthritis, neuralgia (lumbago, sciatica), rheumatoid arthritis, degenerative rheumatism, ankylosing spondylitis, collagen diseases.

3) WOOD — gallstones, headaches.

Terebenthine is used internally, externally and as an inhalation. Pungent and bitter with both warming and cooling properties, its main internal indications are for chronic bronchial infections with abundant sputum and suppurative infections of the urinary tract, such as cystitis, pyelitis and urethritis. It is also used as a vermifuge, to dissolve urinary stones and to treat rheumatic pain.

Rich in terpenes, terebenthine has unusual penetrating power. Externally it is used for rheumatic pain, neuralgia and tendinitis.

THUJA (YELLOW CEDAR) *Thuja occidentalis*

ACTIONS: Astringent, diuretic, vesicant, diaphoretic.

CONSTITUENTS: Pinene, phenone, thuyone.

PRINCIPAL INDICATIONS ACCORDING TO TERRAIN:

1) **WATER** — prostate hypertrophy, pelvic decongestion in females, urinary tract infections, urinary incontinence, uterine tonic.

2) **EARTH** — intestinal parasites, immune deficiency, condyloma, papilloma.

Thuja has a Water yin and Earth yin nature with sour-cooling and sweet-warming flavors. Its most important function is as a pelvic decongestant indicated for prostate hypertrophy and for cervical dysplasia. It is useful in females for genital warts, condyloma, papillomas (HPV) and cancer, and is therapeutic for cystitis and for urinary incontinence. It is an emmenagogue that can stimulate menses in a woman who is weak or has low immunity. Thuja is also used to eliminate intestinal parasites.

THYME *Thymus vulgaris*

ACTIONS: Antitussive, choleretic, respiratory antiseptic, anthelminthic, antibacterial (wide spectrum), antifungal, antiviral (herpes); stimulates thymus activity and white blood cell production.

CONSTITUENTS: Thymol, carvacrol, cymol, terpinene, cymene, borneol, linalool.

NEUROENDOCRINE PROPERTIES: Parasympatholytic; stimulates the adrenal cortex, stimulates the thymus gland.

PRINCIPAL INDICATIONS ACCORDING TO TERRAIN:

1) METAL — bronchitis, asthma, colds, influenza, pneumonopathy, chronic bronchitis, emphysema, respiratory mycosis, immune deficiency, leukopenia, colitis, intestinal parasites.

2) WATER — urinary infections, hypotension, furuncles, chronic rheumatism, immune deficiency.

3) EARTH — gastric atony, diarrhea, nightmares accompanying digestive problems, swelling, typhus, parasites, anemia, leukopenia, immune deficiency, intestinal parasites, colitis.

Thyme is Metal yin, Earth yin, Water yin and Metal yang in nature. Its bitterness and pungent warmth benefit the lungs when damaged by cold or dryness. It could be said that sage affects the Spleen; rosemary, the Kidney and Liver; and thyme, the Lung. Thyme is also a powerful urinary antiseptic and parasiticide. It is essentially indicated for colds, influenza, bronchitis, sore throat, acute pneumonopathy, asthma, emphysema, respiratory mycosis, low immunity, leukopenia, anemia, diarrhea, typhoid fever, gastric atony and parasites. Thyme dries and cleanses mucous secretions and soothes irritated mucous membranes. It is excellent for controlling and treating rectocolitis, simultaneously building immune resistance.

Culpepper recommended it for headaches, hysteria and other nervous disorders and to strengthen the lungs. As a folk remedy it has been used as a stomachic for colic, flatulence, colds, dyspepsia and pertussis. In Russia, its traditional usage is for pertussis and bronchitis.

VERVAIN *Verbena officinalis*

ACTIONS: Astringent, vulnerary, febrifuge, bitter tonic, diuretic, oxytocic, stimulant.

CONSTITUENTS: Essential oil, mucilage, saponins, tannins, bitter principle and glycosides verbenaline and verbenine.

NEUROENDOCRINE PROPERTIES: Parasympathomimetic, stimulates oxytocin and prolactin production, gonadotropin antagonist.

FIVE PHASE CATEGORIES: Earth yang, Earth yin.

PRINCIPAL INDICATIONS ACCORDING TO TERRAIN:

1) EARTH — dysmenorrhea, galactic insufficiency, malaria, chronic rheumatism, weakness of the heart, cellulitis, febrifuge; antigonadotropic action; benefits childbirth labor, stimulates the parasympathetic nervous system.

2) WOOD — sciatic neuralgia, neuralgias, tinnitus, nervousness.

Traditional use of vervain recommends it as an astringent, diaphoretic and antispasmodic for numerous complaints. It is said to be useful in intermittent fevers, ulcers, ophthalmia and pleurisy. As a poultice, it is said to be good for headaches, pain in the ear and rheumatism, and can be applied externally for piles. Its flavors are bitter-warming and sour-cooling.

Therapeutically, it is used to induce labor and to treat insufficient lactation. Its actions of dispersing wind-cold and dampness explain is use in the treatment of chronic rheumatism, malaria and splenomegaly. As a febrifuge, it has an action comparable to quinine. Vervain is slightly parasympathomimetic, and therefore has the properties of calming sympathotonic conditions, such as migraine or nervousness. As an analgesic, it is indicated for sciatic and other neuralgias, especially for trigeminal neuralgia, and for headaches in the temples. It has applications in treatment of tinnitus, and is useful for expelling mucus from the lungs and for treating pleurisy.

YLANG YLANG *Unona odorantissima*

Actions: Hypotensive, antispasmodic, antiseptic, aphrodisiac.

Constituents: Free and estrified linalool, safrol, eugenol, geraniol, pinene, cadinene, benzyl benzoate, sesquiterpenes, organic acids – acetic, benzoic, formic, salicylic and valerianic.

Neuroendocrine properties: Sympatholytic, calms adrenal function.

Five phase categories: Water yang, Metal yang and Fire yang.

Principal indications according to terrain:

1) Water — tachycardia, hypertension, intestinal infections, excessive sexual excitation.

2) Fire — tachycardia, cardiac arrhythmia, hypertension.

3) Metal — pulmonary infections, infections of the Lung and Large Intestine.

Ylang ylang regulates cardiac rhythm, having a sweet and cooling flavor and a smooth, agreeable aromatic fragrance comparable to hyacinth or clove. It calms hypertension and tachycardia, and treats intestinal infections with purulent secretions that originate from repletion heat in the Small Intestine or the upper digestive tract. It actually has an anaphrodisiac activity, which is useful in cases of impotence and frigidity from excessive excitation.

ESSENTIAL OILS: BRIEF PROFILES

Angelica	Bay Laurel	Benzoin	Bergamot
Birch	Black pepper	Borneol	Calamus
Camphor	Cardamom	Carrot	Cedarwood
Celery	Chenopodium	Clary Sage	Cumin
Cymbopogon	Frankincense	Great Mugwort	Hypericum
Jasmine	Lemon Verbena	Mugwort	Neroli
Nutmeg	Onion	Palma Rosa	Patchouli
Petit Grain	Rose	Serpolet	Spike Lavender
Tangerine	Ti Tree	Yarrow	

ANGELICA *(Angelica archangelica)*: Wood yin, Metal yin, Earth yin, Fire yin. Eupeptic, carminative, antispasmodic, sympatholytic, vagolytic, estrogenic. Angelica is a refreshing and revitalizing tonic that brightens mental activity, stimulates appetite and digestion and is diaphoretic. It is used for digestive cramps, postprandial headaches, asthenia, anemia, anorexia nervosa, asthma, pulmonary tuberculosis, dysmenorrhea and lymphadenopathy. It supplements Liver, Lung and Spleen function.

BAY LAUREL *(Laurus nobilis)*: Earth yin, Metal yin, Fire yin. Eupeptic, carminative, mild diuretic, expectorant, diaphoretic, emmenagogue, mild narcotic. Useful for stomach pain, stomatitis, tooth pain, neuritis and exceptionally good for the pain of arthritis and rheumatism, bay laurel is also a pulmonary antiseptic administered in cases of bacterial bronchopulmonary infections. It is a wide spectrum antibacterial, a strong mucolytic and expectorant. As a lymphatic stimulant, it is both cleansing and therapeutic for Hodgkin's lymphoma. It clears damp heat and is good for the cyclic fevers of malaria. Antiparasitic and antiprotozoal, bay laurel also has antiviral (viral hepatitis) and antifungal properties (several types of candida). It is anticoagulant and a coronary dilator. Bay laurel is not often used topically.

BENZOIN *(Styrax benzoin):* Metal yin, Metal yang, Water yin. Astringent, expectorant, mucolytic. Benzoin is useful for clearing phlegm congestion, especially in the respiratory tract, but also in the urinary tract. It can be taken orally, by inhalation, or externally, where it is especially helpful for dermatitis. It has a warming and mildly euphoric effect.

BERGAMOT *(Citrus bergamia):* Fire yang, Metal yang, Earth yin. Bergamot is a central nervous system sedative and calms the heart. It stimulates digestion and is especially recommended for treating intestinal parasites (and scabies topically) and intestinal spasms. As a douche, it treats leukorrhea and gonococcus. It is used to treat bronchitis and has been found lethal *in vitro* to tubercle bacillus, diphtheria bacillus, staphylococcus, *E. coli* and meningococcus.

BIRCH *(Betula alba):* Fire yang, Water yang, Earth yang. Diaphoretic, diuretic (volumetric, azoturic, uricosuric, antialbuminuric), antalgic, antimicrobial, anti-inflammatory. Used to treat arterial hypertension, pyelonephritis, arthritic and rheumatic disorders, oliguria, uremia, hyperuricemia, kidney stones (oxalic and phosphatic), gout and edema. Birch has also been used to expel intestinal parasites.

BLACK PEPPER *(Piper nigrum):* Earth yin, Water yin. Black pepper strengthens the digestive smooth muscle tone. It stimulates appetite, cleanses mucus from the digestive tract, relieves gas pains and stimulates mucous membranes throughout the body (hence its use to clear phlegm from the respiratory system). It has long been known as an aphrodisiac and for its utility in the treatment of impotence and gonorrhea.

BORNEOL *(Dryobalanops camphora):* Fire yin, Water yin. Cardiotonic, adrenal cortex stimulant, antiseptic. Used externally and internally as a general tonic and heart tonic. It is used to treat depression and infectious diseases. It is a very powerful antiseptic.

CALAMUS *(Acorus calamus):* Earth yin, Water yin, Wood yin. Digestive tonic, diuretic (volumetric and antispasmodic), diaphoretic. Calamus is used for anorexia, gas pains and digestive spasms. It clears out phlegm in the gastrointestinal tract and calms nervous problems such as vertigo and tension headaches. In folk medicine it has been used to treat agues (intermittent fevers) and as a vermifuge. Calamus also has an intoxicating property and was said to be used by witches to help induce out of body experiences.

CAMPHOR *(Cinnamomum camphora):* Fire yin, Metal yin, Water yin. Cardiotonic, diuretic (volumetric), respiratory antiseptic, antidepressant, analgesic. Camphor is a powerful cardiotonic and is used for heart failure, shock, hypotension and depression. By inhalation it treats bronchitis, colds and pulmonary tuberculosis It can be used externally for all of these applications, for itching and for rheumatic pain.

CARDAMOM *(Elettaria cardamomum):* Earth yin. Stomachic, carminative. Cardamom is used for aerophagia, flatulence, anorexia, nausea and heartburn, for postprandial headaches and for intestinal cramps.

CARROT *(Daucus carota):* Wood yang, Wood yin. Choleretic, cholagogue. Carrot is used to nourish the liver and to drain the bile ducts in cases of jaundice or other types of hepatobiliary disorders. It has also been used as an emmenagogue, as an internal cleanser, and in France in skin care to promote skin elasticity and tone.

CEDARWOOD *(Juniperus virginiana):* Water yin, Metal yin. Red cedarwood *(Juniperus virginiana)* and atlas cedarwood *(Cedrus atlantica)* are both referred to as cedarwood. Both have effects similar to sandalwood in medicinal application. A urinary antiseptic for turbid urine, burning pain and gonorrhea, it is used in urinary tract infections including pyelonephritis and urethritis. Cedarwood is applied as a massage oil to the neck and shoulders along with cypress and niaouli to drain the nose and sinuses in respiratory infections. It is also used externally for chronic rheumatism and for seborrheic skin conditions. Although it has been used as an abortifacient, it is extremely hazardous for this purpose.

CELERY *(Apium graveolens):* Water yin, Wood yin. Diuretic (volumetric, salid-iuretic), eupeptic, stomachic. Wild celery seed oil is used to treat oliguria and albuminuria. It stimulates general kidney function for the treatment of albuminuria, uremia, edema and ascites. It has a mild choleretic influence and is also used for chronic respiratory insufficiency, such as in asthma or emphysema. Since the Middle Ages it has gained repute as a treatment for depression.

CHENOPODIUM *(Chenopadium ambrosiodes, var. anthelminticum):* Earth yin, Metal yang, Fire yang. Commonly called wormseed, chenopodium is a powerful anthelminthic agent. It is used for all kinds of worms, especially round worms, but also hookworms, eelworms, tapeworms, pinworms and protozoa. It is used both for children and adults, but it should be administered with caution. Symptoms of overdose are vertigo and sensory disturbances. The maximum adult dose is 25 drops at a time up to 50 drops a day. For children, the daily dose should not exceed one drop per day for each kilogram (2.2 pounds) of body weight, with the daily amount divided into two doses. In case of toxic symptoms, induce vomiting. Chenopodium is mucolytic, stimulates digestive secretions, lowers fevers, calms anxiety and lowers blood pressure.

CLARY SAGE *(Salvia sclaria):* Fire yin, Earth yin, Water yin. Estrogen stimulant, antispasmodic, sedative, anticoagulant. The alcohol sclareol in clary sage has strong estrogenic properties, rendering it useful for the treatment of sexual asthenia in both sexes. It is both euphoric and sedative for timid, nervous types. Clary sage lowers blood cholesterol levels. It is prescribed for amenorrhea, anxiety, depression, poor digestion and to stimulate labor; for phlebitis, varicose veins, hemorrhoids and venous aneurysms; and is excellent for amenorrhea or oligomenorrhea. Topically, it is effective for fungal infections.

CUMIN *(Cuminum cyminum):* Earth yin. Antispasmodic, vagolytic, carminative, estrogen stimulant, thyroid inhibitor. Cumin is used to treat gastritis, intestinal spasms, amenorrhea and dysmenorrhea.

CYMBOPOGON *(Cymbopogon citratus):* Earth yin. Stomachic, parasympathomimetic, galactagogue. Used to treat digestive problems from loss of smooth muscle tonus: gastric atony, flaccid constipation, colitis, gastroenteritis, nervous disorders related to digestion, insufficient lactation. Used externally for scabies, lice and as an insect repellent.

FRANKINCENSE *(Boswellia carterii):* Metal yang, Metal yin, Water yin. Astringent, antiseptic, expectorant, carminative, epitheliogenic. Mostly external use. Also called olibanum, frankincense has been in use for nearly 5000 years. It has an astringent effect on mucous membranes and as an expectorant treats cough, bronchitis and laryngitis. It clears phlegm from the urinary tract or digestive tract and can be used to treat urinary tract infections, gonorrhea or gastrointestinal irritation. Its astringent properties also make it useful for leukorrhea, uterine hemorrhage or hemoptysis. Externally it disinfects and speeds up the healing of wounds. It has an agreeable fragrance, as befits its use as an incense.

GREAT MUGWORT *(Artemisia arborescens):* Metal yang, Earth yin. For topical use. Contains chamazulene and has very similar properties to German chamomile, but is less expensive.

HYPERICUM - ST. JOHN'S WORT *(Hypericum perforatum):* Metal yin, Water yin. Anti-inflammatory (especially for mucous membranes), pelvic decongestant. Hypericum is used both externally and internally for all traumas. Because it is so effective in clearing up blood stasis, it is even prescribed for dissolving tumors. It is very effective for stomatitis, gastric and duodenal ulcers, colitis, vaginitis, prostatitis and cystitis. As a pelvic decongestant, it is also very good for pyelonephritis and endometriosis. Hypericum strengthens the immune system and is particularly indicated for infections that are chronic or recurrent.

JASMINE *(Jasminum grandiflorum):* Water yin. Aphrodisiac, vagolytic, antidepressant, uterine tonic, galactagogue. Jasmine is used externally. It has a marked effect on the moods and arouses erotic thoughts and mild euphoria. It can be useful for dysmenorrhea, to promote labor, and to relieve bronchial spasms.

LEMON GRASS: See **CYMBOPOGON.**

LEMON VERBENA *(Lippia citriodora):* Earth yin. Antispasmodic, parasympathomimetic, stomachic. Lemon verbena is used for digestive spasms, especially the upper digestive tract.

MUGWORT *(Artemisia vulgaris):* Wood yin, Earth yin. Emmenagogue, cholagogue, antispasmodic, antiparasitic (ascariasis, oxyuria). Used to treat amenorrhea, dysmenorrhea, irregular menses, digestive spasms, nervous vomiting.

NEROLI *(Flos citrus aurantium):* Fire yang, Wood yang. Central nervous system sedative, sympatholytic, antispasmodic. Neroli is the essence of the flowers of *Citrus aurantium.* It is effective for depression, and calms Heart Fire in insomnia, anxiety, hysteria, vertigo, neuralgia and diarrhea; it calms forceful heart contractions and cardiac arrhythmia, and induces a mild euphoria.

NUTMEG *(Myristica fragrans):* Earth yin, Metal yin, Water yin. Sympathomimetic, gastrointestinal antiseptic, aphrodisiac, euphoriant. Nutmeg in high doses is hallucinogenic, but the effect is accompanied by uncomfortable pounding of the heart. In normal doses (9-12 drops/day), it is useful for nervous and sexual asthenia, gastroenteritis with diarrhea and flatulence, neuralgia and rheumatism (externally).

ONION *(Allium cepa):* Fire yin, Metal yin, Earth yin. Diuretic, anti-inflammatory, anti-infectious (including staphylococcus), expectorant, thyroid stimulant, hypoglycemiant, antisclerotic, antithrombotic. Used for fatigue, edema, oliguria, diarrhea (intestinal fermentation), obesity, impotence, prostate hypertrophy, genitourinary infections, respiratory infections, diabetes, arteriosclerosis, rheumatism and intestinal parasites.

PALMA ROSA *(Cymbopogon martini)*: Earth yin, Wood yin. Digestive tonic, antifungal, antiviral. Used for anorexia and chronic viral or fungal infections.

PATCHOULI *(Pogostemon patchouly)*: Wood yin, Water yin. Central nervous system stimulant, sympathomimetic, fungicide, antiviral. Has aphrodisiac properties, is used to suppress the appetite for food (externally or internally), and is used to treat skin infections such as eczema, seborrhea, dermatitis and herpes (externally). In high dosage it is used as a sedative.

PETIT GRAIN *(Folium citrus aurantium)*: Fire yang, Wood yang. Central nervous system sedative, antispasmodic. Used for many of the same applications as bitter orange or neroli: insomnia, anxiety, hysteria and digestive spasms.

ROSE *(Rosa damascena and Rosa centifolia)*: Fire yin, Fire yang, Water yin. Antidepressant, aphrodisiac. Rose strengthens uterine tonus, stimulates vaginal secretions and stimulates sperm production. It can be used to treat constipation in feeble patients, and is useful for treating anxiety, metrorrhagia and uterine hemorrhage, especially in Water yin and Fire yin constitutions.

SERPOLET *(Thymus serpyllum)*: Metal yang, Metal yin, Water yin. Antispasmodic, vagolytic, antitussive, expectorant, antibacterial (wide spectrum), antiviral, antalgic (mucous membranes), choleretic, eupeptic, diuretic, urinary antiseptic (wide spectrum antibacterial), emmenagogue. Serpolet is used for respiratory infections, especially childhood infections such as red measles and pertussis. In adults it is used for acute bronchopulmonary infections. Serpolet treats infections of the reproductive system, and is used both systemically and locally for such complaints as cervicitis, metritis, vaginitis, salpingitis, orchitis, prostatitis, epididymitis and colitis. In high doses serpolet is stupefying.

SPIKE LAVENDER *(Lavandula spica)*: Fire yang. Antispasmodic, sympatholytic, vagolytic, antitussive, anti-inflammatory, antiallergic. Spike lavender is noted for its sedative and antispasmodic properties. It is effective for severe coughs, even pertussis, and is also used for tachycardia and cardiac arrhythmia.

TANGERINE *(Citrus reticulata)*: Fire yang. Sedative, antispasmodic, hypnotic. Used for nervous tension and insomnia.

TI TREE *(Melaleuca alternifolia)*: Metal yang, Water yang. Antibacterial, antifungal, antiviral, epitheliogenic. Used topically, ti tree is especially good for a wide range of infectious skin conditions, including ringworm, tinea, herpes and cold sores. It also kills head lice. Used as a douche, it is gentle and effective in treating fungal vaginitis. Internally, it is effective for treating urinary tract infections.

YARROW *(Achillea millefolium)*: Water yin, Wood yang. Analgesic. Yarrow is used externally primarily for its soothing, warming and penetrating influence on the muscles. It can be used locally to soothe bleeding hemorrhoids. Internally it is mildly diuretic.

GEMMOTHERAPY PROFILES

ABIES PECTINATA: Remineralizer, parathyroid stimulant, anti-inflammatory. Stimulates osteoblast function. Used for advanced chronic arthritis, rickets, dental caries, alveolar pyorrhea, lymphadenitis, pediatric rhinitis and pharyngitis.

AESCULUS HIPPOCASTANUM: Vein tonic, hemorrhoids, varicose veins.

BETULA PUBESCENS: Adrenal cortex stimulant, anti-inflammatory, antalgic, antirheumatismal, anticoagulant. Secondary stages of arthritis and rheumatism, venous thromboses, general fatigue, physical or psychological.

CRATAEGUS OXYACANTHA: Tachycardia, arrhythmia, precordial pain, angina pectoris, cardiac insufficiency, congestive heart failure, edema in the lower limbs.

FRAXINUS EXCELSIOR: Diuretic (volumetric, uricosuric), anti-inflammatory. Gout, arthritis, high uric acid levels.

JUGLANS REGIA: Anti-inflammatory, stimulates hepatic macrophage and plasma cell activity. Genitourinary infections, skin infections – especially dermatitis, acne, impetigo, eczema and varicose ulcers.

JUNIPERUS COMMUNIS: Hepatostimulating. Advanced liver pathology, such as cirrhosis, jaundice; eliminates urea and uric acid. Also known as a treatment for aerophagia and intestinal gas.

OLEA EUROPAEA: Hypotensive, sympatholytic, antisclerotic, vasodilator (coronary), diuretic (volumetric, azoturic), hypocholesterolemic. Used for arterial hypertension, memory loss and high cholesterol.

PINUS MONTANA: Problems with articular cartilage. Osteoarthrosis (vertebrae, hips, knees), chronic rheumatism, ankylosing spondylitis, cartilage damage, osteoporosis.

PINUS SYLVESTRIS: Respiratory problems. Acute and chronic bronchitis, pharyngitis, rhinitis, sinusitis, colds, asthma, coughs.

QUERCUS PEDUNCULATA: Adrenal cortex stimulant, stimulates bone growth. Advanced forms of arthritis and rheumatism; fatigue, impotence.

RIBES NIGRUM: Sympathotonic, adrenal cortex stimulant (especially gluco-corticoids), anti-inflammatory, diuretic (volumetric, azoturic, urico-suric). Allergic problems, chronic infections, low immunity, respiratory infections, asthma, rheumatic conditions, urticaria, eczema, herpes zoster (shingles); all infections at early stages, and glomerulonephritis throughout.

ROSA CANINA: Rhinopharyngitis and allergic rhinitis, ear infections, tonsilli-tis (especially pediatric), chronic genitourinary infections (especially the mucous membranes), migraines and other headaches, osteoporosis.

ROSMARINUS OFFICINALIS: Cholagogue, choleretic, antispasmodic. Used for hepatic insufficiency, biliary colic, gallstones, chronic allergies, colitis, Crohn's disease, frigidity, dysmenorrhea.

TILIA TOMENTOSA: Sedative, tranquilizer. Insomnia, neuralgia, headache, anxiety, gastric ulcers, heartburn, esophagitis, cardiac arrhythmia.

VACCINUM VITIS IDAEA: Anti-inflammatory, regulates peristalsis. Intestinal transit problems, intestinal absorption problems (leaky gut), diarrhea, constipation, colibacillosis, urinary tract infections, arthritis; reduces urea, uric acid and cholesterol.

VIBURNUM LANTANA: Vagolytic, antispasmodic. Eczema, dyspnea, asthma, rhinitis, smoker's cough; strengthens respiratory system.

VISCUM ALBUM (MISTLETOE): The only glycerin macerate in gemmotherapy used in the centesimal (1C) dilution. All others are diluted to the deci-mal (1D). Hypertension, gout, diuretic (volumetric, azoturic, albumin-uria), sympatholytic, parasympathomimetic.

VITIS VINIFERA: Stimulates leukocyte formation, anti-inflammatory, antalgic. Leukocytosis (especially lymphocytosis), deforming arthritis, bone tumors, benign tumors.

Oligoelement Profiles

ALUMINUM (A<small>L</small>): Psychological disorders, learning disorders, hyperactivity, memory disorders, anxiety, insomnia due to mental hyperactivity, viral or vaccinal encephalitis, Mongolism, fatigue from mental strain. Contraindicated for Alzheimer's disease.

BISMUTH (B<small>I</small>): Acute stages of tonsillitis, rhinitis or pharyngitis (bacterial infections). **Do not use for more than three days.**

COBALT (C<small>O</small>): Sympathotonic spasmodic disorders, lumbar pain, circulatory antispasmodic, headaches, palpitations, anxiety, hypertension, hot flushes of menopause.

COPPER (C<small>U</small>): Bacterial and viral infections, especially influenza; warts, hepatic detoxification, chronic inflammations, laryngitis, spasmodic colitis, pancreatitis, diarrhea, rheumatism, lumbar pain, anemia, acute bronchitis, candidiasis, premenstrual syndrome. Contraindicated for Wilson's disease.

COPPER-GOLD-SILVER (C<small>U</small>-A<small>U</small>-A<small>G</small>): Acute and recovery stages of infectious diseases, prevention of problems of aging, mental fatigue, adrenal cortex insufficiency, fatigue, staphylococal and streptococcal infections, chronic rheumatism, pharyngitis, hypertension or hypotension, cystitis, constipation, arteriosclerosis, herpes zoster (shingles), periodontal disease.

FLUORINE (F): Stabilizes calcium metabolism, treats osteoarticular disorders, osteoporosis, dental caries, laxity of the ligaments, hyperparathyroidism, scoliosis, osteomalacia or osteochondritis of the spine, hypocalcemia of pregnancy, rheumatoid arthritis, chronic rheumatism.

GOLD (A<small>U</small>): Infections and febrile conditions, vascular sclerosis, hypotension.

IODINE (I): Hyper- and hypothyroid problems, goiter, obesity, arterial hypertension (stress or essential), vertigo, mycoses, viral diseases, amenorrhea, poor libido (male), seborrhea, sciatica.

IRON (F<small>E</small>): Anemia, hyperadrenalism, male infertility, intestinal parasites, disorders of menopause, poor libido (female).

LITHIUM (L<small>I</small>): Anxiety, aggressiveness, irritability, insomnia, depressive disorders, hallucinations, neurotic and psychotic states, anorexia nervosa, dysmenorrhea, gout, lumbar pain, tension headaches, bedwetting. Contraindicated for hyperthyroidism.

MAGNESIUM (MG): Generalized spasms and cramps (spasmophilia), constipation, problems of growth, arthrosis, osteoporosis, rheumatic pain, memory problems, neuritis, edema, myocardial insufficiency, cardiac arrhythmia, arterial thrombosis, low immunity (leukocytosis), sympathotonic constipation, intestinal parasites, premenstrual syndrome, anovulation, amenorrhea, hepatic insufficiency, gallstones.

MANGANESE (MN): All manifestations of allergic problems, fatigue, eczema, urticaria, asthma, headaches, arthrosis, arthritis, collagen and connective tissue disorders, chronic rheumatism, memory loss, hyperthyroid, vertigo, somnolence, hypermenorrhea, impotence.

MANGANESE-COBALT (MN-CO): Psychogenic illnesses, skin disorders, herpes, osteoporosis, inflammatory diseases, amenorrhea, anxiety, arthrosis, depression, impotence, diabetes, colitis, gallstones, gout, headaches, hemorrhoids, hypertension, obesity, osteoporosis.

MANGANESE-COPPER (MN-CU): Chronic infectious diseases, sinusitis, laryngitis, allergic disorders, psychosomatic disorders, menstrual problems, hypothyroidism, goiter, obesity, anxiety, anorexia nervosa, arthritis, arthritic pain, lumbar pain, osteomalacia, chronic bronchitis, cirrhosis of the liver, dysmenorrhea, dysovulation, male infertility, prostatitis, periodontal disease, scoliosis, sciatica, urinary tract infections, eczema, emphysema.

MANGANESE-COPPER-COBALT (MN-CU-CO): Anemia, hypotension, neurasthenia, colitis, immune depletion, thyroid insufficiency, decalcification, seborrhea, acne, periodontal disease, gastritis, hypertension.

NICKEL (NI): Obesity, diabetes, pancreatic insufficiency, intestinal gas, postprandial somnolence.

NICKEL-COBALT (NI-CO): Functional digestive disorders, obesity, constipation, diabetes and prediabetes, pancreatitis, dermatoses, urinary tract disorders.

PHOSPHORUS (P): General spasms and cramps (spasmophilia), tetany, paresthesias, circulatory problems at the extremities, spasmodic cough, spasmodic crying, asthma, mental fatigue, lumbar pain, hypothyroid obesity, scoliosis, osteomalacia, osteoporosis, osteochondritis, rheumatism.

POTASSIUM (K): Chronic rheumatism, sciatica, hyperadrenalism, polyarthritis, arthritic pain, lumbar pain, mental fatigue, alcoholism, obesity (from water retention or hypothyroidism), hyperthyroidism, premenstrual syndrome, diarrhea, gallstones, hepatobiliary insufficiency.

SELENIUM (SE): Cardiovascular problems, hypertension, coronaropathy, cerebrovascular accidents, diseases of aging, autoimmune disorders, cancer protection, cervical dysplasia, toxic liver symptoms from alcohol or medications, coeliac disease, all types of mycoses, skin and mucous membrane disorders, dermatitis, eczema, psoriasis, ulcerated skin.

SILICON (SI): Demineralization, arthroses, growth disorders, arterial protection, connective tissue problems, periodontal disease, weak nails, hair, teeth; osteoporosis, rheumatoid arthritis.

SILVER (AG): Infections and febrile illness, particularly ear, nose, throat, bronchial and pulmonary, such as rhinitis, pharyngitis, sinusitis, tonsillitis, influenza, neuralgias, articular pain.

STRONTIUM (SR): Osteoporosis and problems in bone development.

SULPHUR (S): Rheumatic disorders, gout, allergic and dermatologic manifestations of hepatobiliary dysfunction, hypercholesterolemia, acne, eczema, psoriasis, hay fever, dysmenorrhea, asthma, bronchial and pulmonary diseases, chronic bronchitis, emphysema, laryngitis, hypertension, vertigo, herpes zoster and simplex, arthrosis, osteoporosis, arthritis pain, lumbar pain, spinal discopathy, sciatica, neuralgia, prostatitis.

ZINC (ZN): Functional problems of the endocrine system, retarded growth, dermatoses, acne, cutaneous ulcers, hair loss, problems of nervous equilibrium, adrenal insufficiency, asthma, candidiasis, alcoholism, arteriosclerosis, impotence, prostatitis, frigidity, infertility (male or female), lumbar problems, high cholesterol, hyperthyroidism.

ZINC-COPPER (ZN-CU): Functional problems of puberty and menopause, low immunity, depression, growth disorders, impotence, bedwetting, psoriasis, dermatoses, alopecia, polyuria, enuresis, hyper- and hypoinsulinism.

ZINC-NICKEL-COBALT (ZN-NI-CO): General fatigue, impotence, hyperadrenalism, pancreatitis, gallbladder dysfunction, sluggish digestion, nausea, colitis, subcostal pain or discomfort, diabetes, prediabetes, postprandial somnolence, bedwetting.

AFFINITIES AND ANTAGONISMS AMONG THE TRACE ELEMENTS		
TRACE ELEMENT	**AFFINITIES**	**ANTAGONIST(S)**
Aluminum	Lithium, Magnesium, Copper-Gold-Silver	Phosphorus
Cobalt	Copper, Iodine, Manganese, Nickel	Iron, Calcium
Fluorine	Gold, Zinc, Silver, Manganese	Calcium, Aluminum, Magnesium, Copper, Phosphorus, Lithium, Iodine
Iodine (and iodides)	Manganese, Copper, Zinc, Cobalt, Potassium	Fluorine, Lithium, Magnesium
Iron	Copper, Nickel	Cobalt, Phosphorus, Calcium, Fluorine, Manganese
Lithium	Copper, Gold, SIlver, Zinc, Sulphur	Potassium, Magnesium
Magnesium	Copper-Gold-Silver, Zinc, Potassium, Sulphur	Calcium, Manganese, Phosphorus, Copper, Bismuth, Lithium, Fluorine
Manganese	Copper, Nickel, Zinc, Potassium, Sulphur	Calcium, Phosphorus, Zinc, Iron, Fluorine
Nickel	Zinc, Cobalt, Phosphorus, Calcium, Magnesium	Sulphur, Copper
Phosphorus	Iodine	Calcium, Sodium, Magnesium, Copper, Zinc, Fluorine, Manganese, Bismuth, Iron
Potassium	Manganese, Copper, Iron, Magnesium	Sodium, Calcium
Sulphur	Magnesium	Copper, Cobalt
Zinc	Nickel-Cobalt	Calcium, Phosphorus, Copper

PART THREE
THERAPEUTIC GUIDELINES
ACCORDING TO TERRAIN

THE USE OF BOTANICALS IN HEALING

Knowledge of both the properties of herbs and their derivatives is equally important to an understanding of the terrain. There are a multiplicity of substances in any given herb. The essence of lemon, for example, neutralizes typhoid bacillus in five minutes *in vitro*, staphylococcus also in five minutes and diphtheria bacillus in twenty minutes. A febrifuge, cardiotonic, hemostatic and diuretic, it calms gastric hyperacidity, reduces blood viscosity and stimulates the veins. And that is only its internal usage. As another example, thyme is a tonic, hypertensive, antispasmodic, balsamic (especially to respiratory mucosa), antiseptic, emmenagogue and vermifuge.

In the fragmented Cartesian universe of the Doctrine of Specificity, however, a single drug with two separate applications is an anomalous concept. Reductionistic science attempts to isolate the various components and determine to which substances various properties are attributed. Yet attempting to isolate biologically active substances from a plant such as thyme and assign specific therapeutic functions for each component is not likely to succeed. The broad spectrum of the usefulness of thyme is homologous with what we might think of as a food, rather than a collection of distinct therapeutic agents. Indeed, where do we draw the line between foods and herbs? In traditional East Asian culture the distinction between foods and herbs, even medicinal herbs, is faded and indistinct.

A fundamental challenge in the practice of botanical medicine is a global understanding of plants and their properties. From this we can develop a qualitative understanding sufficient to apply our knowledge of plant influences to our understanding of the physiological terrain. When we deal with herbs classified into categories of physiological spheres of influence and their effects on terrains, we have graduated from the micro-universe of atomized fact as represented by molecular biology into a realm where visible structures and manifestations can be observed in operation. But to cultivate this understanding we must develop a new level of insight, and this requires patient and close observation of clinical signs and their changes.

Practitioners must also strive to develop good clinical methods, viable research protocols and experimental procedures which could lead to new scientific methods for investigating natural substances. Conventional scientific thinking assumes that a disease entity, such as hepatitis, somehow has an autonomous existence apart from the individuals who provide the actual liver along with all their other individual attributes and idiosyncrasies. Clearly a nosology based on specificity in this regard is too simplistic to encompass the complexity of these interactions of plant-derived substances and human or animal physiology.

In classical Chinese medicine, this problem is approached by individualized differential diagnosis of diseases or complaints. Clinical research on the herbal treatment of hepatitis, for example, would be performed by dividing the patient population into terrain-based categories of Liver qi congestion, Spleen qi vacuity, Liver-Kidney yin vacuity, Spleen-Kidney yang vacuity and Blood stasis type, rather than according to microbe populations or other parameters. However, blood analysis of liver enzymes and other significant parameters would also be measured. Then different formulas would be used for each of these terrains and all results for each group collated together.

Although this approach would draw criticism in the West as being unscientific, it is this type of approach that begins to satisfy certain deficiencies of scientific research protocols which, despite significant individual differences among patients, still maintain the tacit assumption that all physiologies are created equal. Taking scientific research out of the laboratory and back into the clinic, and developing research methods that respect biological individuality, will create a scientific atmosphere in which botanical medicine and other natural therapies can flourish.

The Issue of Dosage

One of the most vital factors in botanical medicine, the importance of which is often overlooked by conventional medical thought, is the issue of dosage. We already know that there is a vast range of tolerance among individuals to such common substances as ethyl alcohol, morphine or even table sugar. Medications have different types of effects at different dosages. A strong dose of ipecac is emetic and antidysenteric whereas a mild dose is expectorant, decongestive and hemostatic. The intensity of the action of a plant likewise can vary according to the terrain of the individual and can even induce opposite reactions. Linden extract, well known for its sedative properties, provokes insomnia in certain subjects. This can also occur occasionally with passionflower.

The Arndt-Schulz law states that weak stimuli increase physiological activity whereas strong stimuli abolish or inhibit it. An extension of this law is called the type-effect hypothesis. The German physician Karl Koetschau described how the same substance at a small dose stimulates, a moderate dose stimulates then inhibits, and with a large dose gives a short-lived stimulation followed by a strongly depressive effect. The net result is a stimulus followed by the response of the living system. The stimulus consists of the substance itself whose properties cannot be considered apart from the response. We can say, however, that according to this law of dosage a single substance can have different, often opposite properties at different levels of dosage. Therefore a single substance has no stable, unchanging, predictable qualities.

Conventional medicine uses this principle in the vaccination concept, in which micro-organisms that have the properties to break down the immune defenses are thought to create protection and immunity at low doses. Many patients have paradoxical responses and side-effects to pharmaceuticals. There are countless examples of this phenomenon. Anxiety is a side-effect of the tranquilizer Valium. Many antianxiety drugs, including the well-known and controversial Prozac, elicit side effects of suicidal longings. Aspirin, a febrifuge, can at high doses induce hyperthermia. It is well-known that most anticancer drugs are carcinogenic, as are X-rays, also used for cancer treatment. For over a century strychnine has been known to have stimulant properties in very small doses. To fully appreciate this, one may browse through the *Physicians' Desk Reference* and note the repeated occurrence of "side-effects" of drugs being identical to the condition they are supposed to treat. The controversy over Prozac is only a recent example.

The terrain, or the typology of the recipient of the substance, also can have a highly variable response. The scale by which dosage has traditionally been determined is body weight. Yet one individual can have tolerances for substances that in many cases go far beyond another individual's tolerance levels. Anesthesiologists are familiar with patients who can tolerate many times the lethal dose of some anesthetics.

Further, the intended level of activity of the treatment must be considered with respect to dosage. For example, for an extremely anxious patient, oil of lavender is often much more effective at a low dose. In such a case, a tiny amount (one drop, even applied externally, or one drop orally in a capsule with a base, or three or four drops of a solution of six drops of lavender in 15 ml of propolis tincture or elixir of papain) can effectively bias the intense level of physiological activity. A larger dose might create sudden changes, which, even if corrective, are disconcerting to the enervated patient. On the other hand, if a patient who suffers from chronic toxicity (sluggish bowel or liver function, for example) has an acute infection, it may be necessary to use a higher dose of an essential oil or drainage herb to shift the terrain out of a condition that could quickly deteriorate into a dangerous condition or acute crisis.

There is further evidence, as we will see later, that many herbs do not have properties that exist in any meaningful way outside the context of their field of activity, qualitatively or quantitatively. Quantitatively the dosage must be matched to the vital capacity of the organism's immune response. Qualitatively, the activity of a substance is modulated by the nature of the terrain, the chemical make-up of the individual according to his constitutional type and living habits. The terrain is a concept in which biological individuality is the fundamental law, rather than an exception to the rule.

Precautions in essential oils dosage

Essential oils should be used with caution for a number of reasons. Pharmaceutical grade essences can be safely used orally or rectally. If pharmaceutical or food grade oils are not available, they should be used only externally. The dosage range of essential oils is very wide. The dose of an oil for an acute infection can be as little as 0.2 g per day (1 gram = about 20 drops), usually encapsulated along with flax oil or honey. In a typical ambulatory patient with an acute sinus infection or cold, a simple combination would be three drops of oil of niaouli and two of lemon in capsules to be taken two or three times a day. Three drops of lavender twice a day can control a hypertensive patient (sympathotonic) with a fairly good diet. It is often advisable, as mentioned previously, to give a lower dose of one drop of lavender as needed, either orally or externally, if a patient is in an acute state of extreme anxiety. For a chronic condition in a weak patient, eight drops of cinnamon in 15 ml of a tincture can be used for weeks at a dosage of six drops of the solution three times a day.

There is not as much agreement on toxicity as one might expect. Some writers insist that rosemary not be given to epileptics. Other practitioners claim to use rosemary as a therapeutic agent for epilepsy. One practitioner's therapeutic drainage response or healing phenomenon is another practitioner's toxic reaction. Some practitioners insist that strongly estrogenic herbs, such as sage, should not be used in cancer patients. Others maintain that sage simply alters the terrain, and the body's response will be appropriate to its needs. In other words, sage will not force the body to produce estrogen it does not want. Naturally, caution should always be observed for any type of life-threatening condition. On the other hand, the natural health care practitioner should also weigh the risks and benefits of using botanicals with the risks patients take when they use large doses of pharmaceuticals.

Prolonged use of certain essential oils should be avoided with certain types of medical conditions, unless there are strict specific indications. It always depends on the individual case, so there are simply areas where one should observe caution. An oil or extract that is contraindicated for a condition does not mean that it cannot be used strategically at certain times. It is also possible to use many of these herbs in the form of a tea, or some other less concentrated form. Treatment should be applied cautiously or avoided with the plants noted for the conditions listed below:

CONDITION	OILS TO AVOID
Hemorrhage	*lavender*
Chronic respiratory problems	*oregano, rosemary, marjoram, yarrow, hyssop*
Upper digestive tract problems	*cinnamon, clove*
Circulation problems	*lemon & hyssop* (hypertension), *thyme, serpolet, cypress, hyssop, tarragon, oregano* (glaucoma)
Thyroid problems	*garlic, onion* (hyperthyroidism), *cumin, fennel* (hypothyroidism)
Urinary tract problems	*eucalyptus, juniper* (chronic infections), *thyme, serpolet* (retention of urine)
Prostate problems	*angelica, cypress, hyssop, serpolet* (cancer)
Female reproductive problems	*sage, cypress, fennel, anise, angelica, cumin* (high estrogen, female organ cancers)
Nervous system problems	*lemon, peppermint, pine, phenolic oils* (insomnia), *sage, hyssop* (epilepsy*)
Malignant tumors	*sage, fennel, angelica* and other estrogenic oils

*Note: controversy surrounds numerous essences regarding epilepsy. Some oils contraindicated for epilepsy may increase the number and length of seizures, but greatly reduce their severity.

The phenolic oils (cinnamon, clove, oregano, savory, etcetera) should only be used on the skin or rectally when well buffered and diluted so that they do not irritate the skin or mucous membranes. These oils are best used at very low doses until the patient's tolerance has been tested. Oil of bergamot is photosensitizing and can cause the sun to leave permanent spots on the skin. We feel that most toxicity of the essential oils profiled in this book are issues of dosage rather than innate toxicity, if the purity and quality level is high. Most phytotherapy doctors in Europe use pharmaceutical grade oils. These are oils that are tested not only for quality and purity but also for their therapeutic properties.

The following oils should be used with more caution, and at a lower initial dosage level:

Juniper	can detoxify the kidneys
Lavender	do not take with anticoagulants
Calamus	narcotic
Cinnamon	phenolic
Clove	phenolic
Savory	phenolic
Oregano	phenolic

THE FUNDAMENTALS OF THERAPY

In observing the diverse biological activities of a single plant, we can recognize the complexity of vegetal substances. Having a multiplicity of components, a plant extract can serve various functions in different organs. Yet it is also important to underscore the fact that, by means of these numerous properties, plants can offer the therapist the ability to operate at several therapeutic levels simultaneously. Different schools of thought tend to emphasize treatment at one level in preference to any other, but there are three levels of activity that comprise a systematic approach to patient care, and actually complement each other, allowing a patient to be treated at the stage of the healing process which is appropriate for their condition. These three stages are drainage, symptomatic treatment and altering the terrain.

Drainage, the first level of activity, is the unburdening of the eliminative system relevant to an afflicted organ or structure. The result helps reinforce the second activity, which is to relieve the immediate subjective complaint. The degree of effectiveness of these first two levels of usage depends on the extent to which the terrain can be successfully altered at the third level of treatment. Ideally, modifying the terrain affects the principal cause of the malady – the disequilibrium of the cells' fluid environment and the resulting malfunctions of the endocrine and neurovegetative systems of Western medicine or of the classical Chinese medical channel systems.

Altering the terrain is a process of activating a physical or chemical compensation mechanism. Physiological mechanisms always compensate for a change in the environment, but do not alter the actual chemical or ionic makeup of the fluid system. Physiological thermoregulation mechanisms do not fundamentally alter the biochemical makeup of the cellular environment and create changes that can easily return to a previous equilibrium. Within a physiological range, blood sugar regulation and discharge of cellular waste products, such as urea or carbon dioxide, do not require material resources from the tissues to prevent disequilibrium. With greater or more sudden physical or chemical stimuli, compensation mechanisms may be activated in order to attempt to restore the previous equilibrium. Constant or frequent activation of these mechanisms are usually only able to recreate a semblance of the former equilibrium. Eventually these compensations are inadequate to prevent the pathological changes that result in chronic disease and the aging process. When the organ systems weaken and malfunction, the cellular environment deteriorates so that cellular function is impaired, eventually leading to death.

DRAINAGE

Drainage is the stimulation of the excretory functions of the eliminative organs or ducts, which include the liver, gallbladder, large intestine, kidney and skin. These organs manage the discharge and to some extent the breakdown of the waste products of metabolism. Incomplete evacuation can play a major role in the development of some types of pathology due to the accumulation of waste material – urea, uric acid, cholesterol – which causes either local irritation or disequilibrium upstream along the metabolic chain.

Drainage assists symptomatic treatment allowing the system to return to an unclogged condition, thwarting possible relapses by discharging toxic or morbid material. Often skin problems such as herpes or even eczema can be eliminated by simple hepatic drainage along with symptomatic treatment of the skin.

These different properties – providing vital nutrients, regulating disturbed functions (symptomatic activity) and draining the organs of elimination – constitute the foundation of phytotherapy, the first level of usage. In choosing therapeutic herbs, the practitioner makes selections based on which herbs have properties to counteract as much of the immediate pathology as well as any associated pathology, its antecedents and the patient's predispositions and weak points. This is an important point of divergence from conventional practice based on the doctrine of specificity wherein a medication is considered to have a "specific" activity. Due to their complexity and diverse constituents, plants possess multiple properties. Each plant has a personality, a unique profile of its uses and indications. This is what makes the practice of botanical medicine an art. Understanding the complexity of the activity of plant substances allows the practitioner to match the complexity of a pathological profile and the terrain, thus allowing the greatest possible degree of personalization of treatment.

By way of illustration, we can note that among the herbs for hepatic drainage, the choice of one over another depends on its other properties and how they interface with the other manifestations of disordered hepatic function. Plants used for hepatic drainage include artichoke, black radish and nettle. Artichoke facilitates biliary secretion and counteracts cholesterol buildup, but is also an effective diuretic. Thus, artichoke is preferred when there is an excess of cholesterol and the need for a diuretic. Nettle is chosen especially for its diuretic effects, particularly for uric acid elimination or for its astringent action as a hemostatic, vasoconstrictor or antidiarrheic. Black radish, a powerful cholagogue, has a less marked diuretic activity, but supplies sulphur and vitamin C. It is indicated particularly when there is dermatosis associated with a pulmonary infection. These types of considerations influence the choice of the plant.

As another example, the patient with diarrhea clearly does not, in most cases, require drainage. This patient will benefit from symptomatic treatment according to the terrain and often disinfection, which is also dependent on the terrain.

Thus even at the levels of symptomatic treatment and drainage it is necessary to synthesize various elements of the overall clinical picture. We can treat effectively at this level of practice, but even in spite of effective symptomatic treatment and successful drainage of eliminative organs, the essential pathology may not change; if the patient's individual make-up is ignored, the cystitis can return, the acne or eczema can reappear.

Symptomatic phytotherapy

Each disequilibrium in the organism manifests in characteristic patterns by which the malady is diagnosed. For example, if the presence of bacteria in the bladder results in a local inflammatory reaction, difficulty in urination, pain in the pelvic or lumbar region, sometimes fever etcetera, the combination of clinical signs along with biological testing would lead to a diagnosis of cystitis. Symptom relief would be paramount at this stage. A proper choice for symptomatic treatment might include a febrifuge, an analgesic and a pelvic decongestant in addition to a bactericide. Thus an agent or agents would be used to assuage the symptoms as well as to remove the direct cause. In conventional medicine, by contrast, the approach would be to inhibit the proliferation of bacteria by antibiotic treatment. However, this would not address the primary cause – the organic disequilibrium and local conditions that encourage the flourishing of the bacteria.

The activity of the plant substance at this level can be explained in several ways. There is the contribution of nutrients such as vitamins, minerals, catalytic agents or trace elements. Horsetail, for example, is rich in minerals including silica, calcium carbonate, potassium, magnesium, manganese and iron, and plays an important role in the treatment of demineralization and problems in the balance of phosphorous, calcium and magnesium as seen in osseous pathology, rheumatism and spasmophilia. Plants also influence symptomatology by means of components such as the salicylic acid derivatives found in white willow, meadowsweet or ash, which all have anti-inflammatory, febrifuge and analgesic properties. Clove contains eugenol, well-known to dentists for its anesthetic and antiseptic properties. We know of the formidable antiseptic properties of many essential oils. There are cardiac regulating agents like hawthorn and lily-of-the-valley, appetite stimulants such as gentian, centaury and fumitory, intestinal astringents such as walnut and geranium, and expectorants like mullein and coltsfoot. Indeed much of what has been written about medicinal plants in the classical herbals is about their symptomatic properties.

THERAPEUTICS ACCORDING TO TERRAIN

Practitioners in Europe use different tools to evaluate patients according to the terrain. Some practitioners in France use the aromatogram. Other practitioners use conventional blood tests to give insights into the patient's typology or terrain. The most reliable method of determining the patient's terrain, however, is experience and judgment based on taking a careful history, understanding the patient's medical history, family history, personal habits, likes and dislikes, physical type and personality type. In addition, careful physical examination can reveal the most important data. Methods of palpation and the information derived differ among practitioners of acupuncture, physical therapies and conventionally trained physicians, but the information derived from the physical examination is the most conclusive with respect to the patient's immediate complaints.

An understanding of the classical Chinese medical channel system can assist the practitioner in ascertaining the five phase type. Conventional physicians' training can prepare one to understand the typology according to endocrine and nervous system parameters. Both systems can shed light in areas where the other is less detailed. It is useful to "collect" different systems because each has particular characteristics and correspondences and elucidates phenomena that are ignored by other systems. The study of more than one whole-system model allows the student to be aware that each model, although it is "universal," like any language or software, it has its limitations.

The practitioner should feel free to hybridize systems. Study of conventional methods of physical diagnosis and pathology is useful to the acupuncturist. The conventionally trained practitioner will benefit from knowledge of the five phases and other systems of classical Chinese medical diagnosis. Hand morphology and personality types can help determine constitutional type (see Requena, *Character and Health*). Blood pressure and heart rate may help to identify a patient who is sympathotonic and hyperthyroid, thus distinguishing the Wood type from the Fire type for choosing therapeutic agents. The practitioner might first identify a patient as Wood, but discover an atypical vagotonia that, when addressed, brings about relief of the patient's immediate condition.

Pathology matches the constitutional type about 60 percent of the time. For example, even in a "pure" Fire type (a fairly rare occurrence), Fire-related symptoms and signs appear at a 60 percent rate of frequency. It becomes necessary to blend the influences because each clinical situation presented is unique, and may require a unique blend of therapeutic influences. A person who is Wood yin and Metal yin will usually respond to Wood yin and Metal yin herbs. If this patient presents clinical signs that are Earth in nature, such as diarrhea, Wood yin and Metal yin herbs with an Earth nature should be tried first. If the patient presents a Fire symptom, such as tachycardia, Wood yin or Metal yin herbs with a Fire nature should be considered first. Likewise, one could consider treating tachycardia with Fire yang or Fire yin herbs that have a Wood yin or Metal yin nature. In most cases, the patient will have other symptoms or characteristics that match the clinical picture associated with these Wood yin or Metal yin herbs.

In sum, these levels of utilization and their mechanisms of action comprise the subtlety, variety and depth of efficacy of treatment in botanical medicine. The flexibility of this approach places a method of therapeutic promise at our disposal that can revolutionize medical treatment. A framework encompassing classification of terrains permits the practitioner to make allowances for the uniqueness of each individual and to understand a deeper level of psychological and emotional factors as coherent functions of physiological activity. A whole-system model of the terrain provides a template through which the practitioner's intuition can develop and clinical practice can be mastered in a shorter period of time without sacrificing rigor or conventional examination techniques. In short, it adds a new dimension to the science of human health, expanding its borders and creating a new perspective for the orthodox scientific heritage of the last century.

DETERMINING A TERRAIN DISEQUILIBRIUM USING THE AROMATOGRAM

Many types of examination can be used as supplementary methods of diagnosis. The first step toward a diagnosis is a complete history. Next, examination by conventional means can be extremely useful in therapeutic decisions. All available methods should be sought to obtain useful data including radiological, ultrasonic, biochemical testing — blood, urinalysis and the like. The third step is complementary diagnosis specific to the therapeutic method. The aromatogram is of great importance to botanical medicine in determining disequilibrium of the terrain.

The aromatogram is analogous to the antibiogram of conventional medicine. A sample of blood, urine, feces, vomitus, vaginal discharge, the skin, etcetera is cultured in the appropriate medium and placed on a dish. Pastilles containing essential oils are placed around the perimeter of the dish to test the reaction of the microbes to the oils. After 24 hours at 37 degrees centigrade, the dish is observed to evaluate the inhibition of growth of the micro-organisms by the essential oils. In this way a measurement in millimeters, the diameter of inhibition, is obtained for each essence tested to determine its activity *in vitro*. The interpretation is specific.

The aromatogram was first described in 1949 by Schroeder and Messing. It wasn't until 1970 that Dr. Maurice Girault had the idea to use it in the local treatment of leukorrhea. Working in collaboration with M. Bourgeon and Dr. Jean Valnet, they christened the technique. In 1972, under the guidance of Dr. Valnet, the Association for the Study and Research of Aromatherapy and Phytotherapy extended the use of the aromatogram to systemic infections for which oral prescriptions were made. The Association decided to call the technique the antibio-aromatogram to draw the parallel with the new methodology and its origin in the antibiogram. In 1976, however, the name reverted to "aromatogram" when it became clear that the therapeutic results of essential oils taken orally are not because of their antibiotic or antiseptic action, but because they act on another level.

Results of aromatograms present challenges to the theory of specificity. For example, the essential oils that are revealed by the aromatogram to be the most active – those with the greatest diameter of inhibition on the disc – are not necessarily those with the reputation of being antiseptic or containing active principles that are antiseptic in nature. Also, the minimum inhibitory concentration, (MIC) was found to be dramatically different *in vivo* from *in vitro*. The minimum inhibitory concentration is the least amount of a substance that produces complete inhibition of the growth of a micro-organism. For an antibiotic to be effective, the dose used *in vivo* must be greater than or equal to the MIC of the antibiotic under consideration. With antibiotics the concentration of dosage is the same both *in vitro* and *in vivo*. This is because antibiotics control microbe populations by killing them through direct contact. In the case of essential oils, however, the dose of the essential oil needed to inhibit the growth of microbes *in vitro* is much greater than the concentration of oil that arrives at the tissue level *in vivo* at the time of treatment by a factor of about 100 to 1! Nevertheless, it is therapeutically active as proven by clinical results. In the body, the essential oils seem to operate by a different type of mechanism. Rather than killing microbes by direct contact, they seem to somehow alter the terrain so that it is no longer hospitable to the infecting microbes.

Thus, if antibiotic therapy requires the same level of the tested dosages *in vitro* for therapeutic usage *in vivo*, according to the minimum inhibitory concentration, this appears not to be the case with the essences. Furthermore, a single type of micro-organism is not necessarily sensitive to particular essential oils and, conversely, essential oils are not necessarily specific to certain micro-organisms *in vivo*, regardless of how they behave in a glass dish. Therefore, one cannot say, as with antibiotics, that eucalyptus essence is active against infection of pneumococcus or streptococcus. The same type of microbe presents different aromatograms as well as manifests different types of pathological reactions. The sensitivity of the microbe to the essential oil is thus a function of the host organism, that is, the condition of the patient's terrain.

As an additional advantage, there is no phenomenon of acquired resistance of a microbe to an essential oil. For a given micro-organism, isolated as a temporal factor in the diagnosis, a given essence will completely retain its efficacy over an extended period of time. This illustrates that essential oils do not inhibit the growth of micro-organisms in the manner of an antibiotic, by direct contact, but rather by modifying the conditions that favor and support the microbes' development. The aromatogram permits the practitioner to conduct a precise, thorough and refined diagnosis of the terrain which also contributes to lines of further investigation through interrogation, or further clinical examination.

In summary, the aromatogram elucidates several unexpected phenomena:

1. A microbicidal effect is produced despite the fact that the concentration *in vivo* is far too low to kill micro-organisms by direct contact.

2. The most active essential oils in the aromatogram are not always those reputed to have antiseptic properties or those that contain antiseptic active principles.

3. A single type of microbe possesses no specific sensitivity to a particular essential oil and vice versa. The same type of microbe appearing in different tests in contact with essential oils is affected differently in each

aromatogram. The sensitivity of the microbe to essential oils is thus a function of the host organism, i.e., a function of the terrain.

4.   There is no phenomenon of acquired resistance of micro-organisms to essential oils. For a given microbe isolated at a given moment, the essence will retain all of its efficacy.

Doctors practicing botanical medicine after adjusting their treatments with the aromatogram have found that they can heal refractory illnesses that they had previously been treating blindly. For the first time, it became possible to obtain a laboratory profile of the terrain.

Dr. Paul Duraffourd, senior laboratory chief at the Faculty of Medicine in Paris, described a case of chronic urethritis with a prostate focus that was diagnosed with the aromatogram. According to the aromatogram, the bacterial culture was shown to be extremely sensitive to eucalyptus, juniper and geranium, all oils known for their antidiabetic activity. Fasting blood sugar was normal and glycosuria was negative. Prescription of these essential oils and an antidiabetic dietary regime prevented the recurrence of the symptomatology, which had recurred repeatedly for years. The oils did not act by directly inhibiting the growth of the micro-organisms, but by treating the prediabetic terrain, that is, by altering the conditions that were the origin of the bacterial proliferation.

Understanding the mechanisms involved in the relationship between essential oils, microbes and the terrain requires a new hypothesis. Dr. Paul Duraffourd proposed that the membrane wall, which is the locus of adaptation and nourishment of the microbe, allows the antiseptic properties of a specific essential oil (and none of the others) to be transported to the interior of the micro-organism *in vitro*. The implication is that essential oils act by means of polymerization and depolymerization of the membrane, a sort of chain reaction. This technique may have uncovered an important phenomenon that could have powerful implications for therapeutics.

The aromatogram helps the therapist to specify clearly the nature of the terrain in addition to allowing precise therapeutic decisions. A valuable tool in the growth of this new science, it is the type of test that promises to help construct a new scientific model for botanical medicine in the future.

SYMPTOM LISTINGS OF THERAPEUTIC GUIDELINES ACCORDING TO TERRAIN

The following therapeutic index is designed to provide guidelines in making decisions related to the patient's treatment. It can be useful for matching the patient's terrain to the symptomatic treatment. Differential diagnosis and dosage are the two medical arts that require the most experience and mastery for success. No protocol will ever satisfy all of the practitioner's clinical needs. A guide such as this can be only an aid to stimulate thought and intuition, as well as help the practitioner structure clinical experience so as to accelerate the learning curve.

In the therapeutic guidelines, italicized plant names refer to essential oils. In some cases the plant name, for example, fennel, will be listed both with and without italics. In the description in non-italic listing, fennel could be used as an infusion, a tincture or other type of extract. Italicized, *fennel* refers specifically to an essential oil. Sometimes a plant substance will be listed for both. If a plant such as sage is listed as an essential oil for a certain condition, this does not preclude its use as a tincture or decoction. It merely indicates a preference or a customary use. In the case of acute infections or other types of acute care application, the use of essences would usually be more desirable to obtain a strong impact on the patient's condition.

ACUTE RESPIRATORY INFECTIONS

What can physicians offer to patients with no tolerance for antibiotics? With growing reluctance to take antibiotics, patients are increasingly seeking relief for acute infections from other sources. It is somewhat erroneous to refer to essential oils as being antibiotic when in fact their action as microbicidal agents is twofold.

As mentioned earlier in the section on the aromatogram, there are two modes of action by which essential oils manifest their potency against microbes. One mode is by direct contact by a concentration of oil above the M.I.C. This is the case with cutaneous sores or abscesses treated locally with salves or compresses containing essential oils. Antibiotics work by killing microbes through direct contact when used locally or systemically.

However, in the process of killing anaerobic flora, they reduce the body's immune potential and fatigue the adrenal glands. The other mode of microbicidal activity, which is manifest by essential oils, is indirect.

The typical daily dosage of oils used in infections for systemic treatment is sometimes less than 100 mg (about 4 drops), such that the concentration at the level of contact with the microbe proliferation is always less than the M.I.C. The equivalent dosage of antibiotic for the same level of efficacy is closer to 1000 mg. To achieve the maximum result using essential oils, it is necessary to refer to all qualitative data regarding the nature of the terrain as well as to quantitative factors. The hypothesis proposed earlier is that the species of microbe involved reflects certain aspects of the terrain of the illness and that the essential oils active with these microbes have a relationship to the type of terrain rather than to the species of microbes. Essential oils contain constituents that are mucolytic and immunostimulating as well as constituents that are microbicidal, and these factors can also contribute to the microbicidal effect by making the terrain inhospitable to pathogens.

The chemotype of essential oils (See Chemotypes in Section One) is determined by gas chromatography. Within the same plant, isolated constituents can vary in quality and in their relative proportions. The variations are a function primarily of their soil environment and the time of their harvest. Chemotypes are characterized according to their principal constituent. Thus in thyme, for example, there is thymol, carvacrol and phenol. The bactericidal activity of an essential oil is always associated with the presence among its principal constituents of certain ones classically recognized as strong antiseptics – phenol, carvacrol and thymol in particular.

According to all of the clinical studies done over the last twenty-five years, it appears that the reality is more complex. Neither the bactericidal activity or intensity can be linked exclusively to the grade of the extract as determined by the concentration of phenols or any other constituents – aldehydes, monoterpenic alcohols or esters. In one series of experiments, the essential oils with the highest concentrations of bactericidal components were used. In another series, seventeen chemotypes of oil of thyme were used. In both studies, each time an essential oil was active on the microbe in question, all variations or chemotypes of that same essential oil were active regardless of the level of bactericidal components. On the other hand, if an oil did not manifest any activity with the germ, none of the chemotypes of that oil manifested the slightest bactericidal effect. It is important to remember that a single component can vary in its proportion within an oil from 10 to 60 percent. Thus it appears as follows:

1.   The bactericidal activity of an essential oil is not determined by its concentration of phenols or other antiseptic active principles.

2.   An increase in the level of concentration of phenolic components never increases the antiseptic intensity of an essential oil in a linear fashion. Rather, the variations in intensity of the essential oil using antiseptic components as an index is contradictory and unpredictable.

3.   The activity of a pure essential oil is always superior to that of one enriched with active principles.

It is important, therefore, for the practitioner to understand qualitative aspects of the disease terrain as well as qualitative aspects of the plant materials. Contrary to the conventional scientific method, a quantitative assessment of disease phenomena lacks the necessary precision for effective treatment. Likewise, *in vitro* evaluations of the effects of oils on microbes may have nothing to do with how that oil will affect a living system.

Basic principles of treatment
for acute respiratory infections

1. Determine the target organ, whether it is the same as the disease focus, or the relationship it has to the disease focus. This is determined by interrogation and physical examination.

2. Establish normal balance of the organs involved. This is performed by calming or draining hyperfunctioning organs and stimulating or nourishing hypoactive organs.

3. Re-establish equilibrium of the terrain.

4. Modify the dietary regime.

For acute infections, treatment consists of drainage (vomiting, catharsis, diaphoresis, diuresis, fever reduction, etcetera) and disinfection. Extracts or oils for disinfection are often used to clear up symptoms. If there is recurrence, however, healing cannot take place without drainage and supplementation of the body's defenses. Local treatment with vaporizers, inhalers and massage with oils may also be necessary. Drainage of the respiratory passages in some cases may result in increased discomfort. To minimize this, it is important to drain properly not only the respiratory mucosa but that of the digestive tract as well.

The time-honored treatment for the early stage of acute respiratory infections is to induce diaphoresis. This is not advisable if perspiration has occurred spontaneously or in cases where there is no fever. Viral infections, such as influenza and herpes, are often afebrile and noncatarrhal, or result in a thin catarrhal discharge as in rhinoviral infections. Apart from these considerations, there are no fundamental differences in how infections are treated, regardless of whether the micro-organisms are bacteria, viruses, fungi or even protozoa.

In classical Chinese medicine, acute respiratory infections are considered to manifest at the body's "front line" – the skin, mucosa of the nose, sinuses, pharynx, stomach and broncho-pulmonary regions. Likewise, disease manifestations at the head and neck area, such as swollen lymph nodes, stiffness in the neck and symptoms including headache and tinnitus, can be considered manifestations of exterior pathology. There is a tradition in some cultures of ceremoniously undergoing hot and cold treatment in order to adapt to the coming of winter, and of course using herbs for the purpose of inducing a sweat to break a fever is the classical treatment for colds.

However, chronic diseases of the respiratory system, such as sinusitis, asthma, tuberculosis and emphysema, are considered to be deeply entrenched and difficult to remove. Lung cancer, for example, is considered to be one of the most deeply imbedded cancers and extremely difficult to cure.

Herbs by Terrain: Otorhinolaryngological, Bronchopulmonary Infections

Phase	Herb	Indications
Wood	PLANTAIN	Antiallergic; good for sinus irritation, common cold; anti-inflammatory, astringent and general stimulant.
Fire Yin	ELECAMPANE	Expectorant, diuretic, diaphoretic. Increases biliary secretions. This herb expresses a marked pulmonary tropism and contains anti-infectious principles demonstrated *in vitro* and *in vivo*. It has a global stimulating effect on the hypophysis and marked antiallergic activity in the pulmonary sphere.
Earth Yang	AGRIMONY	Very effective for tonsillitis if taken in an infusion. Decongestant, astringent, diuretic and antidiabetic
Earth Yin	LICORICE	Antispasmodic, antiulcerative, anti-inflammatory, helpful for colon pain and spasms with constipation in cases of colitis.
Metal Yang	MARSHMALLOW	Indicated for skin, pulmonary and intestinal inflammations. Good for tonsillitis.
	HOREHOUND	Antitoxic, antiseptic; febrifuge, diuretic and expectorant with properties of relaxing cardiac excitability, e.g., tachycardia. Like mistletoe, it contains choline.
Metal Yin	BLUE MALLOW	Diuretic, emollient, laxative. Has a decongestant effect at O.R.L. region and urinary tract.
	BLACK WALNUT	Antiseptic, astringent and hypoglycemiant. Useful for respiratory or O.R.L. infections in patients prone to recurrence, and for a vagotonic terrain with pancreatic problems. Good for tonsillitis.
	TUSSILAGO	Expectorant for bronchitis, cough, asthma, tracheitis, laryngitis, influenza, scrofula, lymphadenitis. Used for allergic diathesis with a tendency to chronic infections such as rhinitis, otitis and impetigo.
Water Yang	REST HARROW	Diuretic good for cystitis. Useful as a gargle for tonsillitis.
	BLACK CURRANT	Sympathomimetic properties. Increases secretion of anti-inflammatory substances by the adrenal cortex. Antirheumatic, improves circulation.

Essential Oils by Terrain with Respiratory Tropism

Phase	Herb	Indications
Wood Yin	ROSEMARY	Improves vagal tone, stimulates adrenal cortex
	CYPRESS	Hepatic regulator, strong antitussive, has estrogenic properties, improves circulation; parasympatholytic. One drop sufficient to stop an infant's cough.
Fire Yin	LAVENDER	Sympatholytic, general anti-infectious properties.
Earth Yin	CINNAMON	Stimulates adrenal cortex.
	LEMON	Sympathomimetic
Metal Yang	EUCALYPTUS	For infusions and inhalations; pancreatic tropism. For respiratory ailments with vacuous pancreatic function.
	CAJEPUT	Antiseptic for lungs and sinuses.
Metal Yin	HYSSOP	Parasympatholytic and sympathomimetic.
	MINT	Antispasmodic.
	NIAOULI	Antiseptic for sinuses in particular.
	THYME	Parasympatholytic, general anti-infectious agent for respiratory system used also in inhalers and infusions.
Water Yin	PINE	Sympathomimetic and adrenal cortex stimulant
Water Yang	CLOVE	Adrenal cortex stimulant, anti-infectious.

HERBS AND ESSENTIAL OILS BY ACTION FOR RESPIRATORY PATHOLOGY	
FEBRIFUGES	borage, barberry (the fever herb in France), birch (extract or essence), echinacea, gentian, petite centaury (fruit contains quinine-like alkaloids), vervain, white willow (bark contains salicylic acid)
ANTITUSSIVES WITH ANTISPASMODIC ACTION	elecampane (extract or essential oil), *everlasting* (essential oil), honeysuckle, ivy, oregano (essential oil breaks up thick phlegm), pulsatilla, rosemary (extract or essential oil), *spike lavender* (essential oil), thyme (extract or essential oil)
ANTITUSSIVES WITH EMOLLIENT ACTION	blue mallow, borage, coltsfoot, foenugreek, marshmallow, lungwort, licorice, linden, plantain, red poppy, violet
BRONCHODILATOR	ephedra (stems) (strongly sympathomimetic)
EXPECTORANTS	*bay laurel* (essential oil), bistort (dries excessive secretions), elecampane, fennel, horehound, hyssop (extract or essential oil), licorice, lungwort, mullein (fluidifies secretions), red poppy, *thyme* (essential oil), violet (flowers, root)
GARGLES	bearberry (leaves) also astringent and antiseptic, blackberry (leaves), eyebright (entire plant), goldenrod (fruit, flowers), heather (flowers, leaves; also astringent, antiseptic), honeysuckle (flowers, leaves), horehound (leaves, fruit, flowers), oak bark

HERBS & OILS FOR VACUITY/REPLETION CONDITIONS OF RESPIRATORY SYSTEM	
EXTERIOR REPLETION COLD (HIGH FEVER, NO PERSPIRATION)	borage, ephedra, lungwort
EXTERIOR VACUITY COLD (LOW GRADE FEVER WITH PERSPIRATION)	coltsfoot, cinnamon, oak bark, pine, plantain, rosemary, sage

FEBRIFUGE FORMULATIONS	
GENERAL FEBRIFUGE	gentian (sympathomimetic) 75%, ginger (vagolytic) 25%
"FRENCH FEBRIFUGE"	gentian, horehound, chamomile, chrysanthemum, parthenium, oak bark
FEBRIFUGE BATH	lavender, chamomile, ginger, sassafras
FEBRIFUGE RUB	250 ml ginger tea + oils of chamomile, sassafras, lemon
FEBRIFUGE, DIURETIC	artichoke, ash, hypericum
FEBRIFUGE, DIURETIC AND DIAPHORETIC	blessed thistle, birch (extract or essential oil)
FEBRIFUGE AND DIAPHORETIC	borage, sassafras, chamomile
OTHER CLINICAL FEBRIFUGES	oak, mouse ear, horehound, cinchona, gentian, centaury

COLDS AND RHINOPHARYNGITIS

There are not as many terrain considerations in the treatment of colds, since the treatment primarily consists of drainage. The practitioner will find, for example, that any of 15 to 20 herbs and essential oils are effective in alleviating symptoms. Cases that are not serious allow the practitioner to become comfortable with the use of the oils, herbs and tinctures.

The practitioner can also help by using herbs that match the patient's type so that the patient can derive long term benefits from having an acute illness. For example, the patient with copious secretions and weak adrenals who suffers from recurring colds or sinusitis will benefit from oil of cypress to dry up the mucous membranes and tincture of black currant to strengthen the adrenal cortex and the overall immune resistance. The patient who has an acute infection provoked by stress would benefit more from the use of oils of lavender and thyme, if there are nervous system symptoms, or perhaps fennel extract with oil of melissa, if there are digestive symptoms. The patient with a cold who also has chronic allergies will respond well to nettle and plantain herb or tincture, and oil of hyssop, for example. The patient with fever and headache with sinus blockage would respond more favorably to oils of hyssop and eucalyptus.

DRAINAGE

DISINFECTION AND CLEANSING OF NASAL PASSAGES

Sea water with copper and silver: The sea water has an anti-inflammatory effect and the copper and silver are bactericidal and anti-infectious. It is useful to use all three for their synergistic effect whether the irritation is an infection, an inflammation, an allergy or a combination of these factors.

Niaouli (Melaleuca viridiflora) drops: Ephedra base: water soluble extract of 30 ml. *Ephedra alava, Ephedra sinica,* 1.5 g niaouli oil, 30 ml olive oil. Ephedra is sympathomimetic and liberates endogenous catecholamines stored at the termination of sympathetic postganglionic neurons. It is used for arterial vasoconstriction and to dilate air passages. Ti tree oil *(Melaleuca alternifolia)* can also be used in place of niaouli.

INHALATION

Essential oils that are safe and effective for respiratory infections include *cajeput, eucalyptus, lavender, niaouli, peppermint, pine, rosemary* and *thyme.*

ORAL ESSENTIAL OILS FOR INFLAMMATORY STAGE

clove, rosemary, lavender, savory, pine, thyme, eucalyptus, cinnamon, spike lavender, bay laurel

PERCUTANEOUS TREATMENT

eucalyptus, pine, mustard

ACUTE RHINOPHARYNGITIS (ALLERGIC)

GEMMOTHERAPY	
Rosa canina	
TREATMENT BY TERRAIN	
BOTANICALS (herb, *oil*)	OLIGOLEMENTS
WOOD YANG	
Allergic terrain, hyperthyroid, sympathotonic, nervous, irritable; allergic rhinitis from pollen, dust, hay, usually worse in spring: sneezing, rhinorrhea, conjunctivitis, sometimes with asthma.	
blackberry, black currant, black horehound, black radish, black walnut, eyebright, gelsemium, nettle, pasque flower, plantain, scarlet pimpernel, valerian, *cypress, hyssop, lavender;* cinnamon (asthenic type with coldness in the limbs), *juniper* (diuresis, blood sugar instability), *niaouli* (symptomatic; to drain sinuses).	Mn, S, Mg, P

Acute Rhinopharyngitis
(Coryza, Influenza, Tracheitis, Laryngitis)

Gemmotherapy	
Pinus sylvestris (general); Abies pectinata (rhinitis in children); echinacea (all types)	
Treatment by Terrain	
Botanicals (herb, *oil*)	Oligolements
Earth yang	
Hypopancreatic terrain. Bacterial rhinopharyngitis, sometimes accompanied by stomatitis.	
agrimony, lady's mantle	Zn-Ni-Co, Cu, Ag
Earth yin	
Poor immune adaptability, influenza symptoms from dampness, bronchorrhea, salivation.	
bistort, blue mallow, germander, ivy, licorice, *cinnamon, cypress, eucalyptus, lavender, lemon, ravensare, sage*	Mn-Cu, Cu, Ag
Metal yang	
Hyposthenic terrain, acute rhinopharyngitis, hyperthermia, absence of sweat, bacterial infections, dry cough.	
agrimony, borage, burdock, horehound, hyssop, lungwort, marshmallow, *cypress, eucalyptus, lemon, niaouli, pine*	Cu-Ag
Metal yin	
Hyposthenic terrain, frequent colds, frequent relapses, head colds, chills, laryngitis, tracheitis, viral infections.	
bistort, blue mallow, bryonia (with hypersecretions), coltsfoot, drosera, ephedra, hyssop, ivy, licorice (laryngitis, tracheitis), nettle, plantain (laryngitis), *cajeput, cypress, eucalyptus, lavender, niaouli, pine, ravensare, sage, thyme*	Mn-Cu, Cu
Water yin	
Extreme weakness, elderly patient, severe or frequent infections because of poor immunity.	
black currant, goldenrod, *rosemary*	Cu-Au-Ag, Cu, Ag

Acute Sinusitis

Treatment by Terrain	
Botanicals (herb, *oil*)	Oligolements
Wood	
Sudden onset, poor eating habits, irritability, headache, nausea, thick discharge, or pressure on frontal bone due to lack of drainage.	
black radish, eyebright, hyssop (poor drainage), nettle, pasque flower, *mint, niaouli; eucalyptus* (sinus headaches), *lavender* (anxiety, bacterial infection); *lemon* (plethoric type with mucus congestion; digestive problems, no appetite in morning, thick tongue fur, postnasal drip), *niaouli* (open and drain air passages of head); *pine* (urinary tract irritation; frequent recurrence of infections); *thyme* (raise immunity, cleanse mucous membranes) *hyssop* (frontal headache)	Mn, Mn-Cu

Chronic Sinusitis

GENERAL TREATMENT	
HERBS: Artichoke (liver drainage), black currant (strengthen the adrenal cortex function), marshmallow (anti-inflammatory to soothe irritated mucous membranes) **OILS:** *niaouli, thyme, lavender, camphor, eucalyptus*	
TREATMENT BY TERRAIN	
BOTANICALS (herb, *oil*)	OLIGOLEMENTS
EARTH YANG	
Frontal and maxillary sinuses jammed, condition provoked or aggravated by heat, digestive and blood sugar problems	
black currant, black elder, borage, lungwort, marshmallow, *eucalyptus, lemon, niaouli, pine*	Mn-Cu, S, Cu
EARTH YIN	
Aggravated or precipitated by cold weather and humidity; recurrence in the fall or winter; weak digestion	
black elder, blue mallow, coltsfoot, eyebright, marine algae, plantain, *lavender, lemon, niaouli, pine, thyme*	Mn-Cu, S, Mg, Cu-Au-Ag
METAL YANG	
Aggravated by heat, recurrent in summer	
black elder, borage, lungwort, marshmallow, *eucalyptus, lemon, niaouli, pine*	Mn-Cu, S, Cu
METAL YIN	
Fatigue, recurs in fall and winter, low immunity, aggravated by cold and dampness	
black elder, blue mallow, coltsfoot, eyebright, marine algae, plantain, *eucalyptus, lemon, niaouli, pine, thyme*	Mn-Cu, Cu-Au-Ag, S, Mg

Bronchitis, Pneumopathy

For acute cases, check for signs of pneumonia, especially asymmetric heaving, deep rales, etc. Insure liver drainage and diuresis when necessary.

GENERAL TREATMENT	horehound, marshmallow, black currant, *eucalyptus, lavender, pine, savory, cajeput, garlic, lemon, hyssop*
SYMPATHOMIMETIC AGENTS	hypericum, black currant, *hyssop, pine, savory, sage*
VAGOLYTIC AGENTS	angelica, red poppy, *cajeput, hyssop, cypress, serpolet, thyme*
FOR COUGH	drosera, pasque flower, ivy, *spike lavender, cypress, oregano, thyme, eucalyptus, serpolet*
ANTISPASMODIC	belladonna, drosera, cherry laurel, melilot, *spike lavender, everlasting*
EXPECTORATION	horseradish, black horehound, elecampane, coltsfoot, mullein (liquifies secretions), drosera (vagolytic), licorice, violet, fennel, onion, *lavender, mint, pine, thyme, laurel, ravensare, oregano* (fluidifies secretions), *bay laurel*
SORE THROAT	propolis, *cajeput, cypress*
DRY EXCESS BRONCHIAL SECRETIONS	coltsfoot, ivy, germander, scarlet pimpernel, bryonia, ginger, bistort, *hyssop, mint, niaouli, myrtle, bay laurel*
ANTIALLERGIC, ANTI-INFLAMMATORY	black elder, black currant, elecampane, blue mallow, licorice, marshmallow, plantain, *spike lavender, hyssop*
ACUTE BRONCHITIS IN THE AGED PATIENT	cinnamon, clove, myrtle, savory. Follow Water yin and Metal yin treatment of chronic bronchitis. *Inhalation: lavender, pine, thyme, eucalyptus*

CHRONIC BRONCHITIS

Considered chronic if excessive secretions due to inflammation throughout the bronchial tubes persist at least three months over three years.
Differential diagnosis: pulmonary tuberculosis or cancer.

GEMMOTHERAPY

Pinus sylvestris, Ribes nigrum

TREATMENT BY TERRAIN

BOTANICALS (herb, *oil*)	OLIGOELEMENTS
EARTH YIN	
Poor adaptation, low immunity, cold-damp afflictions, viral infections, moderate fever, bronchial hypersecretion.	
angelica, elecampane, germander, colchicum, woody nightshade, bladderwrack, laminaria, blue mallow, hypericum, echinacea, bistort, mullein, licorice, *cinnamon, cypress, eucalyptus, lavender, mint, rosemary, sage, thyme*	MN-CU, CU, AG
METAL YANG	
Hyposthenic terrain, hyperglycemic, heat-dryness afflictions, bacterial infections (pneumococcus, staphylococcus, streptococcus), dyspnea, high fever, absence of thirst, yellow tongue fur, red cheeks, purulent expectoration.	
agrimony, borage (anhidrosis, hyperthermia), marshmallow (dryness), horehound (dryness), lungwort (anhidrosis, hyperthermia), *bay laurel, eucalyptus, garlic, lemon, niaouli, ylang ylang*	MN-CU, ZN-NI-CO, AG
METAL YIN	
Hyposthenic terrain, cold or cold-dry afflictions, progressive onset viral infections, chills, shivering, moderate fever, aching, stiffness, sweating, bronchial dilatation, superinfections.	
bistort, bladderwrack, blue mallow, bryonia, coltsfoot, drosera, elecampane, fennel, horseradish, germander, ginger, laminaria, plantain, propolis, sarsaparilla, woody nightshade, *cypress, cajeput, eucalyptus, garlic, lemon, lavender, mint, myrtle, niaouli, oregano, pine, rosemary, savory, sassafras, sage, terebenthine, thyme*	MN-CU, CU, AG
WATER YIN	
Anergic terrain, chills, viral infections, hypoadrenal.	
black elder, bistort, mullein, *rosemary, myrtle, pine*	CU-AU-AG, MN-CU, CU, AG

ACUTE INFECTIONS AND CHILDHOOD ILLNESSES

TREATING THE INFECTION BY TERRAIN	
WOOD REPLETION	marjoram, bitter orange, meadowsweet
WOOD VACUITY	black currant, cypress, tarragon, *rosemary*
FIRE REPLETION	marjoram, bitter orange
EARTH REPLETION	*lemon* (respiratory), *cypress* (respiratory), *eucalyptus, juniper, marigold*
EARTH VACUITY	germander, marigold, *cinnamon, lemon, lavender, sage* (esp. respiratory and urinary)
METAL REPLETION	borage, marshmallow, *eucalyptus*
METAL VACUITY	*cinnamon, lemon, savory, thyme*
WATER REPLETION	meadowsweet, *clove, lavender, pine, savory thyme*

CHILDHOOD DISEASES

GENERAL PRINCIPLES	
The goal of treatment is to promote drainage of secretions through mucous membranes, skin or intestines and to support target organs, e.g. pancreas, adrenals. Diaphoretic agents are used during the incubation and invasion stages of eruptive fevers of measles, rubella, scarlatina and chicken pox.	
BOTANICALS (herb, *oil*)	OLIGOLEMENTS
orange flower, elder flowers, meadowsweet, sweet balm	AG and CU (anti-infectious)

MEASLES

During the early phase the terrain can be altered by administering essential oils; eucalyptus and cinnamon oils are especially useful. Eucalyptus supports the pancreas and cinnamon supports the adrenals. For the full onset of symptoms, Dr. Lapraz recommends the combination formula of coltsfoot flowers, elder flowers and black currant leaves.

TO PREVENT COMPLICATIONS	
Ear canal: 2 drops of lemon juice in each ear morning and evening for 5 minutes, or 5 drops of a preparation containing the juice of a lemon in 30 ml of clay water.	
Bronchitis symptoms: Syrup of black radish	

TREATMENT BY TERRAIN	
BOTANICALS (herb, *oil*)	OLIGOLEMENTS
FIRE YANG	
Extremely high fever at onset. It is necessary to break a sweat to prevent possible neurological complications.	
borage, meadowsweet (diaphoretic for preventing complications), *eucalyptus*	CU
METAL YANG	
Respiratory complications. Hyperthermia in an infant with lymphatic swelling. Prostration.	
burdock, borage, lungwort, *eucalyptus*	CU
METAL YIN	
Lymphatic type of constitution most predisposed. Most common type of measles.	
hypericum, coltsfoot, *cinnamon, eucalyptus, pine, thyme*	CU, MN-CU

CHICKEN POX (VARICELLA)

Follow the general principles of treatment of childhood diseases. For itching, black walnut and plantain can be taken internally. For local application, use 3 g each of mint oil and cypress oil in alcohol sufficient for 125 ml. An infusion of violet flowers can also be used to assure drainage of the skin.

For stubborn cases that are of a more Wood nature, use artichoke, centaury, milk thistle, oak, plantain, *lemon, cypress, ravensare* and the oligoelement CU.

SCARLATINA

TREATMENT

At the first cutaneous outbreak during the early phase of high fever, sore throat and cervical lymph node suppuration, use the following formula. In addition to their symptomatic activity, note the properties of each:

lavender	1 ml	(anti-infectious, sympatholytic)
geranium	1 ml	(supports the adrenal cortex)
clove	1 ml	(anti-infectious)
glycerin	sufficient for 125 ml	

Use 2 drops per year of age in an infusion two or three times per day.

To achieve renal drainage and act as an anti-inflammatory when treating a child with normal constitutional strength, give 2 to 4 cups per day of the following:

meadowsweet extract	10-30 drops (depending on age)
borage extract	10-30 drops (depending on age)
fumitory extract	10-30 drops (depending on age)
linden	mild decoction

The Fire constitution child is the most susceptible to scarlatina, being sentimental, emotionally excitable and predisposed to high fevers and convulsions. Borage, eucalyptus oil and meadowsweet are botanicals most often used, and Cu is the oligoelement of choice.

For the Metal yin constitution child, borage, black currant and fumitory are useful botanicals; Cu is the oligoelement of choice.

For gargling, lemon juice is given. The following combination can also be used:

lavender oil	9 ml
savory oil	6 ml
sage oil	1 ml
clove oil	2 ml
niaouli oil	2 ml
licorice extract	15 ml
raspberry extract	15 ml
methylene blue	sufficient for 125 ml

These essences are used for their direct anti-infectious activity, particularly lavender for its action on streptococcus and licorice for its powerful anti-inflammatory activity.

PERTUSSIS

TREATMENT

In addition to antitussive plants some of the specifically antispasmodic herbs should be used: red poppy, drosera, pasque flower (pulsatilla) and belladonna, among others. Anti-infectious agents should be used in the form of essences: *cypress, marjoram, lavender, thyme, rosemary, serpolet, basil, niaouli* or *ti tree.* Oil of *neroli* or *spike lavender* can be useful as a sedative.

For serious cases, use tinctures of belladonna (5 g) and red poppy (4-5 g) in 125 ml alcohol, at a dosage of 20-25 drops three to four times per day. To prevent secondary ear infection 10 drops of the following preparation should be used daily:

cypress	2 ml
niaouli	2 ml
cedarwood	2 ml
alcohol base sufficient for 90 ml	

Pertussis (Continued)

Remember that bed rest is important and food should be served in small portions, especially at the evening meal. If complications arise, hospitalization is sometimes necessary.

Treatment by Terrain

Botanicals (herb, *oil*)	Oligolements

Wood

Nervous, fretful, tendency to vomit, tightness of shoulders and back.

drosera, pulsatilla, black cohosh, mistletoe, hypericum, *marjoram, ravensare, serpolet*	Cu

Earth

Moist cough, abundant saliva, fleshy or flabby child with sugar cravings.

arnica, belladonna, *cinnamon, cypress, hyssop, lavender oregano, thyme, everlasting, ravensare*	Cu, Mn-Cu, Cu-Au-Ag

Metal Yin

Weak constitution, runny nose, cold symptoms during the day, swollen lymph nodes, especially cervical.

red poppy, *everlasting, niaouli, oregano, ravensare, rosemary, serpolet, thyme*	Cu, Mn-Cu, Cu-Au-Ag

Mumps (Infectious parotitis)

Treatment

Mumps presents the possibility of potentially serious complications, including inflammation of the testes, acute pancreatitis and meningoencephalitis. The hormonal complications of the malady necessitate the use of plants with hormonal tropism in order to prevent its progression. Thus the proestrogenic properties of *sage, cypress,* oat and ivy are important for treatment of boys. Blessed thistle, *sage, cypress, tarragon* and *juniper* are important for both sexes. Fumitory, blackberry, *juniper, eucalyptus,* onion and *geranium* are also important for both sexes for their pancreatic activity.

For general treatment, the following essential oil preparation can be used, at a dosage of 20-30 drops three times daily:

sage	1 ml
cypress	1 ml
tarragon	1 ml
juniper	1 ml
elixir of papain	125 ml

The Earth yang type of constitution is the most susceptible to complications. Useful herbs for this type include angelica, nettle and licorice. Cu is the oligoelement of choice.

In case of orchitis a mixture of tinctures of licorice, sage and nettle should be used. It can be administered rectally twice daily, or 15 to 35 drops orally 3 times a day along with a decoction of horsetail and harpagophytum.

In case of pancreatitis, a combination of tinctures of fumitory and black walnut should be given 25-35 drops, three times a day along with pancreatic enzymes or elixir of papain.

Other Complications

Swelling of breasts or ovaries: use formulas with licorice, lady's mantle and yarrow.

Injury to the liver: dandelion

To prevent damage to the liver and complications in general: combretum

Glossitis (Stomatitis, Gingivitis)

Treatment by Terrain	
Botanicals (herb, *oil*)	Oligolements
Earth Yang	
Heat sensations in the epigastric and pancreas areas. Vagal insufficiency, plethoric terrain, hyperglycemic. **Etiology:** obesity, diabetes, mycosis, infectious diseases from heat and dampness.	
agrimony, burdock, blackberry, marshmallow, maize, *juniper, lemon*	Zn-Ni-Co, Cu, Mg
Earth Yin	
Digestive hypofunction, Spleen qi vacuity; asthenic, hypothyroid terrain with low adaptability. **Etiology:** hypothyroidism, infectious disease, fevers, vitamin deficiency, Hunter's glossitis (pernicious anemia), lead poisoning.	
angelica, bistort, blackberry, oak, eyebright, blue mallow, licorice, *geranium, lemon, sage*	Mn-Cu, Cu, Mg
Metal Yang	
Plethoric terrain, hypopancreatic. **Etiology:** diabetes, infectious diseases (heat), gingivitis.	
agrimony, burdock, marshmallow (gingivitis), *lemon*	Mn-Cu, Cu, Mg
Water Yin	
Anergic terrain, hypoadrenal. **Etiology:** auto-immune problems related to the kidneys.	
raspberry, *geranium*	Cu, Cu-Au-Ag, Mg

Otitis

Drainage
Artichoke, black radish, dandelion capsules along with burdock, especially if the skin in the vicinity of the ear is breaking out. Lymph Drainage: *bay laurel, everlasting* (externally).
Chronic cases
Use the following combination. Take 2 to 4 capsules a day outside of mealtime: *eucalyptus* oil — 1 drop *thyme* oil — 1 drop *savory* oil — 2 drops willow bark (dry) — 0.1 g horsetail (dry) — 0.2 g
Local treatment, acute or chronic
garlic or *oregano* oil — 5 drops *lavender* oil — 8 drops 90% alcohol — 15 ml glycerin — 60 ml
Stronger local treatment
Mix equal parts of the following essential oils. Apply 4 drops into the auditory canal three times daily. *lavender* — 5 ml *cinnamon* — 5 ml *chamomile* — 3-5 ml *niaouli* — 5 ml olive oil — up to 30 ml
Milder local treatment
Apply the following formula as drops in the ear, two or three times daily: *lavender* oil — 5 drops *niaouli* oil — 5 drops glycerin — 1 oz.

Otitis (continued)

Sedatives
passionflower, linden, melilot

Treatment by Terrain	
Botanicals (herb, *oil*)	Oligolements
Metal yin	
Swollen lymph nodes, low grade fever.	
blue mallow, marigold, mullein, *cinnamon, clove, lavender, lemon, niaouli, oregano, thyme, everlasting, ravensare*	Cu
Water yin	
Feeble patient, recurrent infection, hypoadrenal, tinnitus, vertigo	
black currant, black elder, *clove, lavender, lemon, niaouli, ravensare, everlasting*	Cu

Tonsillitis

General treatment
Agrimony, black currant, black walnut, elecampane, licorice, mullein, oak
Sore throat and streptococcus
blackberry, honeysuckle, propolis; grapevine (specific for sore throat); heather (protects the kidneys from secondary infection).
Examine for streptococcal infection. This has a sudden onset with severe throat pain, accompanied by fevers of up to 103 degrees F. The pharyngeal mucosa is bright red, swollen and studded with whitish or yellowish pustules. Cervical lymph nodes are tender and swollen. Waste no time in controlling the acute manifestations of this infection. The systemic complications include damage to the heart valves, rheumatic infections and glomerulonephritis.

Treatment by terrain	
Botanicals (herb, *oil*)	Oligolements
Fire yang	
High fever, extreme thirst	
hawthorn, grapevine (strep), *lavender*	Cu, Ag
Fire yin	
Extreme fatigue, heart palpitations	
briarhip, barberry, grapevine, *lavender*	Cu-Au-Ag, Ag
Earth yang	
High fever, copious exudation, swelling, blood sugar instability, obese or flabby constitution.	
agrimony, marshmallow, blackberry, *lemon*	Cu, Zn-Ni-Co
Earth yin	
Poor adaptation, vagotonic, hypopancreatic; repeated tonsillitis during infancy.	
elecampane, belladonna, licorice, foenugreek, blackberry, black currant, black walnut, oak, propolis, *thyme, niaouli, eucalyptus, cinnamon*	Zn-Cu, Cu, Ag
Metal yang	
Tonsillitis due to pneumococcus with high fever.	
agrimony, marshmallow, periwinkle, *thyme, niaouli, eucalyptus, cinnamon*	Mn-Cu, Cu, Ag

TONSILLITIS (CONTINUED)

METAL YIN
Asthenic type with tonsillitis accompanied by rhinopharyngitis, swollen glands.
elecampane, belladonna, coltsfoot, black walnut, oak,   Mn-Cu, Cu, Ag, Bi black currant, propolis, *clove, hyssop, rosemary,* *thyme, savory*
WATER YANG
Hyperactivity, hyperadrenal. **Etiology:** fever, usually staphylococcus.
barberry, *lemon*   Cu, Ag
WATER YIN
Erythemapultaceous tonsillitis in an anergic patient. **Etiology:** tonsillitis from hemopathies or streptococcus.
honeysuckle (streptococcus), black currant, black elder,   Cu-Au-Ag, Bi black walnut, dog rose, licorice, raspberry, *geranium, hyssop, lemon, red rose, rosemary, sage,* *savory, pine, clove, thyme;* **Local use:** propolis

CHRONIC RESPIRATORY INSUFFICIENCY
(EMPHYSEMA, CHRONIC DYSPNEA OR INFECTIONS)

GEMMOTHERAPY	
Ribes nigrum, Viburnum lantana	
TREATMENT BY TERRAIN	
BOTANICALS (herb, *oil*)	OLIGOLEMENTS
EARTH YANG	
Heat of the Spleen; plethoric terrain, hypopancreatic. Frequent mycotic infections of heat and dampness.	
agrimony, marshmallow, periwinkle, woody nightshade, *eucalyptus*	Zn-Ni-Co, Mn-Cu
EARTH YIN	
Poor immunity, hypothyroid; very flabby or gaunt build; dislikes humidity; emphysema.	
angelica, black walnut, blue mallow, echinacea, oak, gentian, germander, hops, ivy, laminaria, licorice, plantain, bladderwrack (emphysema), woody nightshade, *hyssop, lavender, lemon, hypericum, terebenthine, thyme*	Mn-Cu
METAL YANG	
Heat in the Lung; asthenic terrain, arteriosclerosis; chronic bronchitis, emphysema; infections frequent in summer.	
agrimony, Canadian fleabane, horehound, lungwort, periwinkle, woody nightshade, *eucalyptus, niaouli*	Mn-Cu
METAL YIN	
Coldness in the lung; asthenic terrain, fears the cold; easily infected in autumn and winter; chronic bronchitis, emphysema.	
angelica (emphysema), black walnut, bladderwrack (emphysema), blue mallow, coltsfoot, drosera, gentian, germander, horseradish, ivy, laminaria, oak, plantain, woody nightshade, *hyssop, lavender, lemon, myrtle,* *niaouli, oregano, pine, rosemary, sage, terebenthine, thyme*	Mn-Cu
WATER YIN	
Coldness of the Kidney; anergic type; hypoadrenal, gaunt build, fears the cold; vulnerable to infections in the winter. **Etiology:** emphysema.	
celery, bearberry, black elder, birch, *hyssop, lavender,* *myrtle, niaouli, rosemary, thyme*	Cu-Au-Ag

Bronchial Asthma

Asthmatic patients who have been treated with steroids require supplementation to strengthen the adrenal glands during and after withdrawal of the drugs. Essential oils of *rosemary, thyme* and *pine* are useful for this purpose along with tinctures of sea holly, yarrow and black currant.

Gemmotherapy

Pinus sylvestris, Ribes nigrum, Viburnum lantana

Treatment by Terrain

Botanicals (herb, *oil*)	Oligolements

Wood Yang

Allergic terrain, arthritic, hyperthyroid, wind or wind heat asthma, seasonal asthma without rales between paroxysms, allergies to pollen, dust, chemical pollutants or cosmetics, subcostal tightness, tense shoulders.

black cohosh, black horehound, black radish, celandine, eyebright, fumitory, gelsemium, mistletoe, plantain, pulsatilla, valerian, white lily, woundwort, yarrow, *bitter orange, marjoram, melissa, rosemary*	Mn, S, Mg, P

Fire Yang

. Dystonia, wind and heat asthma; gradual onset, difficulty exhaling

black horehound, mistletoe, valerian, white lily, *bitter orange, garlic, marjoram, melissa*	Mn-Co, I, S, Mn, P

Earth Yang

Hyperglycemic terrain, wet cough, copious sputum, wheezing, audible rales. **Etiology:** asthma from moist heat (mycosis aggravated by heat).

agrimony, bay laurel, hawthorn, *eucalyptus, niaouli*	Zn-Ni-Co, P, S

Earth Yin

Poor immunity. Allergies: mycotic, mildew or dust. **Etiology:** asthma with excess secretion of glairy mucus (bronchorrhea), lymphatic swelling.

belladonna, bladderwrack, colchicum, elecampane, fennel, ginger, hypericum, ivy, laminaria, menyanthe, snakeroot, woody nightshade, *anise, caraway, cinnamon, cumin, hyssop, lavender, sage*	Zn-Cu, Mn-Cu, S, P

Metal Yang

Repletion heat in the Lung; asthenic type. **Etiology:** asthma from dryness or from heat and dryness, aggravated by heat or by central heating systems.

agrimony, borage, horehound, opium, *garlic, lemon, melissa*	Mn-Cu, Co, S, P

Metal Yin

Coldness in the Lung; asthenic type; most typical type for chronic asthma. **Etiology:** Asthma due to cold, coldness and dryness, colds and damp; worse in autumn and winter; rales, difficult inhalation.

angelica, belladonna, bladderwrack, blue mallow, coltsfoot, datura, drosera, elecampane, henbane, horseradish, hypericum, ivy, laminaria, nettle, sarsaparilla, snakeroot, woody nightshade, *eucalyptus, hyssop, lavender, lemon, niaouli, oregano, pine, rosemary, savory, sage, terebenthine, thyme*	Mn-Cu, Cu-Au-Ag, S, P

Water Yin

"Mother-Son" mechanism wherein weakened Metal results in Water being undermined. Water terrain undermined by standard treatment with adrenalin for acute asthmatic episodes or steroid treatment for chronic dyspnea. **Etiology:** chronic fatigue, hypoadrenal, asthma due to cold.

celery, datura, fennel, henbane, *hyssop, lavender, pine, rosemary, thyme*	Mn-Cu, Cu-Au-Ag, S, P

PLEURISY

BOTANICALS (herb, *oil*)	OLIGOLEMENTS
TREATMENT BY TERRAIN	
EARTH YIN	
Coldness of the Spleen; immune deficiency, hypothyroid. **Etiology:** pertussis, viral infection, mycotic infections.	
blessed thistle, bryonia, scarlet pimpernel, woody nightshade, *hyssop, savory*	Mn-Cu, Cu
METAL YANG	
Heat of the Lung; asthenic terrain. **Etiology:** usually asthma, pulmonary abscess, pulmonary embolism, post-pancreatitis episode.	
horehound, marshmallow, red poppy, woody nightshade, *juniper, thyme*	Mn-Cu, Cu
METAL YIN	
Coldness of the Lung. **Etiology:** tuberculosis, sarcoidosis, mycosis, Hodgkin's disease, bronchial dilation.	
blessed thistle, bryonia, celery, red poppy, woody nightshade, *clove, hyssop*	Mn-Cu
WATER YANG	
Heat of the Kidney. **Etiology:** bacterial infection or pulmonary abscess.	
black elder, maize, orthosiphon, *birch, juniper*	Cu-Au-Ag, Cu
WATER YIN	
Coldness of the Kidney; chronic fatigue, hypoadrenalism, immune deficiency. **Etiology:** viral infections, sharp rheumatic joint pains, collagenosis, lipoidic nephrosis, leukemia, neoplasia.	
black elder, broom, celery, cherry, maize, mouse ear, scarlet pimpernel, *birch, clove*	Cu-Au-Ag

INFLUENZA, LOW IMMUNITY, FATIGUE SYNDROME

These conditions are often described as being viral infections, although in the case of fatigue syndrome and low immunity there is frequent concurrence with candida infestation or other types of gastrointestinal dysbiosis such as parasitoses and Salmonella.

SYMPTOMATOLOGY
Fatigue (sometimes chronic), recurrent pharyngitis, enlargement of lymph nodes (especially cervical), low grade fever, malaise (myalgia and arthralgia), headache, gastrointestinal discomfort, food sensitivities, depression or mood swings, blood sugar instability and loss of concentration, leukopenia.
DISEASE NAMES ASSOCIATED WITH DISORDERED IMMUNE SYSTEM FUNCTION
Influenza, candidiasis, Epstein-Barr syndrome, fatigue syndrome, glandular fever, infectious mononucleosis, rheumatoid arthritis, systemic lupus erythematosus, Burkitt's lymphoma, Hodgkin's disease, non-Hodgkin's lymphoma, leukemia, nasopharyngeal carcinoma, AIDS, ARC, multiple sclerosis, myasthenia gravis, ankylosing spondylitis, hypothyroidism.
FACTORS KNOWN TO RESULT IN IMPAIRED IMMUNE SYSTEM FUNCTION
Stress, steroid therapy, antithymocyte globulin therapy, renal failure, renal transplantation, malignant tumors, viral infection, endocrine dysfunction, autoimmune dysfunction, anticancer cytotoxic chemotherapy, vaccines, antibiotic treatment.

Influenza

We might characterize influenza as "acute fatigue syndrome." A typical case manifests many if not most of the symptoms listed above. Its course averages four to five days, but recurrences are common as are persistent respiratory symptoms. No specific pharmaceutical agents are available for treating influenza in conventional medical practice. Administration of antibacterial agents endangers the terrain by strengthening the resistance of microorganisms which could produce secondary infectious foci. Use of antibiotics is contraindicated since complications are typically induced by their "prophylactic" use, such as alteration of the flora of gastrointestinal and rhinopharyngeal mucous membranes. Antipyretic treatment is also contraindicated since fevers seldom approach a high elevation, yet even a low temperature increase is a positive sign of active hepatic function that can considerably shorten the course of symptomatology or convalescence.

Following terrain hypothesis, a virus is a fragment or byproduct of cell disintegration or a throwing-off of excess material that does not support cell integrity. Whether it is perceived as a global phenomenon of detoxification or as a chain reaction caused by an invasion of pathogenic viral material, the approach to altering the terrain is the same.

GENERAL TREATMENT
Elixir of papain or other proteolytic enzymes. Oils of *lavender, thyme, pine, cinnamon;* with extracts of artichoke, elecampane, borage or black currant. Essential oil combination: *lavender, cypress, niaouli, eucalyptus.*

TREATMENT BY TERRAIN	
BOTANICALS (herb, *oil*)	OLIGOLEMENTS
WOOD YANG	
Etiology: respiratory symptoms, spasmophilia, hyperthyroid, hyporparathyroid, nervous excitability, emotional mood swings.	
artichoke, black radish, plantain, *cypress*	Mn-Co, Mn, Mg
WOOD YIN	
Etiology: nervousness, muscle spasm, sinusitis, sore throat, irritability, fatigue, headache.	
elecampane, echinacea, milk thistle, plantain, *cypress, rosemary*	Cu-Au-Ag
FIRE YANG	
Etiology: fever, emotional mood swings, panic attacks, ulcerations in the mouth, muscle spasms.	
echinacea, horehound, *marjoram, spike lavender*	Mn-Co, Mn, Cu
FIRE YIN	
Etiology: cold hands and feet, diffuse headache, dyspnea, sweating (cold sweats), dizziness, anxiety and depression.	
elecampane, eleutherococcus, honeysuckle, milk thistle, *rosemary, spike lavender*	Cu-Au-Ag
EARTH YANG	
Etiology: hyperthyroid, vagotonic, low resistance from physical or mental strain, panic attacks.	
elecampane, foenugreek, germander, *cinnamon, cypress, lavender*	Cu, Mn-Cu
EARTH YIN	
Poor resistance, leukopenia, excessive mental effort, vagotonia, hypothyroid, intermittent fever, abundant secretions.	
cinchona, elecampane, germander, *cinnamon, cypress, lavender, niaouli*	Cu, Mn-Cu

INFLUENZA (CONTINUED)

METAL YANG	
Medium build, higher fever.	
marshmallow, *eucalyptus*	MN-CU, CU
METAL YIN	
Hyposthenic, long, lean build, pulmonary weakness.	
blue mallow, coltsfoot, elecampane, fennel, germander, *cinnamon, cypress, lemon, eucalyptus, hyssop, niaouli, pine, rosemary, thyme*	MN-CU, CU
WATER YIN	
Severe anergy.	
black currant, echinacea, *rosemary, clove*	CU-AU-AG

CHRONIC FATIGUE SYNDROME

In the same way that influenza is acute fatigue syndrome, chronic fatigue syndrome is chronic influenza. The microorganisms that may be involved are an aspect of the terrain which must be treated as a type of "dysbiosis" or imbalance. To attempt to destroy them would place further strain on already beleaguered immune and glandular systems. Furthermore, the nature or extent of the involvement of such agents as the Epstein-Barr virus is unclear and no causal relationship has been established. The conventional theory is that immune "surveillance" mechanisms prevent active manifestations of the viral infection, which is a lifelong infestation of the B-lymphocytes and salivary glands. When immunity is compromised by stress or any other factor, the latent viral infection manifests and proliferates.

The infestation of EBV is usually asymptomatic during childhood, but during adolescence to early adulthood, clinical manifestations begin to appear. Transmission of the virus through shedding from the saliva is considered to be a common route of contagion. It is known that shedding of the virus stored in the salivary glands can occur in asymptomatic individuals, but occurs more readily in the immunosuppressed. Infectious mononucleosis was once popularly referred to as "kissing disease" for this reason. Typical symptomatology includes pharyngitis, lymphadenopathy (especially posterior cervical), headache, malaise, myalgia or fatigue. Gradually such symptoms as maculopapular rash and hepatosplenomegaly appear. Complications such as hepatitis, jaundice, anorexia or gastritis can also occur. Younger or more vital subjects usually manifest more "exterior" symptoms (infectious mononucleosis): cervical lymph node swelling, sore throat and headache, whereas older or more constitutionally deteriorated types do not, but tend toward manifesting deeper symptoms: hepatitis, hepatosplenomegaly (cytomegalovirus).

Some theorize that based on abnormal EBV serological tests, SLE, myocarditis, neuritis and Guillain-Barre syndrome, Hodgkins disease, non-Hodgkins lymphoma, nasopharyngeal carcinoma, leukemia, AIDS and ARC are possibly outgrowths of EBV or that perhaps EBV and the entire list are in some way different forms or functions of compromised immunity and/or dysfunction.

The viral fatigue syndrome terrain generally corresponds to the yin terrains. The syndrome is sympathotonic and/or vagal insufficiency, meaning that there is an insufficiency of exocrine and often endocrine secretions. From the Chinese medicine viewpoint, it is necessary to strengthen the yin. The practitioner will often find that when patients are strengthened by means of endocrine restoration, they may experience discomfort. This is due to detoxification that occurs as a result of increased metabolic function. When metabolic function is increased, particularly adrenal and thyroid function, the body typically first throws off its toxic burden. After this has taken place, the patient will experience well-being and a renewed sense of commitment to the regeneration process. During this difficult detoxification period, liver drainage and soothing nervous system irritation are necessary to minimize discomfort. Herbs for liver drainage and Wood yin herbs are extremely helpful for this purpose, regardless of the patient's fundamental typology.

Fungal Terrain Fatigue Syndrome

This usually occurs in a sthenic "yang" type, especially the Wood yang and Earth yang types. The "viral" fatigue syndrome usually has a more delicate constitution. The fungal terrain requires a certain amount of internal dampness, though symptoms are often aggravated by environmental heat and humidity. Digestive symptoms are common: constipation, gas, bloating, extreme food sensitivities, etcetera. Irresistible sugar cravings are also common.

The fungal types often have anxiety attacks with the feeling of "going out of their minds." These are accompanied by crying spells, feelings of irritability and being "spaced out." Chronic sinus infections, which are almost always symptomatic, are often found. Spasmophilia is a common feature, even though there is usually hypothyroidism and weight gain. A typical case can get relief only very temporarily from pain with treatment such as acupuncture, chiropractic or physical therapy. Recurrent and intractable urinary tract infections are often reported. Vaginitis with leukorrhea, itching, burning and anal pruritus are frequent occurrences.

In women, most of the symptoms are worse premenstrually. In men, prostate congestion and prostate hypertrophy are common. Sometimes there are spontaneous episodes of itching in other areas of the skin, or even all over. A butterfly rash is sometimes seen on the face. There are sometimes fungal patches on the skin or the nails, thrush, and more often than not, a white or yellowish-white fur on the tongue.

The fungal fatigue syndrome is often a case of decreased energy from congestion rather than an actual global deficiency of energy. The strategy for this type typically corresponds to the yang type of terrain. From the neuroendocrine model, the terrain is vagotonic and/or sympathetic insufficiency. From the Chinese medicine point of view, the patient suffers from qi congestion and Spleen dampness. Emotions run high with this type of patient, and the practitioner must attempt to gently relieve the liver and bile duct congestion.

The fungal terrain type must be treated with herbs, especially from the Wood yang, Earth yang and Metal yang categories. Agrimony is particularly useful to regulate blood sugar and dry out dampness. Selenium (Se) is used to correct a fungal terrain. Fungicidal agents include bistort, blessed thistle, meadowsweet, madder, scarlet pimpernel, burdock, black walnut and oils of *cinnamon, savory, sage, thyme, peppermint, clove* and *oregano*. It is extremely important to insure adequate liver drainage and bile flow with herbs such as black radish, artichoke, dandelion, boldo or fumitory.

To compare and contrast the two basic types of fatigue syndrome, it is useful to outline the characteristics both share. Often, both types have cervical lymphadenopathy (swollen lymph nodes in the neck). "Brain fog" is common to both types. Chills, low grade fever, weakness, "shaky" muscular activity, a sensation of swelling in the head and the feeling that they are "going crazy" are common features.

COMPARISON OF VIRAL AND FUNGAL FATIGUE SYNDROMES		
Symptom	Viral	Fungal
Fatigue	Intermittent	Progressive
Sugar cravings	Occasional	Irresistible
Gastrointestinal signs	Not many	Constipation, gas, bloating
Skin rash	None	Butterfly rash on face
Food sensitivity	Not obvious	Extreme sensitivities
Postnasal drip	Not much	Constant drip
Hormonal signs	Not cyclic	Aggravated premenstrually
		Menstrual symptoms, e.g., irregularity
Effect of exercise	Aggravation	Improvement
Environmental sensitivities	Not usually	Majority of cases
Effect of dampness	No effect	Worse in cold, damp
Cystitis	Seldom	Often
Itching	None	Anal, vaginal
Tongue	Redness, no fur, red tip,	Yellow or white fur
	cracks in tongue body	in middle of tongue
Anemia	No	Yes

FATIGUE SYNDROME TREATMENT

THERAPEUTIC GUIDELINES

Detoxification, immune support, endocrine reconstruction.

DETOXIFICATION

Cleansing is the first step in raising the patient's vitality. In a weakened patient purgatives are not recommended. It is recommended to detoxify by means of strengthening and supporting eliminative organs, particularly the liver and the bowel. In addition, strength and support to specific systems may be necessary to promote drainage of vicarious channels of elimination: kidneys, lymph, skin, lungs or saturated binding sites, such as connective tissues, joints or fat deposits.

Detoxification is sometimes complicated by gastrointestinal mycosis, particularly *Candida albicans*. This requires a more rigorous approach in bowel elimination and the use of essential oils for disinfection. In weak individuals, this should begin with increased dietary fiber, psyllium seed husks or even herbal enemas.

TREATMENT BY TERRAIN: LIVER SUPPORT

BOTANICALS (herb, *oil*)	OLIGOLEMENTS
WOOD YANG	
Biliary stasis.	
artichoke, black radish, boldo, dandelion, fumitory, *lemon, rosemary*	MN, S, P
WOOD YIN	
Toxic liver, low immunity.	
angelica, barberry, brassica, calendula, centaury, elecampane, germander, hops, milk thistle, *cypress, lemon, mint, hypericum, rosemary, sage*	MN-CU, S, CU, CU-AU-AG
FIRE YANG	
Heart palpitations, anxiety attacks.	
hawthorn, *marjoram, rosemary*	MN-CO, I, LI
FIRE YIN	
Liver enlargement with right-sided cardiac insufficiency.	
milk thistle, *rosemary*	P, LI, MN, K, MN-CU
EARTH YANG	
Congestion at duodenal-pancreatic intersection, pancreatic inflammation or insufficiency, biliary dyskinesia.	
agrimony, artichoke, burdock, fumitory	ZN-NI-CO, S, MG, P, MN-CU
EARTH YIN	
Hepatosplenomegaly, hypoglycemia, gastroptosis.	
centaury, calendula, foenugreek, hypericum, violet; TO PROMOTE LYMPHATIC DRAINAGE: oak, horsetail, laminaria, *bay laurel, ravensare, rosemary*	CU, MN-CU, MN-CU-CO, MG
METAL	
Vagotonia, malnutrition, tubercular type, swollen nodes, cough.	
bladderwrack, coltsfoot, fumitory, laminaria, oak, *ravensare, rosemary, sage*	MN-CU, MN-CU-CO, MG, F

TREATMENT BY TERRAIN: INTESTINAL DISINFECTION

BOTANICALS (herb, *oil*)	OLIGOLEMENTS
EARTH YIN	
Vagotonia, intestinal mycosis, viral enteritis.	
barberry, chamomile, calendula, elecampane, germander, tarragon, *cinnamon, hypericum, lavender, lemon, mint, oregano, savory, thyme*	CU, MN-CU

FATIGUE SYNDROME TREATMENT (CONTINUED)

METAL YIN
Asthenia, vagotonia, mycosis.

Botanicals	Oligolements
calendula, *eucalyptus, mint, hypericum, niaouli, savory, thyme*	Cu, Mn-Cu, Cu-Au-Ag

WATER YANG
Hyperadrenal, sympathotonic.

Botanicals	Oligolements
barberry, meadowsweet, rhubarb	Cu, Co

WATER YIN
Hypoadrenal, frequent secondary infections

Botanicals	Oligolements
bearberry, elecampane, *savory, thyme* TO PROMOTE LYMPHATIC DRAINAGE: black walnut, celandine, coltsfoot, foenugreek, fumitory, horsetail, marine algae, *bay laurel, cinnamon, eucalyptus, everlasting, garlic, hyssop, lavender, lemon, onion, thyme, rosemary, sage*	Cu, Cu-Au-Ag

TREATMENT BY TERRAIN: IMMUNE SUPPORT

BOTANICALS (herb, *oil*)	OLIGOLEMENTS

WOOD
Hepatomegaly, weakness, history of hepatitis.

Botanicals	Oligolements
angelica, artichoke, barberry, black currant, centaury, echinacea, elecampane, germander, hepatica, hops, milk thistle, scarlet pimpernel, tarragon, *cypress, lemon, lavender, mint, rosemary, sage, ravensare*	Cu, S, Mg, Cu-Au-Ag

FIRE
Palpitations, hypopituitarism, sympathetic insufficiency.

Botanicals	Oligolements
angelica, cinchona, echinacea, elecampane, eleutherococcus, marine algae, yarrow, *rosemary, ravensare*	Mg, Cu-Au-Ag

EARTH
Hypothyroid, collagenosis, SLE, slceroderma, post-vaccination or post-infectious anergy.

Botanicals	Oligolements
barberry (bark), bladderwrack, black currant, black walnut, chamomile, centaury, cinchona, echinacea, elecampane, eleutherococcus, germander, gentian, ginger, hops, hypericum, laminaria, menyanthe, oak, plantain, *cinnamon, cypress, lemon, hyssop, sage, ravensare*	Cu-Au-Ag, Mn-Cu, Mg

METAL
Lymphatic swelling, malnutrition, neuropathies, tuberculin type, immunoallergic pneumopathies.

Botanicals	Oligolements
bistort, bladderwrack, black walnut, blessed thistle, centaury, elecampane, eleutherococcus, gentian, germander, ginger, horseradish, horsetail, hops, laminaria, oak, violet, *cinnamon, cypress, hyssop, lemon, mint, savory, sage*	Cu-Au-Ag, Mn-Cu, Mg

WATER
Thin, weak, cold, renal or adrenal insufficiency, nephrotic syndromes, collagenoses, post-infectious anergy.

Botanicals	Oligolements
bistort, bladderwrack, black walnut, elecampane, eleutherococcus, horsetail, marine algae, sea holly, yarrow, *clove, lemon, sage, thyme*	Cu-Au-Ag, Zn-Cu, Cu, Mg

Fatigue Syndrome Treatment (continued)

Endocrine reconstruction
Adrenal insufficiency and atrophy is the common feature of fatigue syndrome. It is considered by some to be a more significant feature than thymus atrophy or hyperplasia. When adrenal strength returns, stamina, appetite and libido improve. Cravings for sugar and alcohol sometimes reappear even after years of absence. Herbs for building the hormone reserve include the following:

Gemmotherapy
Quercus pedunculata, Ribes nigrum

Treatment by terrain

Botanicals (herb, *oil*)	Oligolements
Wood yang	
Nervousness, irritability, hyperthyroidism, difficulties with libido due to hyperexcitability or hysteria.	
angelica, chaste tree, *cumin, ylang ylang*	Mn, Mn-Co
Wood yin	
Libido problems due to nervousness; headaches, depression, sympathetic insufficiency.	
angelica, echinacea, garlic, milk thistle, mint, mugwort, *rosemary, ylang ylang*	Mn, Mg
Fire yin	
Hypogenitalism, global hypopituitarism, sympathetic insufficiency, Heart qi vacuity.	
angelica, bladderwrack, elecampane, laminaria, lonicera, *sage*	Mn-Co, Cu-Au-Ag, Zn-Cu, Al
Earth yin	
Vagotonic terrain, malnutrition, obesity with chill, hypothyroidism, hypogenitalism, Spleen qi vacuity.	
bladderwrack, calendula, elecampane, eleutherococcus, fennel, foenugreek, gentian, ginger, laminaria, mint, *cinnamon, lavender, sage, savory*	Zn-Cu
Metal yin	
Easily chilled, weakness, hypopituitary, hypothyroid, long convalescence, vagotonic terrain.	
bladderwrack, elecampane, eleutherococcus, foenugreek, gentian, ginger, laminaria, mint, plantain, *lavender, sage, savory, thyme*	Mn-Cu, Zn-Cu, Zn, Al
Water yin	
Coldness, impotence or frigidity from hypoadrenalism or hypogenitalism, sentimental, platonic, renal insufficiency, low back pain, Kidney yang vacuity.	
bladderwrack, fennel, eleutherococcus, ginger, honeysuckle, laminaria, *clove, pine, rosemary, savory*	Cu-Au-Ag

GYNECOLOGICAL-OBSTETRIC DISORDERS

In making a diagnosis for disorders of this type, the diligent physician naturally will evaluate the results of Pap smears, pelvic examinations, hematological evaluations and the like in order to determine the exact role that the use of herbs will play in the course of treatment. Here are some of the herbs commonly used in gynecological cases according to some of their properties:

GENERAL TREATMENT	
CONDITION	HERB, *OIL*
EMMENAGOGUES	mugwort, elecampane, chamomile, caraway, fennel, juniper, yarrow, calendula, *lavender, parsley, sage, thyme*
ESTROGENIC PLANTS	angelica, black cohosh, calendula, caraway, coriander, eleutherococcus, elecampane, oat, fennel, ginger, hops, ivy, lovage, scarlet pimpernel, white willow, *angelica, anise, caraway, clary sage, coriander, cypress, fennel, parsley, sage*
ESTROGEN INHIBITORS	chaste tree (vitex agnus castus), *cumin*
LUTEOTROPIC PLANTS	lady's mantle, blessed thistle, sarsaparilla, licorice, yarrow
THYROID INHIBITORS	brassicas, fennel, lycopus, maize, *cumin*
ANTISPASMODICS	angelica, black cohosh, chamomile, lavender, lovage, mugwort, pasque flower, passionflower, white willow, valerian, *melissa, mint, oregano, sage*
UTERINE SEDATIVES	goldenseal, viburnum, white willow, yarrow, *cajeput*
ANTIHEMORRHAGICS AND PELVIC DECONGESTANTS	barberry, bilberry, borage, horsetail, gingko, goldenseal, grapevine, horse chestnut, shepherd's purse, viburnum, witch hazel, *cypress, lavender*
ANTI-INFECTIOUS PLANTS	elecampane, heather, *cinnamon, juniper, lavender, oregano, sage, savory*
ASTRINGENTS	agrimony, bilberry, oak, plantain
REMINERALIZERS	bladderwrack, horsetail, laminaria

AMENORRHEA

TREATMENT BY TERRAIN	
BOTANICALS (herb, *oil*)	OLIGOLEMENTS
WOOD YANG	
Irritability, nervousness, hyperthyroid, hyperestrogenic, functional amenorrhea, Basedow's disease, pituitary overstimulation, sympathotonia in reaction to shock or stress, spasmophilic terrain.	
groundsel, lady's mantle, lycopus, nettle, pulsatilla, stoneseed, woundwort, *cumin*	Mn, Mn-Co, I, S, Mg, P
WOOD YIN	
Nervous women, sympathetic insufficiency, pale, hypotensive, amenorrhea from liver disease, infectious disease, functional hypoestrogenic amenorrhea.	
angelica, elecampane, eleutherococcus, hops, lovage, mugwort, *cypress, lavender, mint, sage*	Mn, S, Mg
FIRE YANG	
Passionate women, hyperpituitary, genital congestion, sympathetic hyperstimulation.	
goldenseal, stoneseed, white willow, *marjoram, ravensare*	Mn-Co, I, S, Co

AMENORRHEA (CONTINUED)

FIRE YIN
Sentimental types, hypopituitary, sympathetic insufficiency, valvulopathy, amenorrhea due to stress, congenital cardiopathy.

elecampane, motherwort, *clary sage, lavender, ravensare, sage*	Cu-Au-Ag

EARTH YANG
Obesity, diabetic or prediabetic terrain. Amenorrhea from hypophyseal or hypothalamic hyperstimulation.

arnica, groundsel, linden *marjoram, ravensare*	Zn-Ni-Co, Mn-Co, Li

EARTH YIN
Young or underdeveloped women, prepubescent obesity, inadequate growth. Deficiency of FSH and LH. Amenorrhea with myxedema, functional hypogonadism or hypopituitarism from stress, trauma or medications (e.g., tranquilizers), acrocyanosis or Raynaud's disease.

bladderwrack, black walnut, calendula, chamomile, elecampane, gentian, groundsel, hops, ivy, laminaria, licorice, menyanthe, mugwort, snakeroot, *cinnamon, caraway, lavender, mint, sage, clary sage, ravensare*	Zn-Cu, Zn, Al, Li

METAL YIN
Hyposthenic women, lymphatic types, underweight, vagotonic, hypothyroid, amenorrhea from malnutrition, anorexia nervosa, lack of concentration, anemia, functional hypothyroidism, hyperhidrosis, functional amenorrhea from local vasoconstriction, acrocyanosis, Raynaud's phenomenon.

angelica, bladderwrack, black walnut, buckthorn, elecampane, gentian, groundsel, horse chestnut, ivy, laminaria, licorice, mugwort, plantain, snakeroot, *lavender, mint, oregano, sassafras, sage, thyme*	Mn-Cu, Mn-Cu-Co, Zn, Al, Li

DYSMENORRHEA

TREATMENT BY TERRAIN	
BOTANICALS (herb, *oil*)	OLIGOLEMENTS

WOOD YANG
Nervousness, irritability, spasmophilia, anguish, migraines, visual disturbances, vertigo, vomiting of bile, pruritus, Quincke's edema, herpes, functional hyperthyroidism, pelvic pain, mastosis following ovulation. Blood stasis, Liver Wind, Liver Fire.

angelica, barberry, black cohosh, broom, calendula, cramp bark, gelsemium, goldenseal, grapevine, groundsel, lady's mantle, mistletoe, mugwort, pulsatilla, stoneseed, witch hazel, white willow, woundwort, yarrow, *caraway, cajeput, everlasting, rosemary*	Mn, I, S, Co, Mg

WOOD YIN
Pallor, hypotension, sympathetic insufficiency, dysmenorrhea related to liver dysfunction, nervousness, restless leg, vertigo, tired eyes, binding depression of Liver qi.

calendula, milk thistle, mugwort, *rosemary, ravensare, everlasting*	Mn, S, Mg, P

FIRE YANG
Sympathotonic, passionate woman, dysmenorrhea with pelvic congestion, hyperpituitarism or corpus luteum insufficiency, flushing, blood stagnation, herpes, vagal insufficiency, true or functional hyperthyroidism.

goldenseal, groundsel, grapevine, stoneseed, white willow, yarrow, *marjoram, melissa, spike lavender*	Mn-Co, Co, I, Mg

Dysmenorrhea (continued)

FIRE YIN	
Sympathetic insufficiency, hypogonadism, insufficient libido, mitral valve stenosis, arrhythmias, menorrhagia.	
cramp bark, milk thistle, *everlasting, ravensare*	Cu-Au-Ag, Co
EARTH YANG	
Obese or prediabetic women, ovarian cysts, PMS with edema, water retention, heavy leg, swelling, abdominal or epigastric pain, vomiting, steatorrhea, damp-heat congestion.	
horse chestnut, lady's mantle, stoneseed, *juniper*	Zn-Ni-Co, Li, Mn-Co
EARTH YIN	
Retarded growth or development, plump with cellulite, cold limbs, sluggish, sleepy, hypoestrogenic or hyperluteal; global steroid insufficiency; edema, swelling, mastosis, hypoglycemia, hypothyroid; blood vacuity, qi vacuity, cold-damp repletion.	
bladderwrack, calendula, fennel, foenugreek, elecampane, groundsel, laminaria, snakeroot, *anise, ravensare, savory*	Zn-Cu, Zn
METAL YIN	
Pale, hyposthenic women, insufficient menstrual flow, hyperluteal or global hypogenitalism, lymphatic congestion, tuberculosis, emaciation, fatigue, weak voice, constipation, hypothyroidism, blood vacuity, qi vacuity.	
bladderwrack, calendula, elecampane, fennel, foenugreek, ginger, hypericum, laminaria, snakeroot, everlasting, *hypericum* (endometriosis), *mint, savory*	Mn-Cu
WATER YANG	
Hypergenitalism, hyperadrenalism, hyperandrogenic, insomnia, flushing, hirsutism.	
bearberry, groundsel, shepherd's purse, white willow	Mn-Co
WATER YIN	
Depression, coldness, cold feet, adrenal insufficiency, hypogenitalism, insufficient pelvic circulation, hypotension, low back pain, weakness at onset of menses, lower leg edema, swelling of the eyes, Kidney yang vacuity.	
bearberry, eleutherococcus, madder, raspberry, yarrow, *cypress, geranium, hypericum* (endometriosis), *lavender, rosemary, sage*	Cu-Au-Ag, Zn-Cu

Metrorrhagia

It is especially important with hemorrhage to examine the possible causes of bleeding. Many women are diagnosed with "functional bleeding" because the true cause has not been determined. Some of the possible causes are pelvic inflammatory disease, uterine fibroma, thyroid problems, threatened miscarriage, diabetes, drainage from IUD irritation, birth control pills, use of anticoagulant medications, steroids, thyroid pills, emotional traumas.

TREATMENT BY TERRAIN	
Botanicals (herb, *oil*)	OLIGOLEMENTS
WOOD YANG	
Hyperthyroid, hyperestrogenic, metrorrhagia of fibroids, endometritis or menopause	
barberry, broom, chaste tree, cramp bark, goldenseal, grapevine, horse chestnut, horsetail, lady's mantle, nettle, witch hazel, woundwort, *cypress, lemon*	Mn-Co, Co

METRORRHAGIA (CONTINUED)

WOOD YIN	
Women with hepatic insufficiency, hypofolliculine terrain.	
angelica, lovage, milk thistle, mugwort, *cypress*	Cu, S, Mg, P
FIRE YANG	
Fibroid metrorrhagia, endometritis, vasomotor metrorrhagia, psychogenic anovulatory metrorrhagia, premenopause.	
goldenseal, grapevine, mistletoe, witch hazel, yarrow	Mn-Co
EARTH YANG	
Overweight, prediabetic type, metrorrhagia from adnexitis, endometritis, metrorrhagia of pituitary origin, ovarian cysts.	
lady's mantle, *lemon*	Zn-Ni-Co, Mn-Co
EARTH YIN	
Metrorrhagia from malnutrition, cancer, metabolic disorders, psychogenic metrorrhagia.	
bistort, Canadian fleabane, oak, plantain, *cinnamon, cypress, geranium, rose*	Zn-Cu
METAL YIN	
Hyposthenic women; abundant blood, breakthrough bleeding, often psychogenic at the first stage, metrorrhagia due to corpus luteum insufficiency, chronic illness or malnutrition (metrorrhagia occurs most frequently in Metal yin types).	
bistort, plantain, *cypress, geranium*	Mn-Cu
WATER YANG	
Hyperadrenal, hypersympathetic terrain, premenopausal or psychogenic metrorrhagia; metrorrhagia due to Stein-Leventhal syndrome.	
Canadian fleabane, horsetail, shepherd's purse	Mn-Co
WATER YIN	
Hypoadrenal terrain, cold body, psychogenic metrorrhagia, metrorrhagia from steroid side effects, chronic disease (especially kidney disease).	
bistort, Canadian fleabane, yarrow, *geranium, rose*	Cu-Au-Ag

UTERINE FIBROIDS

HEMORRHAGE FROM UTERINE FIBROIDS	
BOTANICALS (herb, *oil*)	OLIGOLEMENTS
barberry, chaste tree, goldenseal, shepherd's purse, witch hazel, *everlasting, hypericum*	Mn-Co, I, S

Infections (Ovaritis, Salpingitis, Endometritis, Leukorrhea, Vaginitis)

Treatment by Terrain	
Botanicals (herb, *oil*)	**Oligolements**
Wood yang	
Cervicitis from staphylococcus, streptococcus, gonococcus.	
angelica, lady's mantle, grapevine, pulsatilla (orchitis, ovaritis), woundwort (ovaritis), yarrow (uterine spasm), *lavender*	Cu (2x day), Mn, S
Wood yin	
Chronic leukorrhea of hepatic origin.	
angelica, grapevine, lovage, mugwort, *lavender*	Mn, Mg, Cu (2x day)
Fire yin	
Cervicitis, proteus, streptococcus.	
angelica, elecampane, honeysuckle (staphylococcus), raspberry, *lavender*	Cu (2x day)
Earth yang	
Mycoses aggravated by heat; trichomonas; yellowish-orange leukorrhea, damp-heat congestion, candida in its heat manifestations (aggravated by pregnancy, diabetes, antibiotics).	
agrimony, arnica (mycosis), burdock (mycosis), groundsel, lady's mantle, licorice, white hellebore, white lily, *juniper*	Cu (2x day), Zn-Ni-Co
Earth yin	
Especially enterococcus and Candida albicans; leukorrhea of tuberculosis.	
bilberry, bistort, blessed thistle, blue mallow, chamomile (mycosis), groundsel, hops, horseradish, hypericum, ivy, oak, plantain, scarlet pimpernel, *hyssop, lavender, myrtle, thyme*	Cu (2x day), Mn-Cu
Metal yin	
Especially enterococcus and Candida albicans; leukorrhea of tuberculosis.	
bilberry, black walnut, blessed thistle (mycosis), blue mallow, elecampane, groundsel, hops, horseradish, hypericum, ivy, periwinkle, plantain, oak, *birch, hyssop, lavender, mint* (mycosis), *rosemary, terebenthine, thyme*	Cu (2x day), Mn-Cu
Water yang	
Cervicitis of streptococcus, staphylococcus, gonococcus.	
shepherd's purse (metritis), *eucalyptus*	Cu (2x day)
Water yin	
Cervicitis, especially proteus, and streptococcus; candidiasis aggravated by cold.	
bearberry, bistort, briarhip, Canadian fleabane, heather, honeysuckle (staphylococcus), madder (mycosis), mouse ear, scarlet pimpernel, sea holly (mycosis), *eucalyptus, geranium* (streptococcus), *hyssop, lavender, savory* (mycosis), *sandalwood, terebenthine, thyme*	Cu (2x day)

CERVICAL DYSPLASIA

The general approach is the same as for uterine fibroids regardless of whether there are actual fibroma present. The use of estrogen antagonists such as chaste tree and/or progesterone stimulants like lady's mantle is an important part of the overall treatment. Local treatment is an indispensable part of the treatment. There are several essential oils that can be used for douching with specific properties for correcting cervical dysplasia, HPV (Human Papilloma Virus), and condyloma: *thuja, myrtle, everlasting, geranium* and *lavender*. Pelvic decongestant herbs taken orally are helpful, such as horse chestnut or broom. For local use, oils of *thuja, everlasting, hypericum* and *rosemary* can be used as pelvic decongestants. To restore the vaginal mucosa, *sage* and *everlasting* in an excipient of calendula cream accelerates healing. *Sage* should be used no more than twice a week, and only after full recovery, because of its strong proestrogenic properties.

VAGINITIS

GENERAL TREATMENT	
CONDITION	HERB, *OIL*
VAGINITIS	savory, shepherd's purse, yarrow, *juniper, lavender, thyme*
CANDIDA ALBICANS	Combine 30 ml each of extracts of bistort, goldenseal, nettle and plantain. Separately, combine 1.5 g each of oils of *lavender, savory* and *cinnamon* with wheat germ oil sufficient to 125 ml. Put 45 drops of each concoction in water and drink 10 minutes before each meal. Use *lavender, myrtle* and *geranium* for local treatment. OLIGOTHERAPY: Selenium (mycosis). Take 4-6 capsules of horsetail daily.
TRICHOMONAS	SYSTEMIC TREATMENT: licorice, propolis, *savory thyme*. LOCAL TREATMENT: propolis, *thyme, savory*, calendula extract
NONSPECIFIC VAGINITIS	yarrow, shepherd's purse, horsetail, *thyme, lavender, geranium, myrtle, juniper, hypericum, serpolet*. LOCAL TREATMENTS: calendula ovules; cream of calendula for painful lesions or crevices. One ampule of vitamin A, 0.5 ml extract witch hazel, 2 drops of oil or oils indicated by aromatogram from the local discharge, and green clay to form a bolus or ovule. Green clay cataplasms.
VULVAR PRURITUS (VAGINAL ITCH)	*lemon, sage, thyme* (by terrain) LOTIONS OR COMPRESSES: chamomile, melilot, linden, elder, blue mallow. LOCAL TREATMENT: 50 drops of lady's mantle tincture in a tumbler of water. HERBAL DOUCHE: blue mallow, chamomile, lady's mantle, witch hazel - 50 drops in 12-16 oz water or weak chamomile tea.

DISCOMFORTS OF MENOPAUSE

GENERAL TREATMENT		
BOTANICALS (herb, *oil*)		OLIGOLEMENTS
PERIMENOPAUSE		
Nervous, irritable, short cycles, menses abundant and painful. Adequate liver drainage and amelioration of liver function important for successful treatment.		
chaste tree, dandelion, lycopus, pulsatilla; SEDATIVE: black horehound, hawthorn, melilot, melissa, valerian, passionflower; *bitter orange, chamomile, lavender:* 1.5 ml each in 125 ml elixir of papain		MG, LI (1 x daily, bedtime)

Discomforts of Menopause (continued)

EARLY MENOPAUSE	
Painful menses, abundant or spotting, long and short cycles, breast sensitivity.	
bladderwrack, grapevine, lady's mantle, melilot, yarrow, pulsatilla; SEDATIVE: hawthorn, melilot, passionflower, valerian, white willow; *bitter orange, cypress, juniper, lavender:* 1 ml each in 125 ml wheat germ oil	MG, LI (1 x daily, bedtime)
MENOPAUSE	
Menstruation infrequent, nightsweats, hot flushes, insomnia, emotional instability.	
dandelion, grapevine, lady's mantle, melissa; SEDATIVE: as above; 2-6 capsules horsetail daily; 2 capsules sage at bedtime if hot flushes or night sweats; *angelica, cypress, tarragon:* 1.5 ml each in 125 ml wheat germ oil	LI (1 x daily, bedtime), MG
POST-MENOPAUSE	
black currant, lady's mantle, wild oat, witch hazel; *basil, lavender, sage:* 1.5 ml each in 125 ml wheat germ oil	MG
OSTEOPOROSIS	
horsetail, yarrow, witch hazel; *basil, lavender, sage:* 1.5 ml each in 125 ml wheat germ oil	GEMMOTHERAPY: Rosa canina
HOT FLUSHES	
echinacea, hawthorn, passionflower, witch hazel, *melissa, sage*	

POST-MENOPAUSAL VAGINAL DRYNESS	
oil of sage	2 drops
lady's mantle extract	0.5 ml
oil of calendula	0.5 ml
powdered licorice root	1.25 ml
green clay	1 g
Combine in a gelatinous excipient or cocoa butter to make ovule. Insert one ovule at bedtime three times weekly.	

Mastoses

(Mastodynia, Mastitis, Crevices, Mammary Infections)

TREATMENT BY TERRAIN	
BOTANICALS (herb, *oil*)	OLIGOELEMENTS
WOOD	
Hyperestrogenic, hyperthyroid.	
chaste tree, pulsatilla, stoneseed, *cumin*	MN, S
FIRE	
Hyperestrogenic, sympathotonic, hyperprolactinemia.	
chaste tree, yarrow, stoneseed, *lavender*	MN-CO, I
EARTH	
Hyperestrogenic, overweight, excessive milk, diabetic terrain.	
chaste tree, stoneseed, *melissa, sage*	ZN-NI-CO, MN-CO, ZN

AGALACTICA (BREAST MILK INSUFFICIENCY)

BOTANICALS (herb, *oil*)	OLIGOELEMENTS
black elder, cumin, goat rue, hops, *caraway,* vervain, *anise, coriander, cymbopogon, fennel;* cumin seeds plus fennel seeds: 1 tsp. each per cup: infuse for 10 minutes 3 times daily.	

TO STOP LACTATION

BOTANICALS (herb, *oil*)	OLIGOELEMENTS
periwinkle, artichoke, *clary sage, mint, sage.* Oil of *sage* plus oil of *mint* 1.5 ml with 125 ml elixir of papain. Artichoke extract, 30 drops 3 times daily.	MN-CO

ENGORGEMENT
To drain milk, make a compress with decoction of chamomile flowers. Apply camphorated oil of *hypericum* or oil of *chamomile.* For crevices, use cream of calendula.

INDUCTION OF LABOR

HERB FUNCTION	Herb, *Oil*
OXYTOCIC HERBS	black cohosh, blue mallow, elecampane, fennel, goldenseal, honeysuckle, lady's mantle, madder, motherwort, shepherd's purse, snakeroot, vervain, woundwort, *clove, cajeput, cinnamon, sage*
UTEROTONIC HERBS	motherwort, *juniper, thuja*
ANTIOXYTOCIC HERBS	lovage, pasque flower, viburnum, white willow

TREATMENT BY TERRAIN
BOTANICALS (herb, *oil*)

WOOD YANG OR FIRE YANG
Muscle spasm, hyperthyroid terrain, strong contractions, but delayed dilation.
black cohosh, goldenseal, lady's mantle, woundwort

FIRE YIN
Sympathetic insufficiency, slow pulse rate, congenital cardiopathy.
agrimony, honeysuckle

EARTH YANG
Obese or overweight women with difficult labor.
lady's mantle

EARTH YIN
Hypogenital, overweight or asthenic, habitual slackness of abdominal muscle.
blue mallow, vervain, calendula, snakeroot, *cinnamon*

METAL YIN
Lymphatic congestion, hypogenital
blue mallow, snakeroot

WATER YIN
Hypoadrenal, asthenic, cold body, cold limbs.
lady's mantle, madder, *clove*

Pregnancy disorders

Condition	Herb, *Oil*
THREATENED ABORTION	pulsatilla, viburnum, white willow
NAUSEA OF PREGNANCY	ginger, fresh or in capsules (avoid using essential oil)
CONSTIPATION OF PREGNANCY	raspberry, preferably an infusion of the leaves
PREPARATION FOR LABOR	essential oil of rose prepares the uterus for expansion. Use topically when stretching of lower abdominal tissue begins. Snakeroot for delayed or protracted labor.

HERBS TO AVOID DURING PREGNANCY

belladonna, bistort, blessed thistle, borage, broom, buckthorn, Canadian fleabane, cherry laurel, cypress, digitalis, drosera, ephedra, false hellebore, gelsemium, goat rue, grapevine, groundsel, hellebore, hepatica, henbane, hops, horse chestnut, ivy, khella, licorice, lily, lily-of-the-valley, lotus, lycopus, mistletoe, opium, red poppy, rauwolfia, shepherd's purse, stoneseed, white hellebore, yarrow

HERBS TO AVOID DURING PREGNANCY (ABORTIFACIENTS)

arnica (internally), black cohosh, calendula, chaste tree, cinchona, goldenseal, honeysuckle, lady's mantle, madder, motherwort, rhubarb, scarlet pimpernel, senna, snakeroot, vervain, woundwort

ESSENTIAL OILS TO AVOID DURING PREGNANCY

basil, birch, calamus, chenopodium, cumin, hypericum, hyssop, marjoram, myrrh, oregano, parsley, rosemary, sage, savory, serpolet, tarragon, thyme, wintergreen, yarrow, ylang ylang

ESSENTIAL OILS TO AVOID DURING PREGNANCY (ABORTIFACIENTS)

cedarwood, cinnamon, clary sage, clove, cypress, everlasting, mugwort, sassafras, thuja

Infertility

TREATMENT BY TERRAIN	
BOTANICALS (herb, *oil*)	OLIGOLEMENTS
WOOD YANG	
Anovulatory sterility from excessive stress or trauma, hyperthyroid terrain.	
chaste tree, stoneseed, yarrow	MN-CO, I
EARTH YIN	
Pituitary factors important; FSH, LH insufficiency, hypophysogonadic dysadaptation.	
caraway, cypress, elecampane, eleutherococcus, gentian, ginseng, lady's mantle (hypoluteal), licorice, mugwort, *geranium, savory, sage*	ZN, ZN-CU
METAL YIN	
Hypothyroid, malnutrition, lymphatic congestion, corpus luteum insufficiency.	
cypress, elecampane (+++), eleutherococcus, gentian, ginseng, lady's mantle (hypoluteal), mugwort, sarsaparilla, wild oat, *clary sage, geranium, savory, sage*	MN-CU, ZN
WATER YIN	
Gonadal insufficiency, steroid insufficiency, adrenal insufficiency.	
elecampane, licorice, sarsaparilla, yarrow, *geranium, sage*	CU-AU-AG, ZN-CU, ZN

GASTROENTEROLOGICAL COMPLAINTS

HERBS FOR DIGESTIVE DISORDERS AND THEIR FUNCTIONS

BITTER TONICS	artichoke, barberry, chamomile, chicory, dandelion, elecampane, fumitory, germander, gentian, ginger, hops, horehound, lady's mantle, madder, vervain, yellow dock, *juniper*
STOMACHIC HERBS; EUPEPTIC & APERITIF HERBS	blessed thistle, the chamomiles, celery, centaury, fennel, cinchona, coriander, foenugreek, gentian, menyanthe, germander, ginger, tarragon, vervain, *anise, basil, juniper, cinnamon, clove, lemon, mint, hyssop, sage, thyme, savory*
HERBS FOR PANCREATIC DRAINAGE	agrimony, bilberry, blackberry, black walnut, coriander, fennel, foenugreek, fumitory, gentian, ginger, goat rue, yellow dock, onion, periwinkle, plantain, *caraway, eucalyptus, geranium, lemon, sage*
ASTRINGENT AND ANTIDIARRHEIC HERBS	agrimony, bilberry, black currant, black walnut, briarhip, horse chestnut, lady's mantle, oak, plantain, yarrow, *bitter orange, geranium, lavender, lemon, rosemary, sage, sandalwood, savory*
HERBS TO CLEAR THE BOWEL (CATHARTICS)	ash, barberry, birch, blue mallow, buckthorn, heather, senna, rhubarb, solidago, yellow dock
SYMPATHOLYTIC OILS	*chamomile, coriander, lavender, marjoram, melissa, mint, rosemary*
VAGOLYTIC OILS	*basil, caraway, cumin, tarragon, thyme*
ANTI-INFLAMMATORY AND ANTI-INFECTIOUS PLANTS	bilberry, chamomile, garlic, germander, ginger, *cajeput, chamomile, cinnamon, garlic, juniper, geranium, clove, lavender, lemon, marjoram, mint, niaouli, pine, rosemary, savory, sage, ti tree, thyme*
INTESTINAL ANTISPASMODICS	angelica, chamomile, celandine, datura, hawthorn, linden, melilot, mugwort, pulsatilla, vervain, yarrow, *anise, basil, cajeput, caraway, cinnamon, lavender, mint, marjoram, melissa, oregano, savory, sage, tarragon, thyme*
CARMINATIVE PLANTS	*garlic, angelica, anise, caraway, coriander, cumin, tarragon, fennel, ginger, clove, hyssop, lovage, chamomile, sweet balm, mint, oregano, rosemary, savory*
EUPEPTIC PLANTS	*garlic, anise, basil, chamomile, cinnamon, caraway, milk thistle, coriander, cumin, tarragon, fennel, juniper, gentian, germander, ginger, hyssop, lavender, lovage, horehound, melissa, mint, oregano, rosemary, savory, linden, sage, thyme, vervain*
ANTIULCERATIVE PLANTS	brassica (fresh juice), chamomile, licorice, *calendula, lemon, geranium*
ANTISPASMODIC AND STONE-PREVENTING PLANTS FOR THE BILIARY TRACT	artichoke, barberry, black radish, combretum, dandelion, madder, rest harrow
CHOLAGOGIC AND CHOLERETIC PLANTS	agrimony, artichoke, barberry, black currant, black radish, boldo, burdock, calendula, chamomile, celandine, dandelion, elecampane, fumitory, hawthorn, hypericum, madder, meadowsweet, milk thistle, *lemon, lavender, melissa, mint, rosemary, savory, sage*
HERBS FOR HEPATIC DRAINAGE	artichoke, black radish, boldo, celandine, centaury, dandelion, fumitory, nettle, *rosemary, melissa, lavender, mint, lemon, marjoram, sage, thyme*
HEPATOPROTECTIVE PLANTS	artichoke, milk thistle
VERMIFUGES	basil, black currant, black walnut, brassica, chamomile, elecampane, garlic, gentian, tarragon, caraway, *clove, chenopodium, cinnamon, eucalyptus, geranium, hyssop, lavender, savory, terebenthine, thyme*

Gastralgia
(Gastritis, Duodenitis, Gastric Hyperacidity, Gastroenteritis, Gastric Hypertonia, Gastric Hypochlorhydria)

GEMMOTHERAPY	
Tilia tomentosa	

TREATMENT BY TERRAIN	
BOTANICALS (herb, *oil*)	OLIGOLEMENTS

WOOD

Sympathotonic, hyperthyroid terrain, gastralgia from impediment of the bile flow, gastritis, biliary dyskinesia, cholelithiasis.

angelica (hyperacidity), artichoke, celandine (duodenitis), white willow (hyperacidity), *lemon* (ulcers, hyperacidity), *marjoram, bitter orange, rosemary, ravensare*	Mn, S, P, I

FIRE YANG

Vagal insufficiency or dystonia, gastralgia due to excess eating, sedentary lifestyle, hysterical stomach pains.

birch, chaste tree, mullein, white willow, *melissa, bitter orange, ravensare*	Zn-Ni-Co, Mn-Co, S, P, Mg

EARTH YANG

Vagal insufficiency, hypopancreatic terrain, subacute pancreatitis, epigastric tightness, epigastric spasms.

calendula, fumitory, licorice, marshmallow, vervain, *juniper, lemon, melissa*	Zn-Ni-Co, Ni-Co, S, P

EARTH YIN

Hypothyroid, vagotonic terrain, postprandial drowsiness, chronic gastritis, gastric ulcer, hypochlorhydria, autoimmune related gastritis, anorexia from hypothyroidism.

angelica (hypo or hyperthyroidism), calendula, elecampane, fennel, gentian, groundsel, licorice (hypochlorhydria and ulcers), mullein, oak, vervain, yellow dock (hypochlorhydria), *anise, chamomile, cinnamon, coriander* (hypochlorhydria), *geranium, hyssop, lavender* (hypochlorhydria), *mint, ravensare, savory*	Mn-Cu, Mn-Cu-Co, Bi, Mg

METAL YANG

Vagal insufficient terrain, gastralgia with colitis and constipation, hemorrhoids, acute duodenitis, duodenal ulcers.

agrimony, lady's mantle, marshmallow, *eucalyptus*	Mn-Cu, Mn-Co, P, Ni-Co

METAL YIN

Hyposthenic, vagotonic terrain, chronic duodenitis, sensitive to cold, anorexic, gastroptosis.

datura, elecampane (hypochlorhydria), henbane, nettle (duodenal ulcer), oak, *cajeput* (gastric spasms), *eucalyptus, coriander, hypericum, hyssop, lavender* (hypochlorhydria), *mint, rosemary, savory, thyme*	Mn-Cu, Bi

WATER YIN

Emotional sensitivity, fatigue, cold, hypoadrenal constitution, chronic ulcers, chronic gastritis.

licorice, mullein, *geranium, hypericum, rosemary*	Cu-Au-Ag, Mg, Bi

Dyspepsia

(Indigestion, Aerophagia, Pancreatic Insufficiency)

GEMMOTHERAPY		
Tilia tomentosa		

TREATMENT BY TERRAIN		
BOTANICALS (herb, *oil*)		OLIGOELEMENTS
WOOD YANG		
Sympathotonic, hyperthyroid terrain, more or less spasmophilic, sympathotonic spasms sometimes with globus hystericus, thoracic oppression, biliary dyskinesia.		
fumitory, lady's mantle, lovage, *bitter orange, juniper, lavender, lemon, marjoram, melissa*		Mn, P, Co, Ni-Co, I, Bi-I
WOOD YIN		
Sympathetic insufficient terrain, acetonemia, hepatic insufficiency, insufficient biliary secretions, pallor, sequela of liver disease.		
angelica, barberry (biliary insufficiency), lovage, mint, tarragon (biliary insufficiency), rosemary, yarrow; CHOLERETIC HERBS: artichoke, black radish, boldo, celandine, centaury, combretum, elecampane, fumitory; CHOLERETIC OILS: *lavender, rosemary*		Mn, Cu, S, P
FIRE YANG		
Dystonia, psychic distress, esophageal spasms, hiatus hernia.		
meadowsweet, yarrow, *bitter orange, marjoram*		Mn-Co, I, Bi-I, P, Ni-Co
EARTH YANG		
Vagal insufficiency, hypopancreatic terrain, heavyset constitution, reflux, esophageal spasms, postprandial drowsiness, hiatal hernia.		
fumitory, linden, bilberry, celandine (choleretic), *juniper, lavender* (choleretic), *melissa*		Mn-Co, I, Bi-I, P, Ni-Co
EARTH YIN		
Vagotonic, insufficient gastric, pancreatic secretions, atonic dyspepsia, hypochlorhydria, anorexia.		
barberry, belladonna, centaury (choleretic), elecampane (choleretic), fennel, gentian, germander, ginger, hops, hypericum, licorice, *cinnamon, caraway, coriander, hyssop, mint, savory, sage*		Zn-Ni-Co, Bi
METAL YIN		
Vagotonic, hyposthenic terrain, anorexia, anorexia nervosa, lymphatic congestion, atonic dyspepsia.		
belladonna, centaury, coriander, elecampane, fennel, germander, ginger, hops, hypericum, *clove, hyssop, lavender, mint, savory, sassafras, thyme*		Mn-Cu, Zn-Ni-Co, Bi

Gastroptosis

Treatment by Terrain	
Botanicals (herb, *oil*)	Oligolements
Earth yin or Metal yin	
Hypothyroid, hyposthenic, vagotonic terrain, lymphatic congestion, insufficient gastric and pancreatic secretions; malnutrition, exhaustion from illness, cachexia, aged patients, Spleen yang vacuity.	
angelica, elecampane, oak, fennel, gentian, hypericum, *cinnamon, eucalyptus, hyssop, lavender, sage, savory, thyme*	Mn-Cu, Cu-Au-Ag

Colonopathy (Colitis, Megacolon)

Treatment by Terrain	
Botanicals (herb, *oil*)	Oligolements
Wood yang	
Sympathotonic, hyperthyroid, allergic terrain, biliary dyskinesia, migraines, spasmodic constipation, diarrhea, alternating constipation and diarrhea, cramping of bowel, spasmophilia or digestive allergies.	
chaste tree, plantain, pulsatilla, stoneseed, yarrow, *lavender, lemon, marjoram, rosemary*	Mn, S, P, Bi
Fire yang	
Dystonic terrain, nervous, emotional, extreme sympathotonia, stress-related, frequent attacks, diarrhea, colonopathy due to vagotonia in plethoric types.	
shepherd's purse, *lavender, marjoram, melissa*	Mn-Co, P, Bi
Earth yang	
Vagal insufficiency, diarrhea, colonopathy of obesity, hypersecreting type of constitution, pancreatic insufficiency, constipation, right-sided colon pain, damp-heat terrain.	
bilberry, lady's mantle, *juniper*	Zn-Ni-Co, P, Bi, Mn-Co
Earth yin	
Vagotonia, hypophyseal-gonadic dysadaptation, physical or mental strain, excessively sedentary, sensitivity to cold, dysentery, atonic constipation or intestinal fermentation.	
angelica, belladonna, elecampane, fennel, gentian, ginger, licorice, *anise, basil, caraway, coriander, hyssop, lavender, savory, thyme*	Mn-Cu, P, Bi, Co
Metal yang	
Vagal insufficiency, damage from internal heat (sinusitis, coronary disease), constipation, post-antibiotic colitis.	
ash, borage, burdock, marshmallow, rhubarb, senna, *lemon*	Mn-Cu, Mn-Co, P, Bi, Co
Metal yin	
Vagotonic, hyposthenic terrain, apathetic, meticulous, obsession with intestinal function, chronic colitis, sensitivity to cold, megacolon, left-sided colitis or pain throughout colon especially on the left, atonic constipation, chronic constipation, constipation of the aged or from chronic illness, bed confinement.	
belladonna, bladderwrack, datura, elecampane, gentian, laminaria, nettle, *cinnamon, coriander, clove, hyssop, oregano, savory, thyme*	Mn-Cu, P, Bi, Co

INTESTINAL INFECTIONS

TREATMENT BY TERRAIN	
BOTANICALS (herb, *oil*)	OLIGOLEMENTS
FIRE YANG	
Dystonic terrain, damage from heat repletion, hyperthermia, especially staphylococcus.	
meadowsweet, melilot, *marjoram, melissa, niaouli, ylang ylang*	Cu
FIRE YIN	
Sympathetic insufficiency, anergy, viral enteritis, typhoid, shigellosis, salmonella.	
elecampane (virus), *lemon* (typhoid), *thyme, ravensare*	Cu, Cu-Au-Ag
EARTH YANG	
Hypopancreatic terrain, especially fungal enteritis (damp-heat), viral enteritis, colibacillosis.	
agrimony (virus), arnica (mycosis), bilberry (colibacillosis), burdock (mycosis), meadowsweet, woody nightshade, *lemon, melissa*	Cu, Zn-Ni-Co
EARTH YIN	
Vagotonic terrain, pituitary insufficiency, mycosis from dampness or damp-cold, viral enteritis, typhoid, fungal enteritis due to hemopathies.	
barberry, blessed thistle (mycosis), calendula, chamomile, elecampane (virus), germander, hypericum, menyanthe, scarlet pimpernel, *cinnamon* (mycosis), *coriander, myrtle, eucalyptus, lemon, lavender, mint* (mycosis), *ravensare* (virus), *savory* (mycosis, virus), *tarragon, thyme* (virus)	Cu, Mn-Cu
METAL YANG	
Vagal insufficiency, constipation, fungal enteritis, streptococcus.	
agrimony (mycosis), horehound (typhus), woody nightshade, *niaouli, serpolet, thyme* (virus), *ylang ylang*	Cu
METAL YIN	
Hyposthenic, vagotonic terrain, chronic colitis, viral enteritis, mycosis (damp-heat), chronic colibacillosis.	
blessed thistle (mycosis), calendula (virus), elecampane (virus, dermatophylus), horehound (typhus), hypericum, *eucalyptus (E. coli), hyssop* (virus), *mint* (mycosis, virus), *myrtle, niaouli, savory* (mycosis, virus), *serpolet, thyme* (typhus, mycosis, virus)	Cu, Mn-Cu, Cu-Au-Ag
WATER YANG	
Hyperadrenal, sympathotonic terrain, staphylococcus, colibacillus, mycoses (damp-heat).	
bearberry, bilberry (coli), meadowsweet (mycosis), *ylang ylang*	Cu, Co
WATER YIN	
Anergic, hypoadrenal terrain, terrain of choice for secondary infections, chronic infections, viral enteritis, mycotic enteritis, typhoid, chronic colibacillosis.	
bearberry, elecampane (virus), honeysuckle (*E. coli*, staphylococcus), madder (mycosis), sea holly (mycosis), scarlet pimpernel, *cajeput* (virus), *hypericum, hyssop* (virus), *sandalwood, savory* (mycosis, virus), *serpolet, thyme* (virus)	Cu, Cu-Au-Ag

INTESTINAL PARASITES

GENERAL TREATMENT
Oil of chenopodium kills most parasites. Bromelain (from pineapple) and papain (from papaya), or other proteolytic enzymes kill parasites. Intestinal drainage and bile secretion should be normalized. FOR PROTOZOA: oak, ash, gentian, *bay laurel, garlic, lemon, savory*

TREATMENT BY TERRAIN	
BOTANICALS (herb, *oil*)	OLIGOLEMENTS
EARTH YIN	
Most frequent terrain: damp-cold or damp-heat.	
black walnut, chamomile, centaury, elecampane, fumitory, menyanthe, *bay laurel, bergamot, caraway, chenopodium, cinnamon, hyssop, lavender, mugwort, savory, terebenthine, thyme*	Cu
METAL YIN	
Lymphatic congestion, malnutrition aggravated by parasitosis.	
black walnut, cajeput, centaury, chenopodium, elecampane, *cinnamon, clove, hyssop, lavender, mugwort, savory, terebenthine, thyme, thuja*	Cu
WATER YANG	
Excess of glairy mucus, heat, humidity.	
black walnut, chenopodium, mugwort, *thuja*	Cu
WATER YIN	
Hypoadrenal terrain, excess of dampness.	
chenopodium, mugwort, *thuja*	Cu

OXYURIA (PINWORMS)

This is the most frequent type of parasitosis. In France it is estimated that 60 to 90 percent of school age children are affected to some degree. The eggs of the parasite are deposited in the vicinity of the anal margin outside of the digestive tube. From there the infestation sets up the cycle of reinfection and contagion. Symptoms include nervousness, depression, irritability, night terrors, insomnia and clenching of the teeth.

ESSENTIAL OILS TREATMENT
ESSENTIAL OILS FOR KILLING OXYURIA: *chenopodium, garlic, eucalyptus, lemon, thyme*
ESSENTIAL OIL FORMULA FOR OXYURIA:

Combine the following oils:

thyme	1.5 ml
cinnamon	1.5 ml
chamomile	1.5 ml
elixir of papain	125 ml

Or, use oils of thyme, tarragon and geranium, 1 drop each per kilo of body weight, three times daily before meals. Adults may take 45 drops three times per day.

OTHER REMEDIES: Garlic oil suppositories inserted rectally. If necessary, antispasmodic herbs can be used in accompaniment.

ASCARIASIS (NEMATODES)

Nematodes live in the small intestines and grow 15 to 20 cm. long. Their eggs can only germinate outside the body, but can live in soil for five years. The contamination usually occurs from polluted water or from vegetables carrying traces of contaminated soil. Diagnosis is by examination of a stool specimen. Symptoms are typically those of enterocolitis. More serious symptoms can result if they migrate to other parts of the body.

GENERAL TREATMENT

Combine the following essential oils. Children should take 1 drop per kilogram body weight 10 minutes before each meal in a glass of water:

geranium	1.5 ml
eucalyptus	1.5 ml
thyme	1.5 ml
elixir of papain	125 ml

Adults: 45 drops 3 times daily. Garlic capsules orally.

Antispasmodics and sedatives may also be necessary.

OTHER OILS FOR ASCARIASIS: *chenopodium, eucalyptus, thyme, garlic, chamomile*

TAPEWORM (TAENIA)

A parasite of beef or pork, tapeworm can be taken in by eating meats too rare. Its body consists of hundreds of segments, parts of which can be spontaneously discharged in the stool. Symptoms include abdominal pains, nervousness and fatigue.

GENERAL TREATMENT

Roasted pumpkin or gourd seeds are effective for killing tapeworm. Mix a paste of 50 grams of seed paste with an equal quantity of honey. Take in three doses half an hour apart. Two hours later purge with 2 tsp. castor oil in a large cup of senna leaf infusion.

Reduce the dose for children and take the paste mixture for several days before purging.

ESSENTIAL OILS FOR TAENIA: *chenopodium, garlic, terebenthine, thyme*

ANAL PRURITUS

LOCAL ESSENTIAL OIL TREATMENT:

mint	.10 ml
chamomile	.10 ml
lemon	.10 ml
oil of sweet almond.	to mix

FOR LESIONS: calendula cream. Green clay cataplasms are also helpful in many cases

---

Constipation

Gemmotherapy
Vaccinum vitis idaea

Treatment by Terrain	
Botanicals (herb, *oil*)	Oligolements
Wood Yang	
Sympathotonic, hyperthyroid, spasmophilic terrain, hepatic or biliary congestion, biliary dyskinesia, headaches, stomach ulcers, spasmodic constipation.	
artichoke, barberry, black radish, boldo, celandine, combretum, dandelion, fumitory, goldenseal, rhubarb, violet	Mn, S, P
Wood Yin	
Pallor, nervousness, sympathetic insufficient terrain, insufficient bile secretion.	
artichoke, barberry, boldo, combretum, dandelion, fumitory, *rosemary*	Mn, S, P
Fire Yang	
Anxioius, sedentary individual, sympathotonic, emotional.	
ash, marshmallow	Mn-Co, P
Fire Yin	
Sympathetic insufficiency, atonic constipation, depression	
barberry, milk thistle, raspberry	Cu-Au-Ag, Mg, Mn-Cu
Earth Yang	
Vagal insufficiency, diabetic or prediabetic terrain, pancreatic insufficiency, constipation from obesity, excessive sitting, compression of mucus in the bowel.	
ash, burdock, fumitory, marshmallow, rhubarb	Mn-Co, P, Mg, Zn-Ni-Co
Earth Yin	
Vagotonia, flaccid obesity or malnutrition, small-boned frame, abdominal slackness, cold, atonic constipation, hypoglycemia, hypothyroid, megacolon.	
barberry, bladderwrack, blue mallow, buckthorn, fennel, laminaria, licorice, plantain, raspberry, yellow dock	Mn-Cu, P
Metal Yang	
Phlegmatic type, vagal insufficiency, constipation from repletion heat of the Large Intestine, from duodenal ulcers.	
ash, burdock, marshmallow, senna, rhubarb	Mn-Cu, Mn-Co, P
Metal Yin	
Vagotonia, spasmodic constipation, sensitive to cold, megacolon of hypothyroidism, megacolon of opiates addiction, atonic constipation.	
blue mallow, buckthorn, fennel, plantain, raspberry, violet, yellow dock, *rosemary, terebenthine*	Mn-Cu, Cu-Au-Ag, P
Water Yang	
Sympathotonic, hyperadrenal, spasmodic constipation, constipation due to excess heat in the lower abdomen (e.g. cystitis, ovaritis, genital herpes, etc.).	
ash, barberry, marshmallow, senna	Mn-Co
Water Yin	
Adrenal insufficiency, sympathetic insufficiency, cold body, cold limbs, constipation due to dryness, lack of liquid, atonic constipation.	
briar hip, fennel, madder, raspberry, *rose, terebenthine*	Cu-Au-Ag, Mg

DIARRHEA

GEMMOTHERAPY
Vaccinum vitis idaea

TREATMENT BY TERRAIN

BOTANICALS (herb, *oil*)	OLIGOLEMENTS
WOOD YANG	
Sympathotonic, hyperthyroid, allergic terrain, spasmodic forceful diarrhea, diarrhea from biliary dyskinesia.	
lady's mantle, melilot, stoneseed, yarrow, *cypress*	Mn, S, P, Co
WOOD YIN	
Nervous, sympathetic insufficiency, diarrhea from oily food, emotional upset.	
melilot, gentian, hops, *cypress, lemon, lavender*	Mn, S, P, Co
FIRE YANG	
Vagal insufficiency, dystonic, diarrhea from heat in the small intestine, acute severe diarrhea (heat or damp-heat), intestinal infections, sequela of shellfish poisoning, digitalis, antibiotics, stress.	
hawthorn, melilot, rauwolfia, *bitter orange, lavender, marjoram, melissa*	Mn-Co, P-Co, Cu
FIRE YIN	
Liquid, aqueous diarrhea, aggravated by cold, typhoid.	
gentian, *lavender, lemon* (typhoid)	Cu-Au-Ag
EARTH YANG	
Pancreatic insufficiency, diarrhea of indigestion, colchicine poisoning.	
agrimony, lady's mantle, arnica, meadowsweet (mycosis)	Zn-Ni-Co, Mn-Co, Co
EARTH YIN	
Vagotonia, hypothyroid, hypoglycemic, ulcerative colitis, excessive worry, ileocecal tuberculosis, malabsorption, indigestion, steatorrhea, Crohn's disease, chronic injury to the large or small intestine.	
angelica, bistort, black walnut, bladderwrack, blessed thistle, blue mallow, bryonia, chamomile, Canadian fleabane, elecampane, gentian, ginger, groundsel, hops, hypericum, laminaria, licorice, oak, plantain, *cinnamon, geranium, hyssop, lemon, savory, sage, thyme*	Mn-Cu P, Mg, Bi
METAL YANG	
Vagal insufficiency, diverticulitis, sigmoiditis, duodenal ulcer.	
agrimony (mycosis), lady's mantle, marshmallow, opium, periwinkle, white lily, *eucalyptus, niaouli*	Mn-Cu, Mn-Co, Bi
METAL YIN	
Vagotonic, hypothyroid, cold body, ideopathic, chronic diarrhea, Crohn's disease, hemorrhagic rectocolitis, rectocolitis with polyps, rectosigmoid tumors, dysentery.	
bistort, black walnut, blessed thistle, bryonia, gentian, blue mallow, ginger, groundsel, hypericum, nettle, oak, plantain, *cajeput, eucalyptus, clove, niaouli, oregano, savory, thyme*	Mn-Cu, Cu-Au-Ag, Bi
WATER YANG	
Sympathotonic, hyperadrenal, spasmodic diarrhea.	
bearberry (*E. coli, enterococcus*), black elder, goldenrod, meadowsweet, melilot, rauwolfia, shepherd's purse, *lavender, melissa*	Mn-Co, Co
WATER YIN	
Anergic, adrenal insufficiency, chronic colon afflictions, rectal problems, Crohn's disease, hemorrhagic rectocolitis, rectosigmoid tumors, cold body, cold feet.	
bearberry (*E. coli, enterococcus*), black elder, black walnut, bistort, briarhip, Canadian fleabane, goldenrod, nettle, plantain, raspberry, *cajeput, geranium, clove, niaouli, sandalwood, savory*	Cu-Au-Ag, Bi, Mg, Mn-Co

Hepatic congestion, biliary dyskinesia (hepatomegaly, fatty liver)

Gemmotherapy
Rosmarinus officinalis

Treatment by terrain	
Botanicals (herb, *oil*)	Oligolements
Wood yang	
Choleric subject, hyperthyroid, cholestasis, hepatitis, migraines, dyspepsia, digestive spasms.	
artichoke, barberry, black radish, boldo, broom, celandine, combretum, dandelion, fumitory, hepatica, horse chestnut, lady's mantle, nettle, orthosiphon, pulsatilla, stoneseed, woundwort, *bay laurel, lemon, rosemary*	Mn, S, P
Wood yin	
Nervous, sympathetic insufficiency, weak spasms, headaches, toxic liver, toxic hepatitis.	
angelica, barberry, brassica, centaury, calendula, echinacea, elecampane, germander, hops, horse chestnut, hepatica, hypericum, lovage, milk thistle (hepato-splenomegaly, infections, toxic hepatitis), *cypress, lemon, mint, rosemary, sage*	Mn-Cu, S, Cu, Cu-Au-Ag
Fire yang	
Biliary dyskinesia from excess fat consumption, aging.	
artichoke, ash, birch, borage, echinacea, horehound, orthosiphon, shepherd's purse, stoneseed, *lavender*	Mn-Co, S, P, I
Fire yin	
Fatty cardiac liver due to right cardiac insufficiency.	
milk thistle, *lavender*	P, Li, Mg, K, Mn-Cu
Earth yang	
Congestion at duodenal-pancreatic intersection, gallstones, pancreatitis, pancreatic insufficiency.	
agrimony, artichoke, burdock, fumitory, *bay laurel*	Zn-Ni-Co, S, Mg, P, Mn-Cu
Earth yin	
Hepatosplenomegalies, especially due to immune system reactions.	
calendula, centaury, echinacea, hypericum, violet, *lemon*	Cu, Mn-Cu

Cirrhosis of the liver

Gemmotherapy
Juniperus communis (one of the most effective; also good for ascites).

Treatment by terrain	
Botanicals (herb, *oil*)	Oligolements
Wood yang	
artichoke, mouse ear, *juniper, rosemary*	Cu-S, Mg, Li, K, Mn-Co
Wood yin	
angelica, artichoke, brassica, germander, juniper, milk thistle, mouse ear	Cu-S, Mg, Li, K, Mn-Co

ANOREXIA

BOTANICALS (herb, *oil*)	OLIGOLEMENTS
TREATMENT BY TERRAIN	
WOOD YIN	
Nervousness, sympathetic insufficiency, sequela of damage to liver cells.	
barberry, centaury, germander, milk thistle, mint	Cu, P, Mg, Mn
EARTH YANG	
Anorexia from alimentary encumbrance, indigestion, excessive eating.	
birch, fumitory, periwinkle, *juniper, melissa*	Zn-Ni-Co
EARTH YIN	
Anorexia after physical or mental strain, after prolonged illness, impaired immunity.	
angelica, barberry, bladderwrack, chamomile, fennel, foenugreek, gentian, germander, ginger, laminaria, *lavender, spike lavender, lemon, mint, sage, coriander, anise, caraway, tarragon, hyssop, oregano*	Zn-Cu, Cu-Au-Ag
METAL YIN	
Vagotonic, hyposthenic, anorexia of adolescence, anorexia nervosa, anorexia in subjects with lymphatic congestion, tuberculosis, or long convalescence.	
angelica, bladderwrack, calendula, eleutherococcus, foenugreek, gentian, germander, ginger, hops, hypericum, laminaria, wild oat, *clove, hyssop, lavender, sassafras, sage, thyme*	Mn-Cu, Li, F
WATER YIN	
Anergic, hypoadrenal, low vitality, anorexia from chronic illness, weak constitution or nervosa.	
black currant, briarhip, eleutherococcus, *lavender, savory, sassafras*	Cu-Au-Ag, Li, Mg

ARTHRITIS AND RHEUMATISM

GEMMOTHERAPY
Vitis vinifera (anti-inflammatory), Fraxinus excelsior (diuretic, anti-inflammatory), Betula pubescens (anti-inflammatory, antalgic). OSTEOPOROSIS: Abies pectinata, Pinus montana, Quercus pedunculata, Rosa canina

BOTANICALS	
CONDITION	Herb (oil)
ANTI-INFLAMMATORY PLANTS	Ribes nigrum buds, chamomile, ginger, birch, harpagophytum, blessed thistle, meadowsweet, white willow, terebenthine, birch. Proteolytic enzymes are an important feature of treatment. Plant substances most often used are elixir of papain as a base, or extracts of papaya and/or pineapple (bromelia).
DIURETICS (URICOSURIC)	ash, barberry, blessed thistle, ephedra, maize, meadowsweet, orthosiphon, parsley, sarsaparilla, solidago, parsley, lemon, birch, rosemary, sassafras, juniper, cajeput, terebenthine
ANTISPASMODIC PLANTS	angelica, basil, belladonna, chamomile, fumitory, hawthorn, henbane, marjoram, melilot, mint, mistletoe, passionflower, pasque flower, rauwolfia, savory, tarragon, valerian, white willow, yarrow, bitter orange, cumin, lavender, melissa, thyme
SEDATIVES	basil, boldo, chamomile, hawthorn, hops, lavender, marjoram, melissa, passionflower, rauwolfia, valerian, white willow, wild oat
TRANQUILIZERS	angelica, basil, hawthorn, hypericum, lavender, lovage, marjoram, melissa, passionflower, pasque flower, rauwolfia, rosemary, thyme, valerian, white willow
MUSCLE RELAXANTS	colchicum, datura, henbane
ANTALGIC PLANTS:	arnica, black cohosh, black currant, blessed thistle, bryonia, chamomile, Canadian fleabane, ivy, colchicum, harpagophytum, meadowsweet, white willow, birch, chamomile, rosemary, terebenthine
SYMPATHOLYTIC PLANTS	angelica, chamomile, coriander, chaste tree, linden, hawthorn, lavender, lovage, marjoram, melilot, passion flower, white willow
SYMPATHOMIMETIC PLANTS	basil, black currant, cinnamon, geranium, ginger, goldenseal, lemon, pine, savory, sage, witch hazel
PARASYMPATHOLYTIC (VAGOLYTIC)	angelica, belladonna, caraway, cumin, fumitory, gentian, hyssop, lovage, tarragon, cypress, thyme
PARASYMPATHOMIMETIC	chamomile, clove, marjoram, oregano, rosemary, vervain
PLANTS FREQUENTLY USED EXTERNALLY (IN OILS, LOTIONS, LINIMENTS, CLAY COMPRESSES, ETC.)	arnica, calendula, ginger, henbane, hypericum, ivy, juniper, meadowsweet, wintergreen, woody nightshade, yarrow, cajeput, chamomile, cypress, lavender, nutmeg, oregano, rosemary, sassafras, terebenthine

OSTEOARTHRITIS

SYMPTOMS: Morning stiffness, stiffness after periods of inertia, loss of joint function, loss of range of motion, local tenderness, swelling of bony areas. Erosion of synovial membranes, cystic formations, soft tissue and periarticular swelling. Typical osteoarthritic terrain is hyperfolliculine, hypopancreatic and hypothyroid as well as high in somatotropin, with depletion of the osseous reserve.

GEMMOTHERAPY FOR OSTEOPOROSIS	
Abies pectinata, Quercus pedunculata, Rosa canina, Pinus montana, Betula pubescens	
TREATMENT BY TERRAIN FOR ACUTE INFLAMMATORY EPISODES:	
BOTANICALS (herb, *oil*)	OLIGOLEMENTS
WOOD YANG	
Allergic-arthritic terrain, sympathotonic, spasmophilic; transient arthralgia, erratic pain with elevated uric acid levels; arthritis of viral hepatitis (aggravated by the wind).	
artichoke, barberry, bilberry, dandelion, goldenrod, harpagophytum, hawthorn, linden, meadowsweet, nettle, orthosiphon, stoneseed, violet, white willow, yarrow, *birch, lemon*	MN, S
FIRE YANG	
Dystonic terrain, "neuroarthritic," transient pain in articulations without lesions, hyperuricemia, joints "hot" and swollen.	
artichoke (uricemia), bilberry, birch, black currant, harpagophytum, hawthorn, linden, meadowsweet, stoneseed, white willow, *birch, lemon, terebenthine*	MN, MN-CO, S
WATER YANG	
Hyperadrenal terrain, joint erosion, hypercalciuremia, hyperuricemia, transient pains, joint crepitus, infectious arthritis.	
barberry, blackberry, black currant, bilberry, dandelion, goldenrod, harpagophytum, maize, meadowsweet, orthosiphon, *birch, sassafras, terebenthine*	MN, MN-CO, S

RHEUMATISM

GEMMOTHERAPY	
Betula pubescens, Ribes nigrum, Quercus pedunculata	
TREATMENT BY TERRAIN	
BOTANICALS (herb, *oil*)	OLIGOLEMENTS
WOOD YANG	
Arthritic terrain, sympathotonic, spasmophilic. Arthritic gout, coxalgia, knee pain (especially lateral side), arthritis of hepatitis.	
artichoke, ash, barberry, black cohosh, dandelion, harpagophytum, meadowsweet, violet, yarrow, *lemon, cypress, terebenthine*	MN, S, MG, P
FIRE YANG	
Neuroarthritic terrain, dystonia, hyperpituitary, hypermetabolic; arthrosis, arthritis with excess heat, arthritis with elimination problems.	
artichoke, birch, borage, black currant, harpagophytum, meadowsweet, orthosiphon, yarrow (arthrosis), *lemon*	MN-CO, I, S, MG, P, K

Rheumatism (continued)

EARTH YANG
Vagal insufficiency, hypopancreatic, diabetic terrain; arthroses, arthritis of diabetes, psoriatic rheumatism, septic arthritis (heat), chondrocalcinosis, vertebral hyperosteosis.

agrimony, ash, black currant, bilberry, birch, burdock, harpagophytum, horsetail (arthritis), lady's mantle, maize, meadowsweet, vervain, woody nightshade, *juniper, lemon, eucalyptus, terebenthine*	Mn-Co, I, S, Zn-Ni-Co, Mg, P, K

EARTH YIN
Vagotonic, hypothyroid terrain, arthrosis with osteoporosis, arthritis with collagenosis, rheumatoid arthritis, paraneoplastic arthritis, arthritis of hemopathies, arthritis of Whipple's disease, arthritis of Crohn's disease.

bladderwrack, black walnut (arthritis, polyarthritis), blessed thistle, germander, horsetail, hypericum, ivy, laminaria, menyanthe, mouse ear, woody nightshade, yellow dock, *cypress, eucalyptus, oregano, sage, terebenthine*	Zn-Cu, Mn-Cu, Cu-Au-Ag, S, Mg, P, K, F

METAL YANG
Hyposthenic terrain, hyperglycemic, arteriosclerotic, arthroses, arthrosis of diabetes, deforming rheumatism, rheumatoid arthritis.

agrimony, ash, borage, ephedra, harpagophytum, meadowsweet, woody nightshade, *juniper, lemon, terebenthine*	Mn-Co, Mn-Cu, Mg, P, Zn-Ni-Co, K

METAL YIN
Hyposthenic terrain, lymphatic congestion, vagotonic, hypothyroid, hyperparathyroid, scapulohumeral periarthritis, arthrosis with decalcification, arthritis of hemopathy, paraneoplasia, collagenoses, ankylosing spondylitis, rheumatoid arthritis, psoriatic arthritis, arthritis of Crohn's disease.

black walnut, bladderwrack, bryonia, blessed thistle, germander, horseradish, horsetail, hypericum, ivy, laminaria, woody nightshade, yellow dock, *cajeput, cypress, eucalyptus, hyssop, niaouli, oregano, pine, sassafras, sage, ti tree, terebenthine, thyme*	Mn-Cu, Cu-Au-Ag S, Mg, P, K, F

WATER YANG
Hyperadrenal, sympathotonic terrain, infections, arthritis, arthroses, arthritis with problems of urinary elimination.

ash, barberry, black currant, black elder, birch, borage, Canadian fleabane, dandelion, goldenrod, harpagophytum, meadowsweet, maize, orthosiphon, rest harrow, *juniper, sassafras, terebenthine*	Mn-Co, I, S, Mg, P, K

WATER YIN
Anergic, hypoadrenal, vagotonic terrain, demineralized terrain, arthrosis with demineralization, osteoporosis, Paget's disease, malignant osteoses, arthritis of Crohn's disease, arthritis of collagenoses, ankylosing spondylitis, rheumatoid arthritis, calcification of fractures.

black currant, black elder, bladderwrack, gentian, heather, honeysuckle, horsetail, laminaria, lovage, madder, nettle, scarlet pimpernel, yarrow, *cajeput, clove, hyssop, lavender, niaouli, pine, rosemary, terebenthine, thuja, thyme*	Cu-Au-Ag, Mn-Cu, S, Mg, P, K, F

SPASMOPHILIA

Spasmophilia is a syndrome characterized by malaise, irritability and mild to severe "latent tetany," a chronic condition of generalized hypertonicity of tendons and muscles. It is considered to be caused by several factors including chronic stress, impaired calcium metabolism due to insufficient vitamin D and chronic magnesium deficiency. The importance of magnesium has been underemphasized in favor of calcium, but lack of magnesium can have a significant impact throughout the body's physiology. Magnesium deficiency has been cited as a critical factor in PMS, painful menses, mitral valve prolapse, formation of embolisms and possibly even morbidity from cancer. Its role in the nervous, musculoskeletal and endocrine systems is essential. It is the hardness factor in bones and teeth and the flexibility factor in muscles. It promotes bile production by the liver and helps to regulate motility of the intestinal tract and has thermoregulatory, antistress, antiallergic and anti-inflammatory properties.

A hyperexcretion of magnesium in the urine can occur as the result of some kidney disorders, diuretics or medication with lithium. Deficiency can occur also as the result of poor intestinal absorption, abuse of laxatives or alcoholism.

Spasmophilia is usually treated by means of magnesium supplementation as well as magnesium utilization factors: vitamins D3, B6, etc. Beta-blockers are also sometimes used for treatment in addition to nutritional or botanical treatment.

FOODS RICH IN MAGNESIUM: Nuts: cashews, almonds, Brazil nuts, peanuts, pecans, hazelnuts, walnuts. Vegetables: broad beans, soy flour, peas, beets. Grains: bran (especially oat bran), whole barley, whole rye, whole wheat, whole oats, corn, brown rice.

TREATMENT BY TERRAIN	
BOTANICALS (herb, *oil*)	OLIGOLEMENTS
WOOD YANG	
Nervous, hyperthyroid, hypoparathyroid; reacts favorably to calcium-magnesium balancing.	
black cohosh, black horehound, chaste tree, horsetail, nettle, passionflower, pasque flower, valerian, white willow	MN-CO, I, MG, P, CO
WOOD YIN	
Nervous, hyperkinetic, twitches, tics, muscle cramps.	
chaste tree, hellebore, horsetail, nettle, passionflower, valerian, white willow, *lemon, rosemary, everlasting*	MN-CO, I, MG, P, CO
METAL YIN	
Hyposthenic, malnourished, acrocyanosis, sequelae of rickets, hypocalcemia due to malabsorption of vitamin D; calcium supplementation helpful to this terrain.	
elecampane, eleutherococcus, horseradish, horsetail, marine algae, nettle, wild oat, *everlasting*	MN-CU, MG, I, P
WATER YIN	
Anergic, hypoadrenal terrain, cold limbs, low back pain; reacts well to phosphorus supplementation and phosphoric acid, muscular hyperexcitability resulting in muscular weakness, cramps and tetany.	
eleutherococcus, ginger, horsetail, lovage, marine algae, nettle, pine, *geranium, lemon, rosemary, savory, thyme*	CU-AU-AG, P, MG

Genitourinary disorders

Selected diuretic plants	Herb (oil)
Volumetric	garlic, goat rue, gingko, hypericum, raspberry, rest harrow, violet, *lavender, terebenthine, thuja*
Volumetric, Azoturic (removes nitrogen & protein)	burdock, mistletoe, olive, plantain, bilberry, dandelion; (Gemmae: Vaccinium, Vitis idaea)
Volumetric, Salidiuretic (removes sodium and chloride)	bearberry, borage, briar hip, broom, celery, chickweed, heather, honeysuckle, horsetail, lovage, melilot, nettle, scarlet pimpernel, shepherd's purse, *geranium*
Volumetric, Salidiuretic, Azoturic (removes sodium, chloride and nitrogen)	bilberry, dandelion, elecampane, fennel, madder (also phosphaturic), mouse ear, orthosiphon, pellitory-of-the-wall, sea holly, *onion, fennel*
Volumetric, Uricosuric (clears out uric acid)	ash, blessed thistle, Canadian fleabane, germander, nettle, sand spurry, *juniper, rosemary, sassafras*
Volumetric, Azoturic & Uricosuric (clears out uric acid and nitrogen)	artichoke, black currant, goldenrod, *lemon*
Volumetric, Uricosuric, Salidiuretic	barberry
Volumetric, Azoturic, Salidiuretic, Phosphaturic	black elder
Volumetric, Salidiuretic, Azoturic, Uricosuric	maize, meadowsweet, orthosiphon, parsley, *birch*
Volumetric, Antilithiatic (clears stones from the urinary tract)	celery, heather, madder, pellitory-of-the-wall, *birch, celery*
Volumetric, Antispasmodic	garlic, fennel, khella, lovage, madder, *angelica, calamus, garlic, fennel, lavender, parsley*
Antiedematous and pelvic decongestant plants	goldenseal, horse chestnut, shepherd's purse, witch hazel, yarrow, *cypress, lavender, juniper* (ascites) (Gemma: Juniperus communis)
Hemostatics	bilberry, goldenseal, horsetail, shepherd's purse, witch hazel, *cypress*
Urinary tract antispasmodics	black horehound, belladonna
Antalgics for urinary tract	bearberry, heather, maize, rest harrow, *thuja*

RENAL INSUFFICIENCY
(SEROUS EFFUSION, HYDROPS)

GEMMOTHERAPY
Ribes nigrum; Junperus commuis (Wood yin, Water yang, Water yin)

TREATMENT BY TERRAIN	
BOTANICALS (herb, *oil*)	OLIGOLEMENTS
WOOD YIN	
Hepatic insufficiency terrain, sympathetic insufficiency, hepatorenal insufficiency, ascites from cirrhosis or fatty liver, edema, anasarca, uremia.	
black currant, lovage, lespedeza, scarlet pimpernel; CIRRHOSIS: celery, artichoke, germander, maize, milk thistle, mouse ear, *juniper, rosemary*	Cu-Au-Ag, Li, K, Mg
FIRE YIN	
Sympathetic insufficiency terrain, asystole, cardiorenal insufficiency with edema, anasarca, pericardial contact.	
cherry laurel, digitalis, elecampane, false hellebore, lily-of-the-valley, mouse ear, white lily, *birch*	Cu-Au-Ag, Li, K, Mg
EARTH YIN	
Nephrotic syndrome, amylosis, SLE, periarteritis nodosa, retarded growth.	
Canadian fleabane, maize, plantain, scarlet pimpernel, *geranium*	Zn-Cu, Cu, K, Li, Mg, Mg-Cu, Cu-Au-Ag
WATER YANG	
Hyperadrenal, hyperglycemic terrain, interstitial nephropathy of gout, nephropathy of diabetes.	
agrimony, Canadian fleabane, dandelion, maize, olive, meadowsweet, *birch, geranium*	Mn-Co, Zn-Ni-Co, Li, K, Mg
WATER YIN	
Adrenal insufficiency, constitutional kidney weakness, renal insufficiency due to chronic glomerulonephritis, chronic tubulonephritis, interstitial nephritis, nephrotic syndromes, renal amylosis, SLE.	
bearberry, Canadian fleabane, celery, cherry laurel, chickweed, elecampane, goldenrod, horsetail, madder, lily-of-the-valley, lovage, mouse ear, nettle, raspberry, sarsaparilla, scarlet pimpernel, sea holly, yarrow (nephrotic amylosis), *birch, juniper, geranium, clove*	Cu-Au-Ag Cu, Li, K, Mg, Zn-Cu

ORTHOSTATIC ALBUMINARIA

TREATMENT BY TERRAIN	
BOTANICALS (herb, *oil*)	OLIGOLEMENTS
WATER YIN	
Canadian fleabane, celery, goldenrod, heather, horsetail, lovage, maize, sea holly, *birch*	Cu, Cu-Au-Ag, Mn-Cu

Renal lithiasis

Treatment by terrain	
Botanicals (herb, *oil*)	Oligolements
Wood yang	
Sympathotonic terrain, hyperthyroid, arthritic, uric lithiasis, hyperuricemia, excessive fat in diet..	
artichoke, barberry, boldo, dandelion, fumitory, goldenrod, grapevine, hawthorn, hepatica, khella, linden, meadowsweet, nettle, orthosiphon, stoneseed, pellitory-of-the-wall, yarrow, *lemon*	Mn, S, Mg, K, Li
Fire yang	
Dystonic, neuroarthritic terrain, metabolic disorder, gout, lithiasis from hyperuricemia, hypercholesterolemia.	
artichoke, ash, barberry, khella, linden, meadowsweet, orthosiphon, stoneseed, yarrow, *birch*	Mn-Co, S, Mg
Earth yang	
Vagal insufficiency, hypopancreatic, gout, diabetes, uric lithiasis from chronic hyperuricemia, hypercholesterolemia.	
ash, black currant, burdock, fumitory, linden, maize, meadowsweet, olive, orthosiphon, stoneseed, *lemon, juniper*	Zn-Ni-Co, Mn-Co, Mg, K, Li
Earth yin	
Hypothyroid terrain, hypophysogonadic dysadaptation, phosphatic calculi, mixed or oxalic and calcic.	
fennel, ivy, maize, *geranium, hyssop*	Zn-Cu, Mg, K, Li
Metal yang	
Vagal insufficiency, hyperglycemic, hypertensive, oxalic calculi.	
ash, black currant, borage, lungwort, olive, orthosiphon, *birch, lemon, juniper, sassafras*	Mn-Cu, Mn-Co, Mg, K, Li
Metal yin	
Hyposthenic, hypothyroid, hyperparathyroid terrain, phosphatic, oxalic or calcic calculi, problems with vitamin D metabolism, sarcoidosis, myeloma.	
fennel, ivy, *geranium, hyssop*	Mn-Cu, Mg, K, Li
Water yang	
Hyperadrenal, sympathotonic terrain, trouble with urinary elimination, obesity, uric calculi, hyperuricemia, more or less uremic.	
ash, barberry, bearberry, black currant, black elder, broom, dandelion, horsetail, khella, linden, maize, meadowsweet, orthosiphon, pellitory-of-the-wall, rest harrow, sand spurry, shepherd's purse, yarrow, *birch, juniper, sassafras, terebenthine*	Mn-Co, Mg, K, Li
Water yin	
Anergic, hypoadrenal, renal deficient terrain, cold body, phosphomagnesic or phosphatic calculi, phosphaturia due to insufficiency of silica, nephrocalcinosis.	
black elder, briarhip, celery, cherry laurel, heather, fennel, geranium, goldenrod, horsetail, hyssop, maize, yarrow, *geranium, hyssop*	Cu-Au-Ag, Mg, K, Li

URINARY TRACT INFECTIONS

GEMMOTHERAPY
Ribes nigrum, Vaccinum vitis idaea, Juglans regia

TREATMENT BY TERRAIN	
BOTANICALS (herb, *oil*)	OLIGOLEMENTS
WOOD YANG	
Sympathotonic, hyperthyroid terrain, especially cystitis (colibacillus).	
artichoke, boldo, broom, meadowsweet, orthosiphon, pellitory-of-the-wall, tarragon, *lemon, terebenthine*	Cu
FIRE YANG	
Dystonic terrain, high fever, burning urination, cystitis (colibacillus).	
barberry, horehound, orthosiphon, white lily, *lavender, marjoram*	Cu
FIRE YIN	
Hypopituitary, sympathetic insufficient terrain, depression, colibacillus infection, gram-negative bacteria, viral infections, klebsiella.	
honeysuckle (staphylococcus, *E. coli*), *lavender, sage*	Cu, Cu-Au-Ag
EARTH YANG	
Vagal insufficiency, obese or plethoric, diabetic terrain, colibacillus, candida, gram-positive bacteria.	
agrimony, bilberry, blackberry, borage, marshmallow, *eucalyptus, juniper, melissa, niaouli, terebenthine*	Cu
EARTH YIN	
Hypophysogonadic dysadaptation, cystitis, nephritis (colibacillus, gram-negative bacteria, virus).	
bistort, fennel, hypericum, ivy, plantain, *cinnamon, coriander, eucalyptus, geranium, lavender, pine, sage, savory, thyme*	Cu
METAL YANG	
Hyposthenic terrain, more or less hyperglycemic, cystitis (colibacillus, gram-negative bacteria), heat symptoms, fever at 103-104 degrees, pus in the urine.	
agrimony, borage, horehound, marshmallow (urethritis), white lily, *eucalyptus, niaouli, pine, serpolet, terebenthine*	Cu, Mn-Cu
METAL YIN	
Hyposthenic terrain, lymphatic swelling, constipation, chronic colitis, especially chronic colibacillosis.	
bistort, coltsfoot, fennel, ginger, hypericum (cystitis), ivy, plantain (pyelonephritis), *coriander, eucalyptus, hypericum, lavender, myrtle, niaouli* (urethritis), *pine, sage, sassafras* (urethritis), *savory, serpolet, thyme*	Cu, Mn-Cu
WATER YANG	
Hyperadrenal terrain, sympathotonic, difficulty with elimination of urine, cystitis, urethritis, pyelitis with major inflammatory reactions and severe pain, pyuria, retention, thirst, hyperthermia, colibacillus, gram-positive bacteria.	
barberry, bearberry (pyelonephritis, cystitis, metritis), black currant, black elder (pyelonephritis), bilberry, borage (pyelonephritis), broom, chickweed, goldenrod, heather (pyelonephritis, cystitis), horehound, melilot (urethritis), orthosiphon, pellitory-of-the-wall, white lily, *eucalyptus, juniper, lavender* (cystitis), *myrtle, sandalwood, sassafras, terebenthine* (pyelonephritis), *thuja*	Cu

Urinary tract infections (continued)

Water yin
Anergic, hypoadrenal terrain, diathesis most vulnerable to chronic recidivist infections, low back pain, cold body especially cold feet, hypotension, albuminuria low or elevated, potassium low, cystitis, urethritis, pyelonephritis acute or chronic (especially *E. coli*, klebsiella, proteus), also gram-negative bacteria.

Botanicals	Oligolements
bearberry, black currant, Canadian fleabane, cherry laurel, fennel, ginger, goldenrod, honeysuckle; CYSTITIS: horsetail, lovage; PYELONEPHRITIS: elecampane, heather, lovage, nettle, plantain, raspberry, *cajeput* (gram-positive), *eucalyptus, juniper, geranium, lavender, myrtle* (cystitis), *niaouli, pine, sage, sandalwood, sassafras* (urethritis), *savory, terebenthine* (pyelonephritis, urethritis), *thuja, thyme, serpolet, hypericum*	Cu-Au-Ag, Cu

Edema (lower leg edema)

Treatment by terrain	
Botanicals (herb, *oil*)	Oligolements
Wood yang	
Sympathotonic, hyperthyroid terrain, edema connected with venous insufficiency, pelvic congestion.	
artichoke, broom, dandelion, horse chestnut, meadowsweet, orthosiphon, stoneseed	Mn, S, Mg, K, Li
Fire yang	
Dystonic, neuroarthritic terrain, problems with urine elimination, high cholesterol, uric acid, overweight.	
black currant, horse chestnut, meadowsweet, orthosiphon, stoneseed, *birch, lemon*	Mn-Co, S, Mg, K, Li
Fire yin	
Sympathetic insufficiency, asystole, edema from cardiac insufficiency with renal retention.	
elecampane, honeysuckle	Cu-Au-Ag, Mg, K, Li
Earth yang	
Vagal insufficiency, pancreatic insufficiency, diabetes, obese or plethoric condition, edema and cellulite of the waist and buttocks.	
black currant, horse chestnut, maize, meadowsweet, orthosiphon, stoneseed, *lemon*	Zn-Ni-Co, Mn-Co, S, Mg, Li CONTRAINDICATED: K
Water yang	
Hyperadrenal, sympathotonic terrain, difficult urination.	
black currant, cherry laurel, goldenrod, horsetail, lespedeza, maize, meadowsweet, orthosiphon, pellitory-of-the-wall, rest harrow, sarsaparilla	Mn-Co, S, Mg, K, Li
Water yin	
Anergic, hypoadrenal terrain, renal deficiency constitution, low back pain, cold feet, edema of eyelids, condition aggravated by cold, fatigue, menses, prolonged standing.	
celery, cherry laurel, elecampane, goldenrod, heather, horsetail, lovage, maize, mouse ear, sea holly, *birch, juniper, clove*	Cu-Au-Ag, Mg, K, Li

OLIGURIA
(ANURIA, RETENTION OF URINE, HYPERAZOTEMIA)

TREATMENT BY TERRAIN	
BOTANICALS (herb, *oil*)	**OLIGOLEMENTS**
WOOD YANG	
Hepatic, sympathotonic, hyperthyroid terrain, arthritic terrain, oliguria from pelvic or venous congestion, hepatobiliary insufficiency, inflammations from heat or wind-heat.	
broom, dandelion orthosiphon, stoneseed, violet; UREMIA: artichoke, linden, meadowsweet, mistletoe, mouse ear	Mn, S, Mg, K, Li
WOOD YIN	
Oliguria from portal congestion.	
celery, *sage*	Mn, S, Mg, K, Li
FIRE YANG	
Neuroarthritic, dystonic terrain, oliguria due to blood dyscrasias, metabolic encumbrance or deterioration of the mucous membranes.	
broom, violet; UREMIA: ash, borage, broom, linden, meadowsweet, *birch*	Mn-Co, S, Mg, K, Li
FIRE YIN	
Sympathetic insufficiency, hypotension, asystole, oliguria, anuria from cardiac insufficiency, cutaneous eruptions.	
digitalis, elecampane, honeysuckle, *sage*	Co-Au-Ag, Mg, K, Li
EARTH YANG	
Vagal insufficiency, pancreatic insufficiency, diabetes, cellulite, oliguria of obesity, gout or cellulitis.	
black currant, horse chestnut, maize, meadowsweet, orthosiphon, stoneseed, *lemon*	Zn-Ni-Co, Mn-Co, S, Mg, Li CONTRAINDICATED: K
EARTH YIN	
Hypothyroid, moist, cold, obese, water retention, oliguria of cellulitis, oliguria of collagenoses, nephrotic syndromes.	
barberry, calendula, ivy, *sage*	Zn-Cu, Mg, Li
METAL YANG	
ash (uremia), borage, linden (uremia)	Mn-Cu, S, Mg, K, Li
METAL YIN	
Hyposthenic, hypothyroid terrain, hyperparathyroid, oliguria of pleurisy, nephrocalcinosis.	
bryonia, ivy, *sage*	Mn-Cu, Mg, K, Li
WATER YANG	
Hyperadrenal, sympathotonic terrain; more or less hyperglycemic; oliguria with problems of urine elimination due to age or weakness. Nephroses from gout, diabetes, Schönlein-Henoch purpura (rheumatic purpura), congestion of the bladder, lithiases.	
bearberry, bilberry, black elder, briarhip, goldenrod, horsetail, melilot, orthosiphon, pellitory-of-the-wall, sarsaparilla, shepherd's purse; UREMIA: ash, borage, dandelion, meadowsweet; *juniper*	Mn-Co, Zn-Ni-Co, Mg, K, Li
WATER YIN	
Anergic hypoadrenal terrain, renal deficient constitution, terrain most predisposed to oliguria due to renal functional insufficiency, low back pain, albuminuria, edema of eyelids, ankles; oliguria due to chronic renal insufficiency from repeated infections.	
bearberry, black currant, black elder, celery, cherry laurel, elecampane, fennel, goldenrod, horsetail, honeysuckle, lespedeza, lovage, raspberry, yarrow; UREMIA: heather, mouse ear, sarsaparilla, sea holly; *birch, clove, lavender, sage*	Cu-Au-Ag, Mg, K, Li

Enuresis (pediatric urinary incontinence)

Treatment by Terrain	
Botanicals (herb, *oil*)	Oligolements
Wood yin	
Least frequent type; sympathetic insufficiency, hepatic terrain.	
nettle, *sage*	Mn, Al, Li
Earth yang	
Boisterous, happy child in good health; chubby, red-cheeked, fond of sweets.	
agrimony, black horehound, *cypress, juniper*	Zn-Ni-Co, F
Earth yin	
Hypophysogonadic dysadaptation; most frequent type (inherited characteristic), parasitosis can be a factor.	
belladonna, bistort, bladderwrack, hops, hypericum, laminaria, oak, plantain, scarlet pimpernel, *cypress, sage*	Mn-Cu, F
Water yin	
Anergic, hypoadrenal terrain, enuresis in hypersensitive children (look out for infections or structural anomalies); incontinence of cystitis, childbirth and prolapse, neurogenic bladder sensitivity, postconcussion or cerebral damage-related enuresis.	
bearberry, belladonna, bistort, hypericum, oak, plantain, yarrow, *sage, thuja*	Cu-Au-Ag, Al, Li, F

Prostatitis

Treatment by Terrain	
Botanicals (herb, *oil*)	Oligolements
Wood yang	
Acute prostatitis, congestion more than infection, dysuria, pollakiuria.	
broom, horse chestnut, white lily	Mn, Zn
Fire yang	
Acute prostatitis.	
white lily, *thuja, cajeput, lavender*	Cu
Earth yang	
Acute and chronic prostatitis.	
horse chestnut, *thuja, cajeput*	Zn-Ni-Co, Zn, Cu
Earth yin	
Chronic, most frequent terrain.	
bistort, horse chestnut, *thuja, cajeput*	Zn-Ni-Co, Zn, Mg
Water yang	
Mostly acute cases, especially colibacillosis.	
bearberry, broom, white lily, *thuja, cajeput, lavender*	Cu
Water yin	
Chronic or subacute prostatitis.	
bearberry, bistort, *clove, pine, thuja, lavender,* *hypericum, serpolet*	Cu, Cu-Au-Ag

NERVOUS SYSTEM DISORDERS

HEADACHES

GEMMOTHERAPY	
Rosa canina, Tilia tomentosa	
TREATMENT BY TERRAIN	
BOTANICALS (herb, *oil*)	OLIGOLEMENTS
WOOD YANG	
Frontal orbital headaches, or headaches from dystonia, hypertension, hyperthyroid terrain, digestive migraines; subject irritated by the wind; hemicranial or temporal pain, cluster headaches.	
black cohosh, chaste tree, celandine, combretum, lady's mantle, lovage, mistletoe, pasque flower, stoneseed, *marjoram* (cluster), *melissa, bitter orange, terebenthine, neroli*	CO, MN, I, S, LI, MG
WOOD YIN	
Headache on waking up every morning, hepatic and sympathetic insufficiency, frontal or orbital headache with visual disturbance, cluster headaches.	
angelica, artichoke, combretum, elecampane, germander, lovage, milk thistle, *lavender (+++), mint* (external or internal), *rosemary*	CU-AU-AG, MN, CU, S
FIRE YANG	
Sympathotonic, hyperpituitary terrain, plethoric, vagal insufficiency, hyperadrenal, emotional subjects.	
chaste tree, mistletoe, *birch, bitter orange, marjoram* (cluster), *melissa*	MN-CO, S, MG, LI, CO
FIRE YIN	
Anergic, sympathetic insufficiency, heavy head, vertigo, cluster headaches.	
angelica, *lavender*	CU-AU-AG, CO
EARTH YANG	
Hypertensive headache in plethoric, sanguine subject, postprandial "digestive" headache, sensation of head being clamped in a vise.	
agrimony, black cohosh, lady's mantle, linden, vervain (migraine), *melissa*	ZN-NI-CO, MN-CO, CO
EARTH YIN	
Headache aggravated by cold or humidity, malnourished terrain, malabsorption, hypoglycemia, head feels like it is stuffed with cotton, cluster headaches.	
centaury (+++), colchicum, germander, menyanthe (postprandial), vervain	ZN-CU
METAL YANG	
Headache in phlegmatic type, sinus headaches, vertex headaches, cluster headaches, arteriosclerosis.	
agrimony (hypertensive), *eucalyptus, hyssop*	MN-CO
METAL YANG	
Vertex headaches aggravated by cold and humidity, coldness of cranium (like a hat).	
centaury, germander, *eucalyptus, hyssop, mint, rosemary*	MN-CU

Headaches (continued)

Water yang
Headaches from hypertension or uremia; very painful neck (nuchal area) and head, migraine.

shepherd's purse, sarsaparilla, *birch*	Mn-Co, Co

Water yin
Anergic, sympathetic and adrenal insufficiency, usually nuchal pain, heavy head.

sea holly, *clove, lavender, rosemary*	Cu-Au-Ag, Mg, Li, Co

Anxiety
(anguish, hysteria, phobias, aggressiveness, agitation, neurotonia, excitation, neurovegetative dystonia)

Gemmotherapy
Tilia tomentosa

Treatment by Terrain	
Botanicals (herb, *oil*)	Oligolements

Wood yang	
Hyperthyroid, sympathotonic terrain, irritability, anxiety, anguish, phobias, hysteria, spasmophilia.	
black horehound (tachycardia), hawthorn, hellebore, lady's mantle, linden (hysteria), lily-of-the-valley, mistletoe (hysteria), pasque flower, white lily, white valerian (hysteria), white willow, *bitter orange, lavender, rosemary*	Mn, I, S, Mg, P, Li

Fire yang	
Hyperpituitary, sympathotonic terrain, major dystonia, excitable, anxious, hyperemotional, anguish, hysteria, agitation, excessive idealism.	
black horehound (tachycardia), hawthorn, linden, lily-of-the-valley, lotus, melilot, mistletoe, mullein (tachycardia, arrhythmia), passionflower (hysteria), rauwolfia, valerian (hysteria), white lily, white willow, *bergamot, bitter orange, clary sage, lavender, marjoram, melissa, neroli, rose, spike lavender, ylang ylang*	Mn-Co, I, Li

Earth yang	
Vagal insufficiency, hypopancreatic, hypergonadic, giddiness, excessive gaiety, irresponsibility, inconsideration, mania, exhibitionism.	
fumitory, hellebore, lady's mantle, linden, vervain, *melissa*	Zn-Ni-Co, Mn-Co, Fe, Li

Metal yang	
Vagal insufficiency, plethoric terrain, hypomania, mania, inconsideration, perversion	
marshmallow, opium, red poppy	Mn-Cu, Mn-Co, Li

Water yang	
Sympathotonic, hyperadrenal terrain, cerebrospinal hypertonia, aggressiveness, hostility, excessive ambition or jealousy, abusive authority, paranoia.	
black elder, hellebore, passionflower, rauwolfia, shepherd's purse, valerian, white lily, white willow	Mn-Co, I, Li

DEPRESSION

(NEURASTHENIA, PSYCHASTHENIA, OBSESSIONAL NEUROSIS, MELANCHOLIA)

TREATMENT BY TERRAIN	
BOTANICALS (herb, *oil*)	OLIGOLEMENTS
WOOD YIN	
Sympathetic insufficiency, hypothyroid terrain, hypoadrenal, hepatic insufficiency, inhibition, anguish, phobia, pallor, weakness.	
angelica, celery, hellebore, milk thistle, mugwort, *lavender, mint, rosemary*	CU-AU-AG, MN, CU, S, MG, P, LI
FIRE YIN	
Hypopituitary, hypometabolic, sympathetic insufficiency terrain, lack of enthusiasm or motivation, inhibition, anguish, melancholia.	
angelica, briarhip, milk thistle (melancholia), *lavender* (melancholia), *rosemary, rose*	CU-AU-AG, MG, P, LI
EARTH YIN	
Vagotonic terrain, hypophysogonadic dysadaptation, obesity, cold, moist, distracted, lack of intelligence, excessive or obsessive thinking resulting in mental fatigue, obsessions, manic-depressive psychosis, anorexia.	
angelica, bladderwrack, blessed thistle (obsessions), eleuterococcus, foenugreek, gentian, hellebore, hypericum, laminaria, *anise* (anorexia), *cinnamon* (obsessions), *coriander* (anorexia), *caraway, lavender, mint, savory*	ZN-CU, LI
METAL YIN	
Hyposthenic, vagotonic, lymphatic terrain, sadness, melancholy, distraction, abstraction of reality, anorexia, neurasthenia, psychasthenia, schizophrenia, obsessional neurosis.	
angelica, bladderwrack, blessed thistle, datura, eleuterococcus, foenugreek, gentian, henbane, hypericum, laminaria, *cinnamon* (obsession, melancholia), *coriander* (anorexia, melancholia), *lavender* (melancholia), *mint, oregano, rosemary, sassafras, thyme*	MN-CU, LI
WATER YIN	
Vagotonic, hypoadrenal terrain, cerebrospinal hypotonia; subject cold, timid, always tired, inhibited; phobia, anguish, depression, fear of persecution, melancholia, psychosis.	
angelica, black currant, briarhip (asthenia, anguish), celery (melancholia), datura, eleuterococcus, fennel, henbane, madder, sea holly, scarlet pimpernel, *clove, hyssop, lavender* (melancholia), *rose, rosemary, sandalwood, sage, sassafras, savory*	CU-AU-AG, LI

INSOMNIA

GEMMOTHERAPY
Tilia tomentosa

TREATMENT BY TERRAIN	
BOTANICALS (herb, *oil*)	OLIGOLEMENTS
WOOD YANG	
Hyperthyroid, sympathotonic terrain, aggressive, anxious, insomnia from mental restlessness (projects, preoccupations).	
black horehound, boldo, chaste tree, fumitory, hawthorn, lady's mantle, linden, melilot, passionflower, pasque flower, white lily, white willow, valerian, *bitter orange, lavender, marjoram, melissa, neroli, spike lavender*	Mn, S, Al
WOOD YIN	
Sympathetic insufficiency, hyperthyroid, adrenal insufficient terrain, restless sleep, waking up a lot (phobias, anguish).	
celery, hops, mugwort, *ravensare*	Mn, S, Cu-Au-Ag, Al
FIRE YANG	
Sympathotonic, dystonic terrain, hyperpituitary, excitation, tachycardia on waking up during the night, waking up all night, tiring and sleeping again.	
chaste tree, hawthorn, linden, lotus (tachycardia), melilot, passionflower, valerian, white lily, white willow, *bergamot, bitter orange, lavender, melissa, neroli, ravensare, spike lavender*	Mn-Co, I, S, Al
EARTH YANG	
Vagal insufficiency, hypopancreatic terrain, goes to bed late, sleeps late, frequent waking up, gets up for a snack occasionally and goes back to sleep. Total insomnia (mania).	
fumitory, lady's mantle, linden, vervain, *melissa*	Zn-Ni-Co, Mn-Co, Al, Li
EARTH YIN	
Vagotonia, sleeps normally, wakes up late; insomnia all night or from dawn or from 3 to 5 or 6 AM and sleeps till 10 AM or midday; obsession.	
blessed thistle, chamomile, hops, hypericum, *bergamot, ravensare, thyme*	Zn-Cu, Mn-Cu, Al
METAL YANG	
Vagal insufficiency, hyposthenic, goes to bed early, wakes up early, insomnia from dawn (3 AM), preoccupations, projects.	
marshmallow, red poppy, *lavender*	Mn-Cu, Al
METAL YIN	
Vagotonic, hyposthenic terrain, goes to bed early, wakes up early. Insomnia from dawn (3 AM), obsessions, depression.	
blessed thistle, marine algae, wild oat (anorexia), *thyme*	Mn-Cu, Al, Li
WATER YANG	
Sympathotonic, hyperadrenal terrain, goes to bed late, wakes up early, sleeps 4-6 hours a night.	
melilot, passionflower, shepherd's purse, white willow, white lily, valerian, *lavender*	Mn-Cu, Al, Li
WATER YIN	
Vagotonic, hypoadrenal terrain. Goes to bed early, wakes up early. Insomnia of waking up numerous times at night or waking up too early.	
celery, fennel, sea holly, *lavender, thyme*	Cu-Au-Ag, Al

METABOLIC DISORDERS

DIABETES MELLITUS

PLANTS WITH HYPOGLYCEMIANT ACTION
BOTANICALS (herb, *oil*)
agrimony, blackberry, black walnut, bilberry (also good for vascular protection and retinitis), briarhip, burdock, eleutherococcus, eucalyptus, foenugreek, garlic, goat rue, maize, olive, onion, yellow dock, *juniper, geranium, sage*

TREATMENT BY TERRAIN	
BOTANICALS (herb, *oil*)	OLIGOLEMENTS
WOOD YANG	
Diabetes with hepatic factors dominant; high fat, high sugar diet.	
artichoke, lady's mantle, nettle, *lemon*	MN-CO, ZN-NI-CO
EARTH YANG	
Typical diabetic terrain, inherited diabetic tendency, big baby at birth, polyphagia, polyuria, hypertensive, often hiatal hernia, coronaropathy, insufficient carotid circulation, heat repletion of the Spleen	
agrimony, bilberry, blackberry, black mulberry, burdock, goat rue, horsetail, lady's mantle, maize, olive, *eucalyptus, juniper, lemon*	ZN-NI-CO, MN-CO, NI-CO
EARTH YIN	
Diabetes from strain of upper digestive tract, medium cases to insulin-dependent; subjects with poor growth and development, wasting diabetes, cachexia, Zollinger-Ellison syndrome.	
bilberry, bistort, black walnut, cinchona (emaciation), foenugreek, horsetail, *geranium*	ZN-NI-CO, CU-AU-AG
METAL YANG	
Hyposthenic constitution; major signs: thirst, frequent consumption of liquids; hypertension, coronaropathy, colitis, especially left side, slightly overweight, or else long and lean.	
agrimony, olive, periwinkle, *eucalyptus*	ZN-NI-CO, MN-CO MN-CU
METAL YIN	
Hyposthenic terrain, medium case to insulin-dependent, wasting diabetes (weight loss at the outset), scoliotic, demineralized subject.	
bistort, black walnut, foenugreek, horsetail, wild oat (emaciation)	ZN-NI-CO, CU-AU-AG, MN-CU, NI-CO
WATER YANG	
Diabetes from adrenal overload, major sign: polyuria. Excitability, tachycardia	
maize, bilberry, *juniper*	MN-CO, ZN-NI-CO, CO
WATER YIN	
Diabetes from adrenal insufficiency, medium cases evolving to insulin dependency,; wasting diabetes from stress (loss, accidents), demineralization, Kidney qi vacuity low back pain, impotence, diminished Achilles tendon reflex, neuropathy or hypersensitivity in legs near Kidney and Bladder channels.	
black walnut, cinchona (emaciation), eleutherococcus, foenugreek, horsetail, léspedeza, *geranium*	CU-AU-AG, NI-CO

Hypercholesterolemia

GEMMOTHERAPY	
Olea europaea	
TREATMENT BY TERRAIN	
BOTANICALS (herb, *oil*)	OLIGOLEMENTS
WOOD YANG	
Arthritic terrain, sympathotonic, hepatic insufficiency, hypercholesterolemia with biliary dyskinesia, migraines.	
artichoke, barberry, celandine, dandelion, fumitory, grapevine, linden, nettle, orthosiphon, plantain, *everlasting, lemon, rosemary*	Mn, S, Mn-Co, Mg
WOOD YIN	
Sympathetic insufficiency, hypo- or hyperthyroid with adrenal insufficiency, cold body, low cholesterol following liver pathology.	
artichoke, milk thistle, plantain, *rosemary, everlasting*	Mn, S, Mg, P
FIRE YANG	
Neuroarthritic terrain, hypercholesterolemia, more or less associated with uremia and hyperuricemia.	
artichoke, ash, birch, grapevine, linden, orthosiphon	Mn-Co, S, Mg
EARTH YANG	
Plethoric terrain, sanguine, vagal insufficiency, hypopancreatic; hypercholesterolemia associated with hyperglycemia and diabetes.	
ash, fumitory, linden, maize, *birch, lemon*	Zn-Ni-Co, Mn-Co, S, Mg
METAL YANG	
Hyposthenic terrain, vagal insufficiency, cutaneous problems and problems of pulmonary mucous membranes, hyperglycemic terrain.	
ash, linden, *lemon*	Mn-Co, S, Mg, Mn-Cu
WATER YANG	
Hyperadrenal, sympathotonic terrain, hypercholesterolemia more or less associated with hyperuricemia.	
ash, barberry, dandelion, goldenrod, linden, maize, orthosiphon, *birch*	Mn-Co, S, Mg
WATER YIN	
High cholesterol associated with hyperuricemia, hyperadrenal, sympathotonic.	
ash, barberry, dandelion, goldenrod, linden, lespedeza, maize, orthosiphon, *birch*	Mn-Co, S, Mg

Basedow's Disease
(Grave's Disease, Hyperthyroidism)

TREATMENT BY TERRAIN	
BOTANICALS (herb, *oil*)	OLIGOLEMENTS
WOOD YANG OR FIRE YANG	
Choleric, irritable, loss of weight, twitches, trembling, anguish, thermophobia, exophthalmos, profuse sweating.	
brassica, hellebore, lily-of-the-valley, lycopus, passionflower, *cumin*	Mn, Mn-Co, I, S, Cu, Li

HYPOTHYROIDISM (MYXEDEMA)

TREATMENT BY TERRAIN	
BOTANICALS (herb, *oil*)	OLIGOLEMENTS
EARTH YIN	
Obesity or flabbiness on thin frame, tongue flabby, mentally sluggish, global goiter, myxedema	
elecampane, laminaria, bladderwrack, *garlic*	ZN-CU, AL
METAL YIN	
Hypothyroidism with fixed nodules, malnourished subject, hyperparathyroid, problems with calcium metabolism, osseous demineralization, renal calcification.	
bladderwrack, elecampane, laminaria, wild oat, *garlic*	MN-CU, AL

HYPERADRENALISM
(HYPERCORTICOSURRENALISM, CUSHING'S SYNDROME, HYPERMEDULLOSURRENALISM)

TREATMENT BY TERRAIN	
BOTANICALS (herb, *oil*)	OLIGOLEMENTS
WATER YANG	
Hyperadrenalism from Kidney yang repletion, functional hypercortisolism.	
borage, mouse ear, shepherd's purse, vervain	MN-CO, CO, I

HYPOADRENALISM
(HYPOCORTICOSURRENALISM, HYPOMEDULLOSURRENALISM)

GEMMOTHERAPY	
Quercus pedunculosa, Ribes nigrum	
TREATMENT BY TERRAIN	
BOTANICALS (herb, *oil*)	OLIGOLEMENTS
EARTH YIN	
Adrenal insufficiency with insufficient aldosterone and cortisol secretion.	
fenugreek, licorice, *cinnamon, clove sage, savory*	ZN-CU, CU-AU-AG
WATER YIN	
Anergy, cold body, hypotension, impotence, frigidity, Kidney yang vacuity.	
black currant, eleutherococcus, ginger, mouse ear, oak, *basil, geranium, lemon, pine, rosemary, savory, thyme*	CU-AU-AG

RETARDED DEVELOPMENT
(RETARDED GROWTH, RETARDED PUBERTY, SLOW SEXUAL DEVELOPMENT, PSYCHOMOTOR SLUGGISHNESS, DISRUPTION OF FSH AND LH SECRETION CYCLES)

TREATMENT BY TERRAIN	
BOTANICALS (herb, *oil*)	OLIGOLEMENTS
EARTH YIN	
Short, thin, small body, child-like, underdeveloped, exhaustion following strain, post-vaccination, long convalescence, eruptive fever.	
black walnut, bladderwrack, calendula, elecampane, eleutherococcus, gentian, laminaria, licorice, mugwort, plantain, Canadian fleabane, *lavender, sage*	ZN-CU, AL, LI, MG

Osteoporosis
(osseous demineralization, decalcification)

Gemmotherapy
Abies pectinata, Rosa canina, Pinus montana, Betula pubescens, Quercus pedunculata

Treatment by Terrain	
Botanicals (herb, *oil*)	Oligolements
Earth yin	
Retarded development, hypothyroid, hyperparathyroid, osteoporosis from rheumatic infections arising from coldness and dampness, osteosis of anemia, diabetic osteoporosis, osteosis of neuropathies.	
bladderwrack, black walnut, centaury, elecampane, foenugreek, germander, horsetail, laminaria, menyanthe, *sage*	Zn-Cu, Cu-Au-Ag, Mg, K, F, Sr
Metal yin	
Hyposthenic, vagotonic terrain, lymphatic, hypothyroid, hyperparathyroid, hemopathies, apathetic, osteomalacia from vitamin D deficiency, rheumatism from wind, cold, dampness, anemia	
bladderwrack, black walnut, centaury, elecampane, foenugreek, germander, horsetail, laminaria, madder, wild oat, *lemon, thyme*	Cu, Cu-Au-Ag, Mg, P, K, F, Sr
Water yin	
Anergic, hypoadrenal, sympathetic insufficiency terrain, hypogonadal, cold body, timid, inhibited, low back pain, pronounced kyphosis, typical osteoporotic terrain; osteoporosis from aging, Paget's disease, malignant osteosis, hemopathies, slow healing of fractures.	
bladderwrack, black currant, black walnut, celery, heather, horsetail, laminaria, madder, *eucalyptus, sage, thyme*	Cu-Au-Ag, Mg, P, K, F, Sr

Gout

Gemmotherapy
Fraxinus excelsior, Viscum album

Treatment by Terrain	
Botanicals (herb, *oil*)	Oligolements
Wood yang	
Arthritic, hyperthyroid, sympathotonic terrain, hepatic involvement, gout, evolving arthritis.	
artichoke, barberry, broom, dandelion, germander, orthosiphon, goldenrod, stoneseed, yarrow, *lemon*	Mn, S, Mn-Co
Fire yang	
Neuroarthritic terrain, dystonic, hypermetabolic gout of upper limbs (especially hands, notably third and fourth digits).	
artichoke, ash, barberry, black currant, dandelion, linden, mistletoe, orthosiphon, stoneseed, *birch, lemon*	Mn-Co, S
Earth yang	
Vagal insufficiency, hypopancreatic terrain, plethoric or obese condition, "clogged" metabolism. Classic gout on the big toe and the knee areas crossed by the Spleen channel.	
agrimony, ash, black currant, burdock, centaury, colchicum, germander, maize, sarsaparilla, *birch, juniper, sassafras*	Zn-Ni-Co, Mn-Co, S
Water yang	
Hyperadrenal, sympathotonic terrain, gout of lower limbs.	
ash, barberry, black currant, black elder, dandelion, goldenrod, heather, maize, orthosiphon, sarsaparilla, sand spurry, *birch, sassafras*	Mn-Co, S

Gout (continued)

Local treatment
Apply green clay. Mix 1.5 ml each of oils of juniper, thyme, oregano and chamomile with 150 ml alcohol.

Obesity

Condition	Herb (*oil*)
Hypolipemiant plants	artichoke, bladderwrack, dandelion, ephedra, fumitory, germander, grapevine, horsetail, juniper, laminaria, maize, mouse ear
Plants for regulating the pancreas	agrimony, bilberry, fumitory, garlic, horsetail, juniper, maize
Plants for thyroid stimulation	bladderwrack, brassica, ivy, laminaria, onion, wild oat, *garlic*

Treatment by terrain	
Botanicals (herb, *oil*)	Oligolements
Wood yang	
Alimentary overload, hepatic and renal factors, hypercholesterolemia.	
artichoke, broom, dandelion, fumitory, horse chestnut, lady's mantle, orthosiphon, *lemon*	Mn-Co, Mg, I, S
Fire yang	
Metabolic problems due to advanced age or sedentary lifestyle.	
artichoke, broom, grapevine, horehound, horse chestnut, orthosiphon, *birch,* horsetail capsules	Mn-Co, Mg, S
Earth yang	
Constitutional tendency to obesity aggravated by high fat diet, prediabetic terrain, damp-heat terrain.	
agrimony, black currant, fumitory, germander, lady's mantle, marine algae, meadowsweet, woody nightshade, *lemon*	Zn-Ni-Co, Mn-Co, Mg
Earth yin	
Obesity from pituitary dysfunction, vagotonia, marble-like coldness, water retention, small frame.	
elecampane, eleuterococcus, horseradish, marine algae (especially laminaria)	Zn-Cu, Al, Mg
Water yang	
Metabolic problems, water retention linked to problems with clearing the kidney.	
bearberry, black currant, orthosiphon, *birch,* horsetail capsules	Mn-Co, Mg, S

Circulatory Disorders

Angina Pectoris
(Precordial Pain, Sequela of Infarction)

Cardiac Muscle Antispasmodic Plants	
pasque flower, *melissa*	
Gemmotherapy	
Crataegus oxyacantha	
Treatment by Terrain	
Botanicals (herb, *oil*)	Oligolements
Wood Yang	
Sympathotonic, hepatobiliary, hyperthyroid terrain. Frequently associated with digestive signs, subcostal (hypochondrial) pain.	
pasque flower, celandine, *melissa*	Mn-Co, I, S, P
Fire Yang	
Dystonic terrain, hypertension, tachycardia, insidious onset.	
borage, ginkgo, hawthorn, valerian, *bitter orange, melissa*	Mn-Co, Co, I, Bi-I, P
Fire Yin	
Sympathetic insufficient terrain, with sympathotonic attacks, timorous character, bradycardia.	
briarhip, ginkgo, lily-of-the-valley, motherwort, *lavender*	Mn-Co, Cu-Au-Ag, Co, P
Earth Yang	
Hypopancreatic, vagal insufficient terrain, plethoric, sanguine, associated with hiatal hernia, diabetes	
agrimony (weak doses vasodilate, strong doses vasoconstrict), arnica, maize, meadowsweet, periwinkle	Zn-Ni-Co, Mn-Co, Co, P
Earth Yin	
Hypothyroid, hypoglycemic, mild obesity.	
centaury, fennel, *anise*	Zn-Cu, Co, P
Metal Yang	
Hyposthenic terrain, vagal insufficiency, often hyperglycemic.	
arnica, borage, gingko, periwinkle	Mn-Co, P
Metal Yin	
Hyposthenic, pulmonary pathology antecedents, chronic respiratory insufficiency.	
fennel, centaury, gingko	Mn-Cu, Mn-Cu-Co, Co, P
Water Yang	
Insidious onset, hyperadrenal, robust individual.	
borage, periwinkle, *lemon*	Mn-Co, Co, I, P

Hypertension

GEMMOTHERAPY
Olea europaea, Viscum album

HYPOTENSIVE PLANTS
black currant, Canadian fleabane, celandine, garlic, hawthorn, hellebore, melilot, mistletoe, olive, parsley, periwinkle (central), rauwolfia, woundwort, *lavender, spike lavender, ylang ylang*

Treatment by terrain

Botanicals (herb, *oil*)	Oligolements
WOOD YANG	
Tensional lability, hyperthyroid, vertigo, visual disturbances, extreme shoulder stiffness.	
barberry, black cohosh, black horehound (tachycardia), celandine, fumitory, hellebore, khella, lily-of-the-valley (tachycardia), mistletoe, melilot, periwinkle, rauwolfia, valerian, woundwort	Mn-I, then I, Bi-I, S, Cu
WOOD YIN	
Sympathetic insufficiency, more or less hyperthyroid, hypoadrenal, hepatic congestion, cirrhosis, fatty, liver, ascites.	
barberry, celery, elecampane, hellebore, milk thistle, *lavender*	Mn-S, Mg, K
FIRE YANG	
Hyperemotional, extreme stress.	
black horehound (tachycardia), birch, borage, cassis, fumitory, grapevine, hawthorn, hellebore, khella, lavender, linden, lotus (tachycardia), lily-of-the-valley (tachycardia), meadowsweet, melilot, passionflower, periwinkle, rauwolfia, valerian, *lavender, spike lavender, ylang ylang*	Mn-I, then Mn-Co, I, Bi-I, Co-Cu
EARTH YANG	
Plethoric or obese constitution, hypopancreatic terrain, "apoplectic" constitution.	
calendula, fumitory, hellebore, horsetail, linden, maize, olive, periwinkle, *birch, lemon*	Mn-I, then Mn-Co, Cu, Zn-Ni-Co
METAL YANG	
Arteriosclerosis, phlegmatic types most predisposed as well as least predisposed.	
periwinkle, *eucalyptus, lemon, ylang ylang*	Mn-I, then Mn-Co, Mn-Cu, Cu
WATER YANG	
Hyperadrenal, sympathotonic terrain, authoritarian type, hypertension with urinary elimination difficulties.	
barberry, black currant, borage, hellebore, khella, maize, meadowsweet, melilot, passionflower, periwinkle, rauwolfia, rest harrow, shepherd's purse, valerian, *birch*	Mn-Co, I, Co-Cu
WATER YIN	
Anergic, hypoadrenal terrain, renal hypertension, cardiac insufficiency, cardiorenal edema, chronic renal insufficiency, ascites.	
celery, elecampane, horsetail, lily-of-the-valley (tachycardia), lovage, *birch, clove, lavender*	Mn-Co with prudence, Cu-Au-Ag, K, Li, Mg

Acrocyanosis or Raynaud's phenomenon

General treatment	
Botanicals (herb, *oil*)	**Oligolements**
bladderwrack, black walnut, laminaria, lungwort (external)	Zn-Cu, Mn-Cu, Mg, P, Co

Treatment by terrain	
Botanicals (herb, *oil*)	**Oligolements**
Water yang	
Hyperadrenal, hyperandrogenic women, hirsutism, Cushing's disease, Stein-Leventhal syndrome, amenorrhea due to hyperadrenal reaction to trauma	
borage, hops, horehound, lycopus, mouse ear, shepherd's purse, vervain, white willow, *ylang-ylang*	Mn-Co, Co
Water yin	
Timorous women, sentimental, cold body, cold feet, hypoadrenal, blushes easily, amenorrhea due to insufficient adrenal or gonadal steroids. **Etiology:** anergy, depression, stress, trauma, bereavement, terror, tuberculosis, Addison's disease, infectious illness.	
bistort, bladderwrack, elecampane, fennel, horsetail, laminaria, licorice, lovage, madder, sea holly, yarrow, *clary sage, thuja, geranium, lavender, sassafras, sage*	Cu-Au-Ag

Hypotension
(lipothymia, syncope)

Treatment by terrain	
Botanicals (herb, *oil*)	**Oligolements**
Wood yin	
Allergic, sympathetic insufficiency terrain, acetonemia, hepatic involvement, sequela of hepatitis or other hepatopathy, vertigo.	
angelica, mugwort, ephedra, milk thistle, *rosemary*	Mn, S, P, Mg, Cu-Au-Ag
Fire yin	
Cardiac insufficiency, marked sympathetic insufficiency, syncope, vertigo.	
angelica, digitalis, elecampane, ephedra, false hellebore (valvulopathy), milk thistle, mullein (tachycardia and arrhythmia), *garlic, sage, spike lavender*	Cu-Au-Ag, P
Earth yin	
Disorders of growth and development, hypothyroid	
angelica, mullein (tachycardia and arrhythmia), *sage*	Cu-Au-Ag, Mn-Cu-Co, Zn-Cu, P
Metal yin	
Hyposthenic, hypothyroid, cold body, pulmonary factors.	
ephedra, wild oat, *garlic, hyssop, rosemary, sage, thyme*	Cu-Au-Ag, Mn-Cu-Co, P
Water yin	
Adrenal insufficiency, lipothymia, syncope, nightsweats.	
bladderwrack, chickweed, eleutherococcus, lily-of-the-valley, mullein (tachycardia and arrhythmia), *hyssop, rosemary, sage, thyme*	Cu-Au-Ag, P

VARICOSE VEINS
(HEAVY LEG, PHLEBITIS, PARAPHLEBITIS)

GEMMOTHERAPY
Aesculus hippocastanum, Betula pubescens

LOCAL TREATMENT
Witch hazel and/or oils of cypress and mint with alcohol.

TREATMENT BY TERRAIN	
BOTANICALS (herb, *oil*)	OLIGOLEMENTS

WOOD YANG	
Hyperthyroid, sympathotonic terrain; if there is phlebitis, use melilot and violet especially.	
dandelion, goldenseal, grapevine, horse chestnut, melilot, violet, witch hazel, yarrow, *lemon, cypress*	MN, MN-CO, MG, S, CO

WOOD YIN	
Portal congestion, severe hepatic insufficiency, sympathetic insufficiency.	
milk thistle, groundsel, *lavender*	MN, CU, S, F, CU-AU-AG

FIRE YANG	
Dystonic terrain, insufficient elimination, excessively sedentary.	
goldenseal, hawthorn, melilot (+++), witch hazel, yarrow, violet (+++), grapevine, *lemon, cypress*	MN-CO, MG, S, CO

EARTH YANG	
Vagal insufficiency, hypopancreatic terrain, varicose veins from obesity, cellulite, insufficient capillary circulation.	
bilberry (+++), *cypress (+++), lemon*	ZN-NI-CO, MN-CO, S, CO, MG

EARTH YIN	
Obese, hypothyroid, hypercoagulability.	
groundsel, hypericum, ivy, *clary sage, cypress*	ZN-CU, F, CO, CU-AU-AG

METAL YIN	
Hyposthenic terrain, hypothyroid, significant capillary problems, acrocyanosis with chilled limbs.	
hypericum, ivy, licorice, *cypress, myrtle (+++)*	MN-CU, F, CO, CU-AU-AG

WATER YANG	
Hyperadrenal, sympathotonic terrain, dietary excess.	
dandelion, pellitory-of-the-wall, melilot, shepherd's purse	MN-CO, MG, S, CO

Hemorrhoids

GEMMOTHERAPY
Aesculus hippocastanum

LOCAL TREATMENT
Sitz bath with whole plant of pellitory-of-the-wall, licorice root, oak bark and horse chestnut bark

INFLAMMATION
myrrh

BLEEDING
yarrow

TREATMENT BY TERRAIN

BOTANICALS (herb, *oil*)	OLIGOLEMENTS
WOOD YANG	
Sympathotonic, hyperthyroid, arthritic terrain, insufficient venous circulation, varicose veins from labor, constipation with biliary dyskinesia.	
barberry, chaste tree, goldenseal, grapevine, horse chestnut, horsetail, mistletoe, violet, witch hazel, yarrow, *cypress*	Mn-Co, Mn, I, S, Mg
FIRE YANG	
Great dystonia, sedentary lifestyle, insufficient elimination, bleeding hemorrhoids.	
goldenseal, grapevine, horse chestnut, melilot, mistletoe, witch hazel, yarrow	Mn-Co, I, S
EARTH YANG	
Vagal insufficiency, hypopancreatic terrain, obesity, digestive encumberment, encumbrance of duodenal-pancreatic intersection.	
arnica, cypress, bilberry	Mn-Co, Co, S, Mg, Zn-Ni-Co
METAL YANG	
Hyposthenic terrain, susceptible to intestinal colic, chronic colitis, constipation (heat), spicy diet.	
lungwort	Mn-Cu, Mn-Co, Mg
METAL YIN	
Hyposthenia, vagotonia, chronic colitis, atonic constipation from vacuity of the Large Intestine, elderly patient, colon prolapse, rectal prolapse.	
bistort, horse chestnut, hypericum, ivy, oak, *cypress, myrtle*	Mn-Cu, Co, Mg
WATER YANG	
Hyperadrenal terrain, lumbago, acute torticollis.	
black elder, melilot, pellitory-of-the-wall, shepherd's purse	Mn-Co

VERTIGO

LOCAL TREATMENT
Use oils of *everlasting* and *rosemary* around the neck area.

TREATMENT BY TERRAIN	
BOTANICALS (herb, *oil*)	OLIGOLEMENTS
WOOD YANG	
Sympathotonic, hyperthyroid terrain, neurotoxic vertigo, vestibular hypersensitivity, altitude or motion sickness, vertigo with agoraphobia, anguish, Ménière's disease.	
angelica, black horehound, chaste tree, hawthorn, woundwort, *melissa, rosemary, sage*	MN, I, S, MG, P
WOOD YIN	
Vestibular hypersensitivity, sympathetic insufficiency, hepatic insufficiency.	
lavender	MN, S, MG, P
FIRE YANG	
Sympathotonic, hyperpituitary, neurotonic, vascular vertigo.	
hawthorn, chaste tree, *birch, melissa, rosemary*	MN-CO, I, MG
FIRE YIN	
Sympathetic insufficiency, arteriosclerosis and cerebral circulatory insufficiency.	
angelica	CU-AU-AG
EARTH YANG	
Plethoric terrain, vagal insufficiency, arteriosclerosis (enervation).	
linden, vervain, *bay laurel*	ZN-NI-CO, MN-CO
EARTH YIN	
Psychasthenia, mental sluggishness, hypoglycemia.	
vervain, *coriander*	ZN-NI-CO, ZN-CU
METAL YIN	
Hyposthenia, fatigue, swollen lymph nodes.	
coriander	MN-CU
WATER YANG	
Uremia, overweight, hyperadrenal terrain, thirst.	
birch	MN-CO, MG
WATER YIN	
Adrenal insufficiency, hypotension.	
clove, rosemary	CU-AU-AG

Skin disorders
Dermatoses, Eczema, Psoriasis

Gemmotherapy
Juglans regia, Ribes nigrum

External treatment
INFLAMMATIONS: Arnica
PSORIASIS: Drainage infusion: equal parts of lavender flowers, violet flowers, borage flowers and sweet balm flowers.
ECZEMA: green clay; decoction of oak bark or black walnut leaves; 20 ml each of oils of *geranium, lavender, chamomile* and *sage* with 50 ml sweet almond oil.
URTICARIA: calendula cream or fomentation of chamomile decoction.
SKIN DRAINAGE HERBS: burdock, honeysuckle, raspberry, rest harrow, woody nightshade, violet, *birch, calamus*

Treatment by terrain	
Botanicals (herb, *oil*)	Oligolements
Wood yang	
Allergic terrain, contact eczema, photosensitivity, allergic eczema and dermatosis to cosmetics and topical medications, hypersensitivity to insect bites, pruritus, urticaria, pityriasis rosea.	
black radish, boldo, dandelion, goldenrod, nettle, plantain, pulsatilla, violet, woody nightshade, *bay laurel, bitter orange, lavender, marjoram*	Mn, S, P, Co
Wood yin	
Sympathetic insufficiency terrain, psoriasis of scalp, lichen, psoriasis from syphilis, vitiligo, vesicular lesions, dermatoses from hepatic dysfunction.	
hops, woody nightshade, *lavender*	Cu-Au-Ag, Mn, S
Fire yang	
Dystonic terrain, erysipelas, intermittent scarlatina from psoriasis, symmetrical eczema, eczema of palms and soles, Quincke's edema, lichen, Duhring's disease (dermatitis, herpetiformis).	
boldo, borage, orthosiphon, plantain, pasque flower, woody nightshade, *birch,* horsetail capsules	Mn-Co, I, S, P
Earth yang	
Diabetic terrain, gout, sanguine type, hypertensive.	
burdock, fumitory, woody nightshade, *juniper*	Zn-Ni-Co, Mn-Co S, Mn-Cu
Earth yin	
Tubercular terrain, lymphatic, hyposthenic, cutaneous sensitivity, atopic terrain, constitutional eczema and psoriasis, psoriasis of gout, postvaccination eczema, seborrhea, seborrheic dermatoses, collagenoses: SLE, dermatomyositis, scleroderma, eczema of malabsorption, erythema nodosum, cutaneous sarcoidosis, cutaneous tuberculosis, psoriatic rheumatism.	
bladderwrack, black walnut, blue mallow, calendula, centaury, hops, laminaria, oak, *geranium, hyssop, sage*	Mn-Cu, S, P, Cu-Au-Ag, Zn-Cu
Metal yang	
Dermatoses accompanying colitis, enteritis, hyperglycemic terrain, hyperthermia, constipation (heat).	
burdock, borage, woody nightshade, *serpolet*	Mn-Co, S, Mn-Cu

DERMATOSES, ECZEMA, PSORIASIS (CONTINUED)

METAL YIN
Tubercular terrain, lymphatic, hyposthenic, atopic terrain with cutaneous sensitivity, constitutional eczema and psoriasis, psoriasis of gout, postvaccination eczema, seborrheic dermatoses, collagenoses: SLE, dermatomyositis, scleroderma, eczema of malabsorption, erythema nodosum, cutaneous sarcoidosis, cutaneous tuberculosis, psoriatic rheumatism.

black walnut, centaury, dandelion, laminaria, nettle, menyanthe, oak (dampness), sarsaparilla (dryness), violet (keratitis, cradle cap), woody nightshade, yellow dock, *hyssop, myrtle, sassafras, sage, thyme*	Mn-Cu, S, P, Cu-Au-Ag, Zn-Cu

WATER YANG
Hyperadrenal terrain, urticaria, eczema, uremia, burning itch.

borage, lovage, dandelion, *birch,* horsetail capsules	Mn-Co, S

WATER YIN
Anergic, hypoadrenal, sympathetic insufficient terrain, seborrhea, eczema with rheumatism in seborrheic areas, dermatoses with collagenoses, postvaccination eczema, psoriatic rheumatism.

black elder, black walnut, bladderwrack, goldenrod, laminaria, lovage, myrtle, sarsaparilla, scarlet pimpernel (mycoses), *hyssop, myrtle, sassafras, thyme*	Cu-Au-Ag, Zn-Cu, Mn-Cu, S

ACNE

LOCAL TREATMENT
10 minutes green clay mask daily.

Compress with oils:

geranium	.75 ml
lavender	.75 ml
sage	.75 ml
thyme	.75 ml
sweet almond oil	20. ml
alcohol	125 ml of 90% solution

Cabbage leaf compress.

TREATMENT BY TERRAIN	
BOTANICALS (herb, *oil*)	OLIGOLEMENTS

WOOD YANG
Sympathotonic, hepatic terrain, damage from cold, juvenile acne from liver malfunction.

artichoke, dandelion, nettle, pasque flower, *lemon, lavender*	Cu, S, Mg, Cu-Au-Ag, Mn

EARTH YANG
Plethoric, vagal insufficiency hyperglycemic terrain, acne rosacea, acne and furuncles, diabetic secondary infections (staphylococcus), red blotches.

agrimony, burdock, fumitory, *calendula, lemon, sage*	Zn-Ni-Co, S, Cu

EARTH YIN
Lymphatic congestion, hypophysogonadic dysadaptation.

centaury, bladderwrack, black walnut, dandelion, laminaria, *hyssop, lavender, sage*	Zn-Cu, Mn-Cu, S

Acne (continued)

METAL YIN	
Hyposthenic, vagotonic terrain, typical acne type, juvenile acne, rickets, scoliosis, anorexia, depression, crisis of adolescence.	
bladderwrack, calendula, dandelion, laminaria, violet, *hyssop, lavender, sage*	Mn-Cu, S, Mg, Cu-Au-Ag
WATER YANG	
Hyperadrenal, sympathotonic terrain, more or less hyperandrogenic (male or female).	
black walnut, borage, dandelion, white willow (hyperandrogenic women)	Mn-Co, Cu, S, Cu-Au-Ag (if tolerable)
WATER YIN	
Anergic terrain, significant acne on the back.	
bladderwrack, black elder, black walnut, goldenrod, laminaria, lovage, violet, yarrow, *hyssop, lavender, rosemary, sandalwood, sage, thyme*	Cu-Au-Ag, S, Mn-Cu

Herpes

GEMMOTHERAPY	
Ribes nigrum	
TREATMENT BY TERRAIN	
BOTANICALS (herb, *oil*)	OLIGOLEMENTS
WOOD YANG AND WOOD YIN	
Allergic terrain, hepatic and sympathetic insufficiency, genital herpes, herpes of the cornea, peribuccal herpes, premenstrual outbreaks, Liver blood vacuity.	
dandelion, goldenrod, hops, plantain, pellitory-of-the-wall, scarlet pimpernel, violet, woody nightshade, *cypress, lavender, ravensare*	Mn-Cu, S
EARTH YANG AND EARTH YIN	
Poor immunity, adaptation, herpes related to diabetes, genital contact or infectious illness.	
burdock, gentian, hops, propolis, sarsaparilla, scarlet pimpernel, woody nightshade, *cinnamon, cypress, ginger, lavender, lemon, thyme, ravensare, sage*	Mn-Co, S
WATER YIN	
Peribuccal herpes, persistent buttock or genital lesions.	
goldenrod, madder, propolis, sarsaparilla, *clove, geranium, lavender, pine, ravensare, savory, thyme, ylang ylang*	Cu-Au-Ag, Mn-Co, S
LOCAL TREATMENT	
Cabbage leaf compress or lemon juice.	

Compress			
cypress	2 ml	geranium	4 ml
lavender	6 ml	alcohol	90 ml

Compress	
oil of *ravensare*	chamomile tea solution
oil of *thyme*	

As a douche, use one drop of each oil in a pint of weak tea solution.
Propolis for pain, disinfection and antiviral effect.

SHINGLES

GEMMOTHERAPY
Ribes nigrum

TREATMENT BY TERRAIN	
BOTANICALS (herb, *oil*)	OLIGOLEMENTS
WOOD YIN	
Most frequently encountered terrain. Shingles that appear at the change of the seasons, especially Spring and Fall. Intercostal and ophthalmic.	
woody nightshade, plantain, *birch, cypress, lemon, lavender, sage, ravensare*	CU-AU-AG, MG, CU, S
FIRE YIN	
Elbow region, axillary region, median nerve, ophthalmic herpes.	
plantain, woody nightshade, *birch, cypress, lavender, lemon, sage, thyme, ravensare*	CU-AU-AG, MG, S, CU, CO
METAL YIN	
Radial region, Lung vacuity condition or Metal yin constitution.	
chamomile, hypericum, violet, woody nightshade *birch, cypress, lemon, ravensare, sage*	CU-AU-AG, MG, CU, S
WATER YIN	
Often seen in very weak condition, after steroid use, with cancerous conditions or AIDS, in the region of the kidney or bladder channels, or along the sciatic nerve.	
black elder, *birch, clove, geranium, lavender, rosemary, savory, thyme*	CU-AU-AG, MG, CU, S

LOCAL TREATMENTS
Cabbage leaf compress.

Topical application			
lavender	10 ml	*rosemary*	5 ml
geranium	10 ml	*sage*	5 ml
hypericum (extracted)	125 ml		

Topical application			
lavender	10 ml	*ravensare*	5 ml
chamomile	10 ml	*sage*	5 ml
hypericum (extracted)	125 ml		

ACQUIRED IMMUNE DEFICIENCY SYNDROME (AIDS)

According to the concept of the terrain, AIDS is not a viral disease caused by a single microbe, but a general breakdown of immune system activity with a complex microbial terrain. Because of the sluggishness of lymph circulation, different "subterrains" or microenvironments nationalize. For example, a single patient may suffer simultaneously or at different times from herpes outbreaks on the skin (viral), pneumocystis carinii in the lungs (protozoal), cryptosporidiosis in the intestines (protozoa), or candida in the mouth (fungus).

For the immune-deficient patient, generally plants classified as Metal yin or Water yin are nourishing to a weakened system. For lymph stasis, remineralizing herbs like marine algae, especially bladderwrack and laminaria, are useful. Horsetail is also in this category. Any of the lymph draining herbs, especially oils of *everlasting, hyssop* and *rosemary* can help to clear an infected region.

IMPORTANT HERBS FOR AIDS	
PROTEOLYTIC ENZYMES (PINEAPPLE AND PAPAYA EXTRACTS)	anti-inflammatory
ELECAMPANE	dries up phlegm, stimulates pituitary function
FOENUGREEK	dries up phlegm, helps with "wasting," stimulates adrenal cortex function
HORSETAIL	remineralizer, moves stagnant lymph
HYPERICUM	clears out worms, stimulates general immunity, useful for depression
GENTIAN	elevates white blood cell count

OTHER USEFUL HERBS

black walnut (astringent, antifungal), blessed thistle (antifungal, antidepressant), centaury, echinacea, fumitory, garlic, oak (astringent), onion, propolis (immune boosting, antimicrobial) sea holly (antifungal)

IMPORTANT ESSENTIAL OILS FOR AIDS

SAVORY   Anthelminthic, antibacterial (including staphylococcus), antiprotozoal, anti-fungal, antiviral, cerebral stimulant (dementia), antidiarrheic, general tonic, treats skin infections, adrenal cortex stimulant.

THYME   General tonic, adrenal cortex stimulant, clears phlegm, elevates white cell count, stimulates thymus function, antiviral (including herpes), antifungal, antibacterial, treats skin infections.

SAGE   Cerebral tonic, adrenal cortex stimulant, astringent for perspiration (even the nightsweats of tuberculosis), strengthens deficient immunity, stimulates the pituitary gland, moves lymph stasis, good for chronic bronchial infections and splenomegaly.

CINNAMON Adrenal cortex stimulant, antiparasitic, treats digestive infections, diarrhea, fungal infections.

OTHER USEFUL ESSENTIAL OILS

bay laurel (lymph drainage, antiprotozoal), *cajeput, caraway, clove, eucalyptus, everlasting* (lymph stasis), *hyssop, lavender, lemon, myrrh* (bronchial infections), *niaouli, oregano, pine, ravensare* (expectorant, antiviral), *spike lavender, terebenthine, thuja*

GEMMOTHERAPY

Ribes nigrum, Vitis vinifera, Quercus pedunculata

GENERAL TREATMENT

CONDITION	HERB (OIL)
DEMENTIA	*basil, clove, lemon, rosemary, sassafras*
MYALGIA PAINS	blessed thistle, horseradish, hypericum, marine algae, chamomile, *eucalyptus, ravensare*
ANXIETY AND DEPRESSION	angelica, bladderwrack, blessed thistle, foenugreek, hypericum, milk thistle
ANTIFUNGAL OILS	*cinnamon, clove, garlic, oregano, savory, sage, thyme*
ANTIVIRAL OILS	*cinnamon, cypress, eucalyptus, juniper, niaouli, ravensare* (herpes), *sage, savory, serpolet, thyme* (herpes)
PNEUMOCYSTIS CARINII	elecampane, horseradish, foenugreek, germander
TO DISSOLVE PHLEGM	*ravensare, birch, cajeput, clove, cypress, hyssop, lemon, myrtle, myrrh, niaouli, sage, savory, myrrh*
ANTIPROTOZOAL	germander, oak, garlic, savory, *bay laurel,*

CRYPTOSPORIDIOSIS	
Watery diarrhea, cramping abdominal pain, weight loss, flatulence, exacerbation of diarrhea and abdominal cramps after eating; sometimes nausea, vomiting, malaise, myalgia, dehydration.	
CONDITION	HERB (OIL)
DIARRHEA	ash, oak, *geranium, niaouli, savory, sage*
WEIGHT LOSS	foenugreek, *sage*
DEHYDRATION	licorice
ANTIPROTOZOAL	ash, oak, garlic, *lemon, bay laurel, savory*
ASTHENIC CONDITION WITH DIARRHEA	black walnut, blessed thistle, blue mallow, gentian, hypericum, nettle, plantain, *cajeput, clove, oregano, thyme*
KAPOSI'S SARCOMA	black walnut, burdock, sarsaparilla, *geranium, sage, sassafras, thyme.*
TOPICAL TREATMENT	
myrrh	
OLIGOTHERAPY FOR AIDS	
CU-AU-AG, ZN-CU, CU	

GLOSSARY OF TERMINOLOGY[1]

abortifacient - an agent that causes abortion.

abscess - an accumulation of pus in a cavity resulting from tissue disintegration.

acetonemia - excess of acetone in the blood (also called ketonemia).

acrocyanosis (Raynaud's sign) - symmetrical cyanosis of the extremeties with blue or red discoloration of the skin and subjectively cold skin.

adaptogen - increases overall resistance and vitality.

adenopathy - swollen lymph nodes or other glands.

adrenergic - activated by epinephrine or similar substances.

aerophagia - swallowing of air followed by spasmodic belching.

albuminuria - presence of serum albumin in the urine (proteinuria).

alopecia - baldness; absence of hair in areas normally covered with hair.

alveolar (dental) - sockets in the maxilla and mandible in which the roots of the teeth are attached.

amenorrhea - absence of menses.

amylosis (amyloidosis) - accumulation of amyloid in body tissues.

amyotrophic lateral sclerosis (Lou Gehrig's disease) - progressive deterioration of neurons of the corticospinal tract and motor cells of the brainstem and spinal cord.

analeptic - a drug that acts as a restorative.

analgesic - diminishes pain.

anaphrodisiac - diminishes libido.

anasarca - generalized edema.

androgens - masculinizing hormones.

anergy - a diminished reactivity to noxious stimuli.

ankylosing spondylitis - the form of rheumatoid arthritis that affects the spine.

anodyne - eases pain.

---

[1]Botanical functions terms are bold face; general medical terms are italicized bold face.

anorexia nervosa - abnormal loss of appetite; emaciation resulting from a nervous condition in which the patient refuses to eat almost everything.

anosmia - loss of the sense of smell.

anoxia - reduction below normal levels of oxygen in tissues.

antidiarrheic - soothes diarrhea by astringent, adsorbent or antibiotic effects.

antigalactic - inhibits secretion of breast milk.

antihelminthic (anthelmintic) - destroys or expels intestinal worms.

antihemorrhagic - combats hemorrhage by assisting in the transport or manufacture of coagulation factors.

anti-infectious (antiseptic) - kills microbes or impedes their growth.

anti-inflammatory (antiphlogistic) - reduces excessive inflammatory reactions.

antilithiatic - opposes the formation of biliary or urinary calculi.

antiphlogistic - an agent that counteracts inflammation.

antimicrobial - disinfects and kills micro-organisms.

antiparasitic (vermifuge) - expels parasites including amoebae.

antipruritic - relieves itching.

antipyretic (febrifuge) - reduces fever.

antiscorbutic - treats scurvy.

antispasmodic - relieves spasms, particularly of the smooth muscle.

antisudoral - diminishes perspiration.

antitussive - inhibits or relieves cough.

antiemetic - calms nausea and vomiting.

anuria - cessation of urinary excretion.

aperiant - mild laxative.

aperitif (bitter) - stimulates appetite and gastric function.

aphrodisiac - stimulates sexual energy.

aphtha - small reddish or white ulcers found in the mouth.

arrhythmia - an irregularity in heart rhythm.

arteriosclerosis - hardening of the arteries.

arteritis - inflammation of the arteries.

arthrosis - joint disease.

ascites - accumulation of serous fluid in the abdominal cavity.

asthenia - lack of strength.

astringent - contracts tissues, mucous membranes, capillaries, orifices, etcetera to reduce secretions of mucus; often having hemostatic and antidiarrheic properties; sometimes refers to antisudorals.

ataxia - irregularity of muscular coordination.

azotemia - excess of urea in the blood.

balsamic - soothes mucous membranes of the bronchial tubes and respiratory tree.

bathmotrope - the response of a tissue to stimuli.

bechic - soothes irritations of the pharynx.

biliary dyskinesia - irregularity of the filling and emptying of the gallbladder.

blepharitis - inflammation of the eyelids.

blepharospasm - hypertonic spasm of the orbicularis oculi muscle causing closure of the eyelid.

bradycardia - low heart rate (pulse rate below 60 beats per minute).

bronchopneumopathy - disease of the bronchi and lung tissue.

bronchorrhea - excessive fluid secretion of the bronchi.

bulbar - pertaining to the medulla oblongata.

bursitis - inflammation of the bursa.

calculus (calculi) - stone.

capsulitis - adhesive tendinitis or bursitis.

cardiotonic - reinforces, strengthens and regulates cardiac function.

carminative - promotes elimination of intestinal gas, relieves flatulence.

cataract - an opacity of the crystalline lens of the eye.

catecholamines - sympathomimetic substances such as epinephrine, norepinephrine and dopamine.

cellulitis - purulent inflammation of the subcutaneous tissue.

ceruloplasmin - a glycoprotein bonded to copper.

cervicitis - inflammation of the uterine cervix.

Cheyne-Stokes respiration - a pathological sign in which there is rhythmic waxing and waning of the depth of respiration with regular periods of apnea.

chilblain - a painful erythema on the fingers, toes or ears from mild frostbite.

cholagogue - contracts the gallbladder to force the expulsion of bile.

choleretic - stimulates the secretion and production of bile.

cholecystitis - inflammation of the gallbladder.

cholinergic - activated or transmitted by acetylcholine; parasympathomimetic.

chondrocalcinosis - pathological changes in cartilage resulting from deposition of calcium salts.

chorea - rapid, clonic involuntary movements.

chronotrope - the response of the rate, as in the rate of contraction of the heart.

cicatrisant (vulnerary) - promotes healing of wounds and resorption of contusions.

cirrhosis - fibrotic disease of the liver.

CNS - central nervous system.

coeliac disease (malady) - malabsorption syndrome resulting from intolerance to gluten-containing foods.

colibacillus - *Escherichia coli* (*E. coli*) bacterium.

collagenosis - pathological changes in connective tissue.

colonopathy - pathology of the colon.

condyloma - papilloma with a core of connective tissue covered with epithelium, thought to be a viral condition.

conjunctivitis - inflammation of the conjunctiva.

coronaropathy - pathology of the coronary arteries.

Crohn's disease - regional ileitis; an inflammation of the ileum resulting in scarring, thickening and abscess formation in the intestinal wall.

cryptosporidiosis - a protozoal infection which causes watery diarrhea, nausea, vomiting and intestinal cramps.

cutaneous - pertaining to the skin.

cystalgia - pain in the urinary bladder.

cystitis - inflammation of the bladder.

cytophylactic - protects the cells.

demulcent - provides a protective coating and relieves internal inflammation of membranes.

depurative - purifies the blood by means of diuretic, laxative, sudorific action or by improving liver function; often used in cutaneous afflictions.

dermatomyositis - a collagen disease in which there is necrosis of muscle fibers, often associated with malignancy.

dermatosis - skin disease, especially noninflammatory.

diabetes insipidus - failure of tubular reabsorption of water in the kidney from lack of antidiuretic hormone (ADH).

diabetes mellitus - inability to oxidize carbohydrates due to a disturbance of insulin secretion.

diaphoretic (sudorific) - provokes perspiration.

diastole - dilatation period of the heart.

diathesis - a constitutional predisposition to a pathological condition.

diuretic - promotes the secretions and excretion of the kidneys; augments the quality of the filtration and the volume of the urine; salidiuretics eliminate chloride and are used in cases of edema; azoturics eliminate urea (nitrogen) and are antiseptics; uricosurics eliminate uric acid (pain and gout); phosphatics and oxalics eliminate salts of phosphoric and oxalic acid (stone formation).

diverticulitis - inflamed diverticuli.

diverticulum - a pouch resulting from a herniation of the mucous membrane lining of a tubular organ, usually the large intestine.

dyscrasia - a morbid condition caused by an imbalance of components, usually referring to the blood.

dysentery - intestinal inflammation.

dysmenorrhea - painful menstruation.

dyspepsia - impaired digestive strength.

dysplasia - structural abnormality of cells.

dystonia - disorder of the muscular or nervous tonus.

eclampsia - convulsions and coma in a pregnant woman due to hypertension, edema or proteinuria.

eczema - superficial inflammatory process occurring in the epidermis characterized by redness, weeping, crusting and scaling.

edema - fluid accumulation in the intercellular tissue spaces.

electrophoresis - movement of charged particles suspended in liquid under the influence of an electric field.

emetic - induces vomiting.

emmenagogue - facilitates and promotes flow of menses; some emmenagogues also stimulate ovarian secretions.

emollient - soothes inflamed mucous membranes, tissues or skin.

emphysema - pathological accumulation of air in the lung due to dilatation of the alveoli or destruction of the alveolar wall.

endometriosis - accumulation of endometrial tissue attaching to anatomical structures throughout the pelvic cavity.

endometritis - inflammation of the endometrium.

enteritis - intestinal inflammation.

enuresis - involuntary discharge of urine.

epididymitis - inflammation of the epididymus.

epigastric - upper abdominal region between the sternal angle inferior to the xiphoid process.

epistaxis - nosebleed.

epitheliogenic - stimulates the growth of epithelial tissue (cicatrisant).

erythema nodosum - acute inflammatory skin disease with tender red nodules from the exudation of blood and serum.

erythematopultaceous - redness of the skin or mucous membranes from capillary congestion.

eupeptic (stomachic) - promotes digestion, improves peristalsis.

exanthematous - pertaining to eruptions or rashes.

extrasystole - premature contraction of the heart outside the normal rhythm.

expectorant - assists expulsion of bronchial secretions.

febrifuge - antipyretic.

febrile - pertaining to a fever.

fibrillation - small, local involuntary contraction of muscle.

fibroma - a tumor composed of fibrous connective tissue.

fistula - abnormal passage between two organs or from an internal organ to the surface of the body.

flocculation - dispersion of a colloid into discrete particles.

fluidifiant - liquefies bronchial secretions to assist expectoration.

FSH - follicle stimulating hormone.

furunculosis - appearance of furuncles, or painful nodules in the skin, usually caused by staphylococcus.

galactagogue - activates or promotes lactic secretion.

galactic - referring to lactation, the flow of milk.

gastralgia - stomach pain.

gastroptosis - loss of tonus of the smooth muscle tissue of the stomach.

gingivitis - gum inflammation.

glaucoma - increase in intraocular pressure, which results in pathological changes in the optic disk.

globulin - a class of proteins soluble in saline, but insoluble in water.

glomerulonephritis - a type of nephritis characterized by inflammation of the capillary loops in the glomeruli of the kidney.

glossitis - inflammation of the tongue.

glycogenesis - synthesis of glycogen.

glycogenolysis - breaking down of glycogen into glucose.

glucosuria - presence of an abnormal amount of glucose in the urine.

gonadotropins - pituitary hormones that stimulate the gonads.

haptoglobin - group of glycoproteins that bond hemoglobin.

HCl - hydrochloric acid.

hematemesis - vomiting of blood.

hematuria - discharge of blood in the urine.

hemoptysis - expectoration of blood.

hemostatic - controls hemorrhage by vasoconstriction or delivery of coagulation factors (vitamin K , etcetera).

hepatosplenomegaly - abnormal swelling of the liver and spleen.

hirsutism - abnormal hairiness, especially in women.

HPV - human papilloma virus.

hypercholesterolemia - high blood cholesterol.

hypercoagulability - more readily coagulated than normal.

hyperfolliculine - pertaining to an excessive amount of estrogen.

hyperglycemia - high blood sugar.

hyperhidrosis - excessive perspiration.

hyperlipidemia - excess of lipids in the blood.

hypermetabolism - abnormally increased metabolism.

hyperosteosis vertebrale - hypertrophy of the spinal bones.

hyperplasia - abnormal increase in the number of cells.

hypersomnia - excessive sleep.

hypersudation - excessive perspiration.

hypertensive - increases arterial tension.

hyperthermia - abnormally high body temperature.

hyperthyroid - excessive functional activity of the thyroid gland.

hypertrophy - enlargement or overgrowth of an organ or structure.

hyperuricemia - escessive levels of uric acid in the blood.

hyperviscosity - excessive viscosity.

hypnotic - induces sleep.

hypochlorhydria - abnormally low hydrochloric acid in the stomach.

hypocholesterolemia - low level of blood cholesterol.

hypoestrogenic - low level of estrogen in the blood.

hypoglycemiant (antidiabetic) - lowers the blood sugar level.

hypopancreatic - diminished pancreatic function.

hypophysis - pituitary gland.

hypophysogonadic dysadaptation - Ménétrier's term for a constitution that develops at an abnormally slow rate.

hypophysopancreatic dysadaptation - Ménétrier's term for a constitution that tends toward hypofunction of the pituitary-pancreatic axis.

hypopituitarism - low pituitary function.

hypotension - low blood pressure.

hypotensive - lowers arterial tension.

hypovolemia - abnormally low fluid volume in the system.

hypoxia - abnormally low levels of oxygen in the blood or tissues.

icterus - jaundice.

infarct - an area of coagulation necrosis due to localized ischemia.

infectious mononucleosis - an infectious disease associated with the Epstein-Barr virus.

in vitro - in glass; in an artificial environment such as a test tube.

in vivo - in a living organism.

ischemia - deficiency of blood resulting from a localized constriction or obstruction of a blood vessel.

Kaposi's sarcoma - malignant reticulo-endothelial cells, usually involving pink, purple or brown skin lesions often on the feet, but also affecting internal organs.

keratitis - inflammation of the cornea.

laxative - facilitates the evacuation of the stool and increases its volume by increasing peristalsis of the intestine or or by hydrating the stool.

leukocytosis - increase in the number of leukocytes in the blood.

leukopenia - decrease in the number of leukocytes in the blood.

leukorrhea - viscous vaginal discharge.

LH - lutenizing hormone.

lipothymia - syncope; feeling of faintness.

lithiasis - condition of forming calculi.

lumbalgia - pain in the lumbar region of the back.

luteotropic - stimulates the formation of the corpus luteum, stimulates progesterone secretion.

lymphadenitis - inflammation of lymph nodes.

lymphoma - neoplastic disease of lymphoid tissue, usually malignant.

macula - a thickened, discolored area.

macula retinae - yellowish depression on the retina just below the optic disk.

macular degeneration - degenerative change in the macula retinae.

maculopapular - an eruption of both macules and papules.

MAO - monoamine oxidase.

mastitis - inflammation of the mammary gland.

mastodynia - breast pain.

mastosis - swelling and nodules in the breast.

meninges - the three membranes that envelop the brain and spinal cord.

meningitis - inflammation of the meninges.

menorrhagia - excessive uterine bleeding at the time of menses.

metrorrhagia - prolonged uterine bleeding, usually at irregular intervals.

mitral valve prolapse - often asymtomatic condition in which the mitral valve leaflets prolapse into the right atrium during ventricular systole, resulting in some mitral regurgitation.

myalgia - muscle pain.

mycosis - disease caused by fungus.

mycostatic - prevents the growth or reproduction of fungi.

myocarditis - inflammation of the myocardium.

myopia - nearsightedness.

nephritic - pertaining to the kidneys.

nephrocalcinosis - precipitation of calcium phosphate in the kidneys.

nephroangiosclerosis - hypertension with renal lesions of arterial origin.

nephrosis - any disease of the kidneys, especially lesions of the renal tubes.

nervine - relaxes nervous tension or excitement.

neurasthenia - a neurosis characterized by emotional hypersensitivity, depression, loss of appetite, fatigability, lack of energy and inability to concentrate.

neuroarthritic - arthritis related to disease of the central or peripheral nervous system.

neurotonia - instability of the tonus of the autonomic nervous system.

nymphomania - exaggerated sexual desire in the female.

ocular - pertaining to the eye.

oliguria - secretion of a diminished volume of urine.

ophthalmia - inflammation of the eye.

ophthalmic - used for afflictions of the eyes and eyelids.

orchitis - inflammation of the testicles.

osteochondritis - inflammation of bone and cartilage.

osteomalacia - softening of bone tissue.

osteoporosis - mineral loss and rarefaction of bone tissue.

otitis - ear inflammation; otitis media: middle ear inflammation.

oxytocic - an agent that promotes evacuation of the uterus by stimulating myometrial contraction.

oxytocin - hormone of the posterior lobe of the pituitary gland that stimulates contraction of the myometrium; used to induce labor in the gravid uterus.

Paget's disease - osteitis deformans; bone inflammation resulting in deformation of the flat bones.

pallor - absence of skin coloration.

papilloma - branching tumor of the epithelium.

papule - small solid elevation of the skin.

paraneoplasia - in the vicinity of a neoplasm.

parasympathotonia (vagotonia) - hyperexcitable condition of the parasympathetic nervous system.

parasympatholytic (vagolytic) - inhibits activity of the parasympathetic nervous system.

parasympathomimetic - stimulates activity of the parasympathetic nervous system and the vagus nerve.

paresthesia - abnormal sensation such as burning or prickling.

parotitis - inflammation of the parotid gland; epidemic parotitis (mumps).

pericarditis - inflammation of the pericardium.

perineum - space between the anus and scrotum.

peripheral resistance - resistance to the flow of blood through the arterioles.

peristalsis - wave of contraction passing through the alimentary canal to propel its contents.

pertussis - whooping cough.

petechia (ecchymosis) - pinpoint round nonelevated red or purplish-red spots visible on the skin.

pharyngitis - inflammation of the pharynx.

pheochromocytoma - vascular tumor of chromaffin tissue of the adrenal medulla or sympathetic paraganglia.

phlebitis - inflammation of a vein.

phosphaturia - abnormally high level of phosphates in the urine.

pityriasis rosea - pink, oval scales or macules on the skin arranged parallel to the lines of cleavage.

plethora - a generic term for a profusion of blood, or a red florid complexion.

pleurisy - inflammation of the pleura with exudation into the pleural cavity.

pneumocystis carinii - protozoa associated with interstitial plasma cell pneumonia.

pollakiuria - frequent urination.

polyarthritis - arthritis affecting more than one joint.

polyarthrosis - joint disease affecting several joints.

polydipsia - excessive thirst over a prolonged interval.

polymenorrhea - abnormally frequent menstruation.

portal congestion - impaired passage of blood through the portal circulation leading to the liver.

postprandial - after a meal.

precordial - pertaining to the region over the heart.

priapism - abnormal erection of the penis, usually not accompanied by sexual desire.

prostaglandin - naturally occurring substances, first found in prostate gland secretions, that stimulate the contraction of smooth muscle including the uterus.

prostatitis - inflammation of the prostate gland.

proteinuria (albuminuria) - presence of excessive serum proteins in the urine.

pruritus - itching.

psoriatic arthritis - arthritis associated with severe psoriasis.

psychasthenia - a neurosis characterized by obsessions, fear, anxiety, sensations of unreality and depersonalization.

purgative (cathartic) - a strong laxative, accelerating peristalsis.

purpura (hemorrhagic) - purplish or brownish-red skin discoloration caused by hemorrhage into the tissues.

pyelonephritis - inflammation of the kidney and its pelvis.

pyorrhea - discharge of pus.

pyuria - presence of pus in the urine.

Quincke's edema - sudden appearance of edema in areas of the skin or mucous membranes associated with urticaria, erythema and purpura.

rachitism - rickets.

Raynaud's phenomenon - severe pallor, usually of the fingers and toes, brought on by cold or by emotional upset; acrocyanosis.

rectocolitis - inflammation of the colon and rectum.

rectosigmoid - lower portion of the sigmoid and upper portion of the rectum.

refrigerant - lowers body temperature.

remineralizer - brings mineral salts and trace elements to correct the balance of electrolytes and normalize the supply of nutrient minerals.

reticuloendothelial - pertaining to the functional defense system of macrophages, Kuppfer's cells, reticular cells, monocytes and others that perform the function of phagocytosis.

retinitis (pigmentosa) - a disease, often hereditary, marked by atrophy of the retina, clumping of the pigment and shrinking of the visual field.

retinopathy - any noninflammatory disease of the retina.

rhinitis (allergic) - hay fever.

rhinopharyngeal - referring to the nose and throat.

rubefacient - used externally to increase blood supply to the skin surface.

salpingitis - inflammation of the uterine tube.

sarcoidosis - chronic progressive granulomatous abnormal increase in reticuloendothelial cells.

satyriasis - excessive sexual desire in the male.

sclera - tough white outer coat of the eyeball; the white of the eye.

scleroderma - chronic hardening and contraction of connective tissue of the body in which the skin becomes thickened, hard and rigid.

scoliosis - lateral deviation of the spine.

scrofula - tuberculosis of the cervical lymph nodes.

seborrhea - excessive secretion of sebum.

sedative (tranquilizer) - calms nervous system activity.

senescence - aging; pathological processes related to aging.

septicemia (blood poisoning) - the presence of pathogenic microbes or their toxic by-products in the blood.

silicosis - condition of lungs reacting to the presence of dust containing silicon dioxide resulting in nodular fibrotic lesions in the lung tissue.

Sjögren's syndrome - a condition marked by dryness of the eyes, mouth and throat with swollen parotid glands and chronic polyarthritis.

SLE - "systemic lupus erythematosus."

somnolence - sleepiness.

spasmophilia - chronic tendency toward mild tetany, or neuromuscular spasms.

spermatorrhea - involuntary excess discharge of semen without copulation.

spondyloarthritis - arthritis of the spinal column.

steatorrhea - excessive amount of fat in the feces.

Stein-Leventhal syndrome - polycystic ovaries causing anovulation and secondary amenorrhea with indications of excessively high levels of androgens, such as with hirsutism.

stimulant - temporarily excites vigilance, nervous, circulatory or digestive activity.

stomachic - eupeptic.

stomatitis - inflammation of the oral mucosa.

stye (hordeolum) - purulent, inflammatory infection of a sebaceous gland in the eyelid, thought to be caused by staphylococcus.

sudorific - diaphoretic.

suppuration - formation and discharge of pus.

sympathotonia - condition in which the sympathetic nervous system function dominates the functioning of the body.

sympatholytic - inhibits the activity of the sympathetic nervous system.

sympathomimetic - simulates the activity of the sympathetic nervous system.

syncope - temporary loss of consciousness; fainting.

synovitis - inflammation of a synovial membrane.

syringomyelitis - inflammation of the spinal cord.

systole - period of contraction of the heart, especially the ventricles.

tachycardia - excessively rapid heart rate, usually above 100 beats per minute.

tendinitis - inflammation of tendons or tendon-muscle attachments.

terrain - a generic term referring to the interstitial fluid and blood as a whole system; the humoral system.

tetters - eczematous skin disease.

thermophobia - dislike of heat.

thrombophlebitis - inflammation of a vein due to a thrombus formation.

thrombosis - formation or development of a thrombus.

thrombus - aggregation of blood platelets and fibrin which causes vascular obstruction.

tinnitus - a noise in the ears, such as ringing, hissing, buzzing, clicking or roaring.

tonic - improves the overall vital functioning of the body in cases of fatigue.

tracheitis - inflammation of the trachea.

tranquilizer - sedative.

tubulonephritis - a type of nephritis that affects primarily the tubules.

urethritis - inflammation of the urethra.

urticaria (hives) - the appearance of smooth reddish or whitish slightly raised patches on the skin (wheals) that usually itch and burn.

uterolytic - an agent that relaxes the uterine tonus.

uterotonic - an agent that increases the tonus of the uterus.

vagolytic - (parasympatholytic) having an effect resembling inhibition of the activity of the vagus nerve.

vagotonia (parasympathotonia) - hyperexcitability of the vagus nerve.

valvulopathy - pathology of the heart valves.

varices - enlarged veins, arteries or lymph vessels, usually swollen veins.

varicocele - varicose condition of the veins forming a swollen sac in the scrotum and causing a constant dull pulling painful sensation.

vascular - pertaining to the blood vessels or the blood supply.

vasoconstrictor - contracts blood vessels.

vasodilation - dilation of a blood vessel.

vasodilator - dilates the blood vessels.

vermifuge - antiparasitic.

vertigo - an illusory sensation of movement, especially a sensation of revolving or spinning.

vulnerary - cicatrisant.

APPENDIX A:

FIVE PHASE CORRESPONDENCES

TABLE OF FIVE PHASE CORRESPONDENCES					
	WOOD	FIRE	EARTH	METAL	WATER
VISCUS	LIVER	HEART	SPLEEN	LUNG	KIDNEY
BOWEL	GALL-BLADDER	SMALL INTESTINE	STOMACH	LARGE INTESTINE	BLADDER
SENSE ORGAN	EYES	TONGUE	LIPS	NOSE	EARS
VISCUS STORES	BLOOD	SHEN (SPIRIT)	NUTRITIVE QI (CHYLE)	QI	JING (SEXUAL ESSENCE)
TISSUE	TENDONS	VASCULATURE	MUSCLES	SKIN	BONES
QUALITY	COLOR	ODOR	FLAVOR	TONE	FLUID
EXPRESSION	SHOUT	LAUGH	SING	WEEP	GROAN
INDICATOR	NAILS	COMPLEXION	LIPS	BREATH	HAIR
SEASON	SPRING	SUMMER	MIDSEASONS	AUTUMN	WINTER
DIRECTION	EAST	SOUTH	CENTER	WEST	NORTH
COLOR	BLUEGREEN	RED	YELLOW	WHITE	BLACK
ODOR	RANCID	SCORCHED	FRAGRANT	FISHY	PUTRID
FLAVOR	SOUR	BITTER	SWEET	SPICY	SALTY
EMOTION	ANGER	FRIVOLITY	WORRY/OBSESSION	GRIEF	FEAR/FRIGHT
ADVERSE CLIMATE	WIND	HEAT	HUMIDITY	DRYNESS	COLD
STRESS RESPONSE	CLENCHING	DEPRESSION	HICCOUGH	COUGH	TREMBLING
FLUID	TEARS	SWEAT	DROOL	MUCUS	SALIVA
EXERTION	WALKING	WATCHING	SITTING	LYING	STANDING
PLANET	JUPITER	MARS	SATURN	VENUS	MERCURY

CORRESPONDENCES BETWEEN THE FIVE PHASES AND THE DIATHESES OF MÉNÉTRIER

DIATHESIS	PHASE	TRACE ELEMENT	ORGAN SYSTEM CORRESPONDENCE
I ALLERGIC	WOOD	MANGANESE	LIVER-GALL BLADDER
II HYPOSTHENIC	METAL	MANGANESE-COPPER	LUNG-LARGE INTESTINE
III DYSTONIC	FIRE	MANGANESE-COBALT	HEART-SMALL INTESTINE
IV ANERGIC	WATER	COPPER-GOLD-SILVER	KIDNEY-BLADDER
V MALADAPTED	EARTH	ZINC-COPPER ZINC-NICKEL-COBALT	SPLEEN-STOMACH

CORRESPONDENCES BETWEEN THE FIVE PHASES AND NEUROENDOCRINE FUNCTIONS

PHASE AND POLARITY	NEUROENDOCRINE PROFILE
WOOD YANG	SYMPATHOTONIC, HYPERTHYROID, HYPERFOLLICULINE
WOOD YIN	SYMPATHETIC INSUFFICIENCY, HYPOLUTEAL, HYPOPARATHYROID
FIRE YANG	SYMPATHOTONIC, HYPERPITUITARY
FIRE YIN	SYMPATHETIC INSUFFICIENCY, HYPOPITUITARY, OXYTOCIC
EARTH YANG	VAGAL INSUFFICIENCY, HYPOPANCREATIC, HYPERGLYCEMIC, HYPERGONADIC
EARTH YIN	VAGOTONIC, HYPOTHYROID, HYPOGONADAL, HYPOPANCREATIC, HYPERGLYCEMIC
METAL YANG	VAGAL INSUFFICIENCY, NORMOCRINE
METAL YIN	VAGOTONIC, HYPOTHYROID, HYPERPARATHYROID, HYPOLUTEAL
WATER YANG	SYMPATHOTONIC, ADRENAL HYPERMEDULLAR, HYPERCORTICAL HYPERANDROGENIC, HIGH LH
WATER YIN	SYMPATHETIC INSUFFICIENCY, HYPOMEDULLAR, HYPOCORTICAL, HYPOANDROGENIC, HYPERALDOSTERONE, LOW LH

FLAVORS AND THEIR INFLUENCE

FIVE ELEMENTS AND FIVE FLAVORS

> *When the liver suffers constraint, one can release it with sweet food.*
>
> *If the heart is excessively loose, one can retract it with sou. [cardiac insufficiency].*
>
> *If the spleen suffers from dampness, one can dry it with bitter.*
>
> *If the lung suffers from reflux of chi, one can drain it with bitter.*
>
> *If the kidneys suffer dryness, one can moisten them with spicy flavor which opens the orifices, attracts fluids and circulates the chi.*
>
> **Su Wen Chapter 22**

Excessive spiciness destroys Wood (spasmophilia).

Excessive saltiness destroys Fire (arteriosclerosis, HBP).

Excessive sour destroys Earth (collagen disease).

Excessive bitter destroys Metal (dry skin, damages lung).

Excessive sweet destroys Water (arthroses, dental caries).

SOUR NOURISHES THE LIVER - EVACUATION

SOUR-WARMING - Disperses repletion of Liver yin: clears hepatic congestion; stimulates the Liver; diminishes venous pressure; stimulates the thyroid and thermogenesis - sympathomimetic, vagolytic.

BOTANICALS: milk thistle, oak, plantain, *lemon, cypress*

SOUR-COOLING - Its effect opposes Liver repletion heat (fire): sympatholytic, antithyroidean, antiestrogenic; purgative; vagotonic, hypoglycemiant.

BOTANICALS: nettle, goldenseal, eyebright, witch hazel, grapevine, horse chestnut, *rosemary, lemon, cypress*

BITTER NOURISHES THE HEART - ELIMINATION, VOMITING

BITTER-WARMING - "Compresses" the Heart yin and supplements the Heart yang: sympathomimetic, cardiotonic, hyperglycemiant, adrenalin-like (Kidney yang), dries dampness of the Spleen: clears excess phlegm in digestive tract.

BOTANICALS: cinchona, digitalis, lily-of-the-valley, milk thistle, fenugreek, *lavender, rosemary, hyssop, niaouli, thyme*

BITTER-COOLING - Febrifuge, emetic, purgative, disperses Fire of the Heart: sympatholytic, cardiomoderater, tranquilizer.

BOTANICALS: hawthorn, hellebore, rauwolfia, valerian, poppy, artichoke, *bitter orange*

SWEET NOURISHES THE SPLEEN - DISPERSAL

SWEET-WARMING - Supplements the Spleen yang; stimulates pituitary, corpus luteum, hyperglycemiant, sympathomimetic; adrenalin-like, cortisol-like, bone catabolism ("too much sweet destroys the bones").

BOTANICALS: fennel, licorice, sweet balm, *anise, cinnamon, sage, caraway, lemon, sandalwood, thuja*

SWEET-COOLING - Emollient, laxative, harmonizing, moisturizing (saliva, sweat, tears), vagotonic, hypoglycemiant (stimulate insulin secretion), diuretic.

BOTANICALS: burdock, ash, hawthorn, sarsaparilla, *juniper, sandalwood, lemon*

SPICY NOURISHES THE LUNG - SUDORIFIC

SPICY-WARMING - Dries and disperses dampness, warms the Lung, increases the Lung yang, vagolytic and sudorific, adrenalin-like; moistens if Lung afflicted by dryness.

BOTANICALS: mugwort, sassafras, oak, nettle, dandelion, *ginger, niaouli, caraway, eucalyptus, peppermint, savory*

SPICY-COOLING - Disperses heat in the Lung through diaphoresis, antilithiatic, adrenolytic, sympatholytic, hypotensive.

BOTANICALS: horehound, eyebright, horse chestnut, black radish, rhubarb, *eucalyptus, niaouli*

SALTY NOURISHES THE KIDNEY - PURGING

SALTY-WARMING - Evacuant, purgative, laxative and diuretic; supplements Kidney yang: stimulates adrenal cortex and medulla, cortisol, salidiuretc, azoturic, eliminates phosphates and oxalates, cardiotonic, sympathomimetic.

BOTANICALS: laminaria, bladderwrack, cornsilk, horsetail, black elder, *hyssop, sandalwood*

SALTY-COOLING - Moistening, diuretic, inhibits adrenal medulla, sympatholytic, uricosuric, azoturic, salidiuretic, vagotonic, hypoglycemiant.

BOTANICALS: meadowsweet, harpagophytum, bearberry, ash, black currant, *thuja*

APPENDIX B

CLASSICAL CHINESE MEDICINE TERMINOLOGY

The classical Chinese medicine terminology used in this book has been selected to provide the closest approximation to the terminology of Traditional Chinese Medicine. In the U.S., acupuncture is often taught according to the rules of T.C.M., which is fundamentally a modern Chinese system of phytotherapy that has been centralized and standardized. In France, the situation is just the reverse. The use of many herbs from the modern East Asian pharmacopoeia is unknown or obscure to most practitioners in Western Europe; acupuncturists have often applied the rules of acupuncture to their traditional materia medica to create a system of phytotherapy. Most of the terms selected for this book can be interpreted in a way recognizable to the typical U.S. practitioner. This list is neither exhaustive nor definitive, but is intended to give examples of how a new materia medica could be integrated into another system that may be already familiar to the practitioner.

Blood heat - A condition characterized by restlessness, thirst, rapid pulse, extravasation of blood, bloody discharges in sputum, urine, stool, etcetera.

Blood stasis - A condition in which the blood is viscous and extravasated. The patient's skin is dark and lusterless, the pulse is rough, there is often fixed pain, masses or swellings, hemorrhage; there are sometimes petechiae and varicosities.

Blood vacuity - A condition in which there are symptoms of pallor, anemia, palpitations, dizziness, a thin pulse, muscle spasms, tachycardia and insomnia.

Damp-cold - A condition characterized by abdominal fullness, diarrhea, swelling and heaviness of the body.

Damp-heat - A condition characterized by fever, pain, distension in the chest, pain and fullness in the abdomen, nausea, vomiting, dark urine and hard stool or diarrhea.

Heart blood vacuity - A condition of pale complexion, memory loss, pale tongue, tachycardia, palpitations, dizziness and shortness of breath

Heart fire upflaring - A condition of restlessness, insomnia and agitation, with rapid, thin pulse and a red, cracked tongue.

Heart qi vacuity - A condition of poor complexion, shortness of breath, tendency to perspire easily, mental fatigue, tachycardia, dizziness, irregular pulse and palpitations.

Heart yang vacuity - A condition of poor complexion, tachycardia, palpitations, dizziness, shortness of breath, cold limbs, cyanotic facies and cold sweats.

Kidney yin vacuity - A condition characterized by tinnitus, dizziness, dryness of the throat and mouth, low grade fever, lumbar pain and fine, rapid pulse.

Kidney yang vacuity - A condition characterized by coldness of the limbs, loss of libido, lumbar pain, frequent urination, tinnitus, dizziness, loss of enthusiasm for life and pale complexion.

Liver blood vacuity - A condition characterized by sluggish venous blood flow, muscle spasms, insomnia, excessive dreaming, amenorrhea or scant menses, paresthesia of the limbs and dizziness.

Liver fire, upflaming of liver fire - A condition in which there is impatience, anger, irritability, red complexion, bloodshot eyes, headache, dizziness, dry mouth, constipation and rapid wiry pulse.

Liver qi congestion - Also called general binding depression of Liver qi, characterized by subcostal discomfort, depression, mood swings and wiry pulse.

Liver yang repletion - Ascendant hyperactivity of Liver yang is similar to upflaming of Liver Fire along with insomnia, palpitations, lumbar pain and weakness in the lower limbs.

Lung qi vacuity - A condition characterized by cough, rapid breathing, shortness of breath, weak voice, weak pulse, thin watery sputum and pale tongue.

Lung yin vacuity - A condition characterized by dry cough, rapid breathing, dry mouth and throat, emaciation, nightsweats, flushed cheeks, tidal fever and hoarseness.

Shen - Principle of consciousness and healthy mental function.

Spleen dampness - A condition characterized by loss of appetite, thick tongue fur, heavy limbs, abdominal distention, thin stool, nausea, vomiting, jaundice, foul-smelling diarrhea with anal burning and painful urination with dark-colored urine.

Spleen qi vacuity - A condition of weakness in the four limbs, fatigue, pallor, diarrhea, abdominal discomfort, weak digestion and poor appetite.

Spleen yang vacuity- Devitalization of Spleen yang is characterized by fatigue, pallor, diarrhea with undigested food and abdominal pain relieved by heat or pressure.

Stomach heat - A condition characterized by swollen bleeding gums, red tongue, halitosis, constipation, hunger and burning sensation in the stomach.

Wind-cold - A condition characterized by aversion to cold or wind, scratchy throat, general aching, floating pulse, fever and headache.

Wind-heat - A condition characterized by headache, fever, migrating aches and pains, swollen cervical nodes, sore throat and red tongue.

EXAMPLES OF THERAPEUTIC AGENTS
FOR TCM SYMPTOM-SIGN COMPLEXES

Liver blood vacuity - cypress, echinacea, milk thistle, mugwort, hepatica, barberry, raspberry, black cohosh, rosemary.

Liver fire repletion - pasque flower, passionflower, white willow, hawthorn, goldenseal, chaste tree, marjoram, melilot, linden, valerian, water lily, *bitter orange, melissa, lavender.*

Liver qi congestion - barberry (subcostal distress), black cohosh, pasque flower, angelica, rosemary, woundwort, cypress, lady's mantle, marjoram, passionflower, *bitter orange.*

Heart qi vacuity - milk thistle, digitalis, lily-of-the-valley, barberry, broom, lovage, *rosemary, sage, lavender, angelica.*

Heart fire repletion - hawthorn, chaste tree, melilot, *lavender.*

Heart fire vacuity - angelica, lily-of-the-valley, milk thistle, digitalis.

Heart blood stasis - yarrow, melilot, passionflower, *melissa.*

Heart blood repletion heat - witch hazel, grapevine.

Heart blood vacuity - angelica, elecampane.

Supplement Spleen qi - elecampane, angelica, anise, camomille, caraway, centaury, blessed thistle, oak, coriander, barberry, gentian, fennel, fenugreek, fumitory, hypericum, plantain, vervain, *lavender, sage.*

Dissipate dampness in the Spleen - anise, elecampane, cinchona, bladderwrack, colchicum, coltsfoot, laminaria, hypericum, myrtle, nettle, eucalyptus, gentian, germander, *cinnamon, caraway, cumin, hyssop, lavender, sage, terebenthine, cypress, mint, clove, lemon.*

Lung qi vacuity - angelica, elecampane, myrtle, oregano, hypericum, coltsfoot, *terebenthine, hyssop.*

Supplement Lung yin - borage, lungwort, horehound, marshmallow, angelica, licorice, oregano, *lemon, melissa, pine.*

Secure Kidney qi - fenugreek, geranium, madder, dandelion, bearberry, yarrow, *celery seed, niaouli.*

Supplement Kidney yang vacuity - eleutherococcus, madder, sea holly, lovage, wild oat, black currant, *sandalwood, pine, rosemary, sage, lavender, clove, ginger, fennel, geranium, cypress, yarrow.*

Supplement blood - angelica, anise, echinacea, black walnut, rosemary, calendula, fennel, elecampane, mugwort, raspberry leaf, shepherd's purse, sage, savory, yellow dock.

Treat blood stasis - yarrow, lady's mantle, ginkgo, motherwort, chaste tree, pasque flower, arnica (external), melilot, barberry, shepherd's purse, witch hazel, horse chestnut, grapevine, laminaria, stoneseed, groundsel, goldenseal, white willow, raspberry leaf, myrrh, *melissa, thuja, everlasting* (external), *lemon, lavender, cypress, sage, hypericum.*

Clear damp-heat - agrimony, burdock, cinchona, fumitory, rhubarb, senna, horsetail, goldenseal, *eucalyptus, niaouli, cypress, juniper.*

Dispel wind-heat - lungwort, borage, birch, lonicera, eyebright, pasque flower, black horehound, plantain, violet, *bitter orange, rosemary, mint, terebenthine.*

Dispel wind-cold - angelica, rosemary, plantain, sassafras, coltsfoot, *lavender, niaouli, oregano, pine, terebenthine, cinnamon.*

Treat exterior repletion - ephedra, lonicera, blessed thistle, lungwort, borage, birch, violet, camomile.

Treat exterior vacuity - cinnamon, cypress, oak, plantain, rosemary, sage, pine, coltsfoot.

Dissipate cold - datura, henbane, *lavender, pine, rosemary, hyssop, celery seed, fennel.*

BIBLIOGRAPHY

PART I

Ayurvedic Society. *Caraka Samhita.* Ayurvedic Society, Jamunagar, India (1980).

Berger G. *Questionnaire caractérologique.* Presses Universitaires de France, Paris (1950).

Bezanger-Beauquesne, Pinkas, Torck. *Les plantes dans la therapeutique moderne.* Maloine S.A. ed. Paris (1975).

Cazin F. J. *Traité pratique et raisonnée des plantes médicinale indignés et acclimatés.* Asselin et Houseau ed., Paris (1886).

Cloarec M. "Critères d'études d'une médication a base de flavonoides." *Vie Médicale* 50:23-30 (1969).

Corman L. *Nouveau manuel de morpho-psychologie.* Stock Plus, Paris (1966).

Coupin H. *Les plantes médicinales.* Costas A. ed. Paris (1920).

Coxe J.R. *The American Dispensatory.* Carey & Lee, Philadelphia, PA (1830).

Duke James A. *CRC Handbook of Medicinal Herbs.* CRC Press, Boca Raton, LA (1985).

Duquesne J. *Dictionnaire des plantes médicinales selon les traditions populaires.* Editions Morgan, Paris (1973).

Duraffourd C. "L'aromatogramme." *Annales du 1er congrès de la S.F.P.A,* Paris (1976).

Duraffourd C., Lapraz J.C. "Propriétés particulières des plantes dans leur indication de médecine de terrain," in Perspectives en Phytothérapie clinique. *CCLS,* Masson ed., Paris (1983).

_____. "Trâitement du terrain." *Annales 2e congrès international de phytothérapie et d'aromathérapie.* Monte Carlo (1977).

Duraffourd C., D'Hervicourt L., Lapraz J.C. *Cahiers de Phytothérapie clinique no. 1-4.* Masson ed., Paris (1982).

_____. *Les terrains endocriniens.* Masson ed., Paris (unpublished monograph).

_____. *Phytothérapie et dermatologie.* Masson ed., Paris (1982).

_____. "Terrains hypercortico-surrénaliens." *Bulletin de la S.F.P.A.,* Paris (1981).

Ellingwood F. *American Materia Medica, Therapeutics and Pharmacognosy.* Eclectic Medical Pub., Portland (1983).

Evans William C. *Trease and Evans' Pharmacognosy*. 13th edition. Baillier Tindall, London (1989).

Fluck Hans. *Medicinal Plants*. V. Foulsham & Co., Ltd., London (1976).

Franchomme P., Penoël D. *L'aromathérapie éxactement*. Roger Jollois editeur. Limoges, France (1990).

Green James. *The Male Herbal*. Crossing Press, Watsonville, CA (1991).

Grieve Mrs. M. *A Modern Herbal, Volumes 1 & 2*. Dover Publications, New York (1971).

Griggs Barbara. *Green Pharmacy*. Viking Press, New York (1982).

Gunther R.T. *The Greek Herbal of Dioscorides*. Hafner Pub., New York (1959).

Henry P. "Introduction à la gemmothérapie." *Cahiers de Biothérapeutique*, No. 1 (1964).

Himalaya Drug Company. *Therapeutic Index*, Bombay, India (1984).

Kobe Igaku Kenkyukai. *Kampô no Rinshô Ôyô*. Ishiyaku Shuppan, Tokyo (1979).

Kubo Michinori. *Kampô no Rinshô Yakugaku*. Kaigai Pub., Osaka (1978).

Lapraz J.C. "L'aromatogramme, nouvelles conceptions." *Annales du 3e congrès internationale de phytothérapie et d'aromathérapie*, Tours (1978).

Lapraz J.C., Duraffourd C. "Le Vagotonique, 1980," in Perspectives en Phytothérapie clinique. *CCLS*, Masson ed., Paris (1983).

Leclerc H. *Précis de phytothérapie, Thérapeutique par les plantes*. Masson ed., Paris (1935).

Ménétrier J. *La médecine des fonctions*. Ed. Le François, Paris (1974).

Paris M., Hurabielle M. *Abrégé de matière médicale, pharmacognosie*. 2 volumes. ed. Masson, Paris (1980 & 1986).

Pelikan W. *L'homme et les plantes médicinales*. 3 volumes. Triade ed., Paris (1962).

Requena Yves. *Terrains et pathologie en acupuncture, rapport avec les oligoéléments*. 3 volumes. Maloine S.A. ed., Paris (1980-1982).

_____. *Character and Health*. Paradigm Publications, Brookline, MA (1989).

Robinson T. *The Organic Constituents of Higher Plants*, Burgess Pub., Minneapolis, MN (1983).

Ross & Brian. *An Introduction to Phytopharmacy*. Pitman Medical, London (1977).

Sawin Clark. *Hormones: Endocrine Physiology*. Little, Brown & Co., Boston (169).

Svoboda Robert. *The Hidden Secret of Ayurveda*. B.A.M.S. Pub., Puna, India (1980).

Tetau M., Bergeret C. *La phytothérapie renovée*. Maloine S.A. ed., Paris (1971).

Thomson William. *Herbs That Heal*, Charles Scribner, New York (1976).

Tisserand Robert. *The Art of Aromatherapy*. C.W. Daniel Co., Saffron Walden, England (1977).

Tyler, Brady and Robber. *Pharmacognosy*. Lea and Febiger, Philadelphia, PA (1981).

Valnet J. *Aromathérapie*. Maloine S.A. ed., Paris (1975).

_____. *Phytothérapie*. Maloine S.A. ed., Paris (1975).

Valnet J., Duraffourd C., Lapraz J.C. *Une médecine nouvelle: phytothérapie et aro-mathérapie.* Presse de la Renaissance ed., Paris (1978).

Valnet J., Reddet C. "Contribution a l'application pratique d'une nouvelle conception du terrain biologique." *A.M.I.F.,* Paris (April-May 1961).

White, Handler & Smith. *Principles of Biochemistry.* McGraw-Hill, New York (1968).

Witzmann Rupert. *Steroids - Keys to Life.* Van Nostrand Reinhold, New York (1981).

Youngken H.W. - *Textbook of Pharmacognosy.* Blakiston, Philadelphia, PA (1943).

Zysset Ch. "Système nerveux autonome et quelques plantes vises neurovegetatives, 1980," in "Perspectives en Phytothérapie clinique." *CCLS,* Masson ed., Paris 1983.

PART II

Albert-Puleo M. "Fennel and Anise as estrogenic agents." *J. of Ethnopharmacology,* 2:337-44 (1980).

Alfieri R., Sole P. "Influence des anthocyanosides administrés par voie parenterale sur l'adapto-électro-rétinogramme du lapin." *C.R. Soc. Biol* 158:2338-41 (1964).

Bezanger-Beauquesne, Pinkas, Torck. *Les plantes dans la thérapeutique moderne.* Maloine S.A. ed., Paris (1975).

Biggs M.J., *et al.* "Platelet aggregation in patients using feverfew for migraine." *The Lancet,* October 2:776 (1982).

Collier H.O.J., *et al.* "Extract of feverfew inhibits prostaglandin biosynthesis." *The Lancet,* October 25:922 (1980).

Coprean D., *et al.* "Biochemical effects of standardized propolis extract and of silymarin on the liver of ethyl alcohol intoxicated rats." *Agressologie,* 28:831-2, SPEI Medical (1987).

Doll R., *et al.* Clinical trial of a triterpenoid liquorice compound in gastric and duodenal ulcer." *The Lancet,* 2:793-6 (1962).

Du Mee C. "Vitex Agnus Castus." *Aus. J. Med. Herbalism* 5(3): 63-5 (1993).

Duraffourd C., D'Hervicourt L., Lapraz J.C. *Cahiers de Phytothérapie clinique no. 1-4.* Masson ed., Paris (1982).

Fox D.W., *et al.*"Pyrollizidine intoxication mimicking Reye's syndrome," *J. P ed.* p.980-2. December 1978.

Gaultier R. "De l'action physiologique et thérapeutique de l'extrait aqueux de gui; son emploi dans les hemorragies congestives et comme medicament hypotenseur." *Gaz de hop.* 80:1419-24, Paris (1907).

Henry P. "Introduction à la gemmothérapie." *Cahiers de Biothérapeutique,* No. 1 (1964).

Lapraz J., Duraffourd C. "Le Vagotonique, 1980." In Perspectives en phytothérapie clinique, *CCLS,* Masson ed., Paris (1983).

Leclerc H. *Précis de phytothérapie, thérapeutique par les plantes.* Masson ed., Paris (1935).

Ménétrier J. *La médecine des fonctions.* Ed. Le François, Paris (1974).

Nishikawa H. "Screening test for antibiotic action of plant extracts." *Japanese Journal of Experimental Medicine* 20(3):337-349 (1949).

Pharmacopoeia Committee of the Ministry of Health. *Pharmacopoeia of the People's Republic of China, Part 1.* People's Health Publishing House, Beijing (1985).

Quillet Chantal. *Nos plantes médicinales.* Engelhard, Angouleme (1978).

Requena Yves. *Acupuncture et phytothérapie,* 3 volumes. Maloine S.A. ed., Paris (1983).

Salz H. "Activité d'un extraite de ginkgo biloba dans les arteriopathies des membres inferieurs." *Thérapie der Gegenwart* XI:1345-56 (1980).

Tetau M., *et al.* "Un anti-inflammatoire d'origine vegetale: Ribes nigrum bourgeons. " *Cahiers de biothérapie* 63:69-72 (1979).

Tetau M., Bergeret C. *La phytothérapie renovée.* Maloine S.A. ed., Paris (1971).

Valette G., *et al.* "Hypocholesterolemic effect of fenugreek seeds in dogs." *Athersclerosis* 50:105-111 (1984).

Valnet J. *Aromathérapie.* Maloine S.A. ed., Paris (1975).

_____. *Phytothérapie.* Maloine S.A. ed., Paris (1975).

Valnet J., Duraffourd C., Lapraz J.C. *Une medécine nouvelle: phytothérapie et aromathérapie.* Presse de la Renaissance ed., Paris (1978).

Weiss R.F. *Herbal Medicine.* Hippocrates Verlag, Stuttgart (1988).

Weston C.F. M., *et al.* "Veno-occlusive disease of the liver secondary to ingestion of comfrey." *Brit. Med. J.,* p.183, July 1987.

PART III

Bezanger-Beauquesne, Pinkas, Torck. *Les plantes dans la thérapeutique moderne.* Maloine S.A. ed. Paris (1975).

Carillon A. *Pour un bon usage des plantes.* ed. Vie & Sante, Dammarie les Lys (1985).

Duraffourd C., Lapraz J.C. "Propriétés particulieres des plantes dans leur indication de médecine de terrain," in "Perspectives en Phytothérapie clinique," *CCLS.* Masson ed., Paris (1983).

_____. "Traitement du terrain." *Annales 2e congres international de phytothérapie et d'aromathérapie.* Monte Carlo (1977).

Duraffourd C., d'Hervicourt L., Lapraz J.C. *Utilisation thérapeutique de 84 plantes médicinales.* Titrex.

_____. *Cahiers de Phytothérapie clinique no. 1-4.* Masson ed., Paris (1982).

_____. *Phytothérapie et dermatologie.* Masson ed., Paris (1982).

Fauron R., Moatti R. *La Prescription en phytothérapie,* EPMG Diffusion, Paris (1980-1986).

Henry P. "Introduction de la gemmothérapie." *Cahiers de biothérapeutique no. 1* (1964).

Lapraz J.C. "l'aromatogramme, nouvelles conceptions." *Annales du 3e congrès international de phytothérapie et d'aromathérapie,* Tours (1978).

Lapraz J.C., Duraffourd C. "Le Vagotonique, 1980." In Perspectives en phytothérapie clinique, *CCLS,* Masson ed., Paris (1983).

Leclerc H. *Precis de phytothérapie, thérapeutique par les plantes.* Masson ed., Paris (1935).

Meyer, J.B. *Abrégé de phytopratique médicale.* ed. Louis Pariente, Strasbourg (1981).

Ménétrier J. *La médecine des fonctions.* ed. Le Francois, Paris (1974).

Paris M., Hurabielle M. *Abrégé de matière médicale, pharmacognosie,* 2 volumes. ed. Masson, Paris (1980 & 1986).

Pelikan W. *L'homme et les plantes médicinales.* 3 volumes. Triade ed., Paris (1962).

Requena Y. *Acupuncture et phytothérapie.* 3 volumes. Maloine S.A. ed., Paris (1983).

_____. *Terrains et pathologie en acupuncture, rapport avec les oligoéléments.* 3 volumes. Maloine S.A. ed., Paris (1980-1982).

Requena Y., *et al. Les Manuels de thérapeutiques integrées, gastro-enterologie et hepatologie.* edns. Solal, Marseille (1990).

Tetau M., Bergeret C. *La phytothérapie renovée.* Maloine S.A. ed., Paris (1971).

Valnet J. *Aromathérapie.* Maloine S.A. ed., Paris (1975).

_____. *Phytothérapie.* Maloine S.A. ed., Paris (1975).

Valnet J., Duraffourd C., Lapraz J.C. *Une médecine nouvelle: phytothérapie et aromathérapie.* Presse de la Renaissance ed., Paris (1978).

Weiss R.F. *Herbal Medicine.* Hippocrates Verlag, Stuttgart (1988).

INDEX